From the time of birth through the early school years, young children rapidly acquire two complex cognitive systems: They organize their experiences into concepts and categories, and they acquire their first language. How do children accomplish these critical tasks? How do conceptual systems influence the structure of the languages we speak? How do linguistic patterns influence how we view reality? These questions have captured the interest of such theorists as Piaget, Vygotsky, Chomsky, and Whorf, but until recently very little has been known about the relation between language and thought during development.

Perspectives on language and thought presents current observational and experimental research on the links between thought and language in young children. Chapters from leading figures in the field focus on the acquisition of hierarchical category systems, concepts of time, causality, and logic, and the nature of language learning in both peer and adult–child social interactions.

Four major themes are presented. First, children honor constraints or biases that limit the possible meanings they consider when learning new words. Second, the conceptual systems underlying language use are intricately subtle and complex. Third, children's "naïve theories" about the world may be integral to their early word meanings. Fourth, studying the nature of social interaction can be a potent tool for disentangling the roles of parent, child, and context during language learning.

The chapters in this volume provide a detailed discussion of the multiple relations between language and cognition in the course of children's first language acquisition. This book will be of special interest to researchers in developmental and cognitive psychology, linguistics, cognitive science, and education.

Perspectives on language and thought

Perspectives on language and thought
Interrelations in development

Edited by

Susan A. Gelman
University of Michigan, Ann Arbor

James P. Byrnes
University of Maryland, College Park

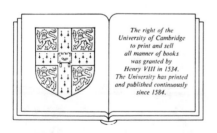

The right of the
University of Cambridge
to print and sell
all manner of books
was granted by
Henry VIII in 1534.
The University has printed
and published continuously
since 1584.

Cambridge University Press

Cambridge
New York   Port Chester   Melbourne   Sydney

Published by the Press Syndicate of the University of Cambridge
The Pitt Building, Trumpington Street, Cambridge CB2 1RP
40 West 20th Street, New York, NY 10011, USA
10 Stamford Road, Oakleigh, Melbourne 3166, Australia

First published 1991

Printed in the United States of America

Library of Congress Cataloging-in-Publication Data
Perspectives on language and thought : interrelations in development /
editors, Susan A. Gelman, James P. Byrnes.

   p.   cm
ISBN 0–521–37497–9
1. Language acquisition.   2. Cognition in children.
3. Categorization (Linguistics)   4. Social interaction in children.
I. Gelman, Susan A.   II. Byrnes, James P.
P118.P42   1991   90-28184
401'.93–dc20   CIP

British Library Cataloguing in Publication Data
Perspectives on language and thought : interrelations in
development
1. Children. Psychology. Psycholinguistics. Cognition
I. Gelman, Susan A.   II. Byrnes, James P.
401.9

ISBN 0–521–37497–9   hardback

To Barbara and Bruce

Contents

vii

Preface

The goal of this book is to explore the multiple relations between language and cognition in the course of first language acquisition. Children learn an enormous amount during the few years between birth and the time they reach school age. Among their accomplishments are the organization of their experiences into categories and the acquisition of a native language. How do they accomplish these critical tasks? How do their conceptual systems influence the structure of the languages they speak? How do linguistic patterns influence how they (and we) view reality? These questions – and the explorations of their answers in this volume – should be of interest to professionals and advanced students in the fields of language development, cognitive development, and cognition more generally.

We are grateful to many people for making this volume possible. The authors of the chapters deserve special thanks and congratulations for their outstanding contributions. Donna Pineau at the University of Michigan spent many hours typing portions of the book and ferrying manuscripts to the post office. Helen Wheeler, Julia Hough, Katharita Lamoza, Mary Racine, and the staff at Cambridge University Press were unfailingly helpful and patient in creating a book out of what had begun as just a thought. We thank Gail Gottfried and Erin Hartman for their careful help with proofreading and preparing the indexes. We also acknowledge the generous assistance of NICHD Grant HD-23378, a Spencer Fellowship from the National Academy of Education, and an award from the W. K. Kellogg Foundation through the Presidential Intiatives

Fund of the University of Michigan for supporting S. Gelman during the preparation of the book. The University of Michigan generously provided resources, moral support, and a semester's leave of absence for S. Gelman during this time.

Contributors

Marylou Boynton
*Graduate School of
Education and Human
Development
University of Rochester*

James P. Byrnes
*Institute for Child Study
Department of Human
Development
College of Education,
University of Maryland*

Maureen A. Callanan
*Board of Studies in
Psychology
University of
California–Santa Cruz*

Eve V. Clark
*Department of
Linguistics
Stanford University*

John D. Coley
*Department of
Psychology
University of Michigan*

Lucia French
*Graduate School of
Education and Human
Development
University of Rochester*

Susan A. Gelman
*Department of
Psychology
University of Michigan*

Dedre Gentner
*Department of
Psychology
Northwestern University*

William S. Hall
*Department of
Psychology
University of Maryland*

Rosemary Hodges
*Graduate School of
Education and Human
Development
University of Rochester*

Frank C. Keil
*Department of
Psychology
Cornell University*

Ellen M. Markman
*Department of
Psychology
Stanford University*

Katherine Nelson
*Developmental
Psychology
City University of
New York*

Mary Jo Rattermann
*Department of
Psychology
University of Illinois*

Ellin Kofsky Scholnick
*Department of
Psychology
University of Maryland*

Marilyn Shatz
*Department of
Psychology
University of Michigan*

Sandra R. Waxman
*Department of
Psychology
Harvard University*

Sharon A. Wilcox
*Department of
Psychology
University of Missouri–
St. Louis*

I. Introduction

1. Perspectives on thought and language: Traditional and contemporary views

JAMES P. BYRNES AND SUSAN A. GELMAN

Introduction

Each of the contributions to this volume began from a simple insight: If we are to understand fully either language or thought, we must understand how they develop and interact in children's minds. Philosophers have long speculated about the origins of our distinctly human abilities to speak and reason complexly. Only relatively recently, however, has the issue been the subject of serious scientific study. We are now in the midst of an explosion of such research. In the past twenty years we have witnessed many exciting advances in the study of language and cognitive development. Now more than ever before, the utterances of small children are being gathered, scrutinized, and incorporated into broader theories of human cognition. The purpose of the present volume is to report and reflect on these advances. The product is a set of detailed and compelling models of language–thought relations (specifically, meaning–concept relations) as reflected in the developing mind of the child.

There are two quite different motivations for focusing on development as a window onto language–thought relations. One motivation is that children's behaviors provide clues to constraints on language and on thought. We can determine how languages and conceptual systems are constrained by examining the forms and meanings that children construct, and which errors they *fail* to make. All natural languages must be learnable by children; thus, children

The preparation of this chapter was supported by NICHD Grant HD-23378 to the second author and an award from the W. K. Kellogg Foundation through the Presidential Initiatives Fund of the University of Michigan. We are immensely grateful to Bruce Mannheim, John Coley, and Sandy Waxman for their thoughtful comments on a previous draft.

provide clues to what is universal, not only in syntax but in semantics as well.

A very different motivation for taking a developmental approach is that it can provide valuable clues to the complexities of the system eventually acquired. A developmental approach is inherently concerned with process, and so is especially suitable for detecting the relations among the ingredients of a complex system (including input, learning conditions, and conceptual requirements). Studying development is thus a powerful methodological tool and potentially more revealing about the organization of the system than any attempt to infer it from the adult end product. Harsanyi (1960) argues that knowledge about how transitions are structured provides insight into how states are structured, but not vice versa. Thus, developmental models are inherently more powerful and predictive than static models.[1]

The three succeeding parts of the book address these concerns, each examining a different content area. Part II concerns the interplay between category learning and the acquisition of individual words. The focus is primarily on the development of object terms at the beginning stages of the acquisition period (i.e., before age 5). Part III focuses on the acquisition of language for complex and abstract systems of time, logic, and causality. Here more extended developments are traced throughout childhood. Part IV examines the interpersonal environment in which language is learned, including peer and parental discourse, which, by implication, clarifies the nature of the child's role.

Shatz and Wilcox aptly observe that "the relations between language and thought [are] neither simple nor unidirectional. Indeed, what makes the study of linguistic and cognitive development intriguing is that it is not" (Chapter 9, this volume). Accordingly, the chapters in this book do not provide a simple conclusion such as "Language comes first" or "Concepts are primary." They decidedly do not present global theories; rather, they forge more particular language–thought links, showing respect for the richness and complexity of the relations.

Nonetheless, each chapter owes an intellectual debt to the great theorists of language–thought relations, including Chomsky, Piaget, Whorf, and Vygotsky.[2] Allusions are made throughout the chapters to the provocative notions endorsed by these grand theorists (such as *linguistic determinism* and *internalization of communi-*

cative speech). However, we asked the authors not to dwell on such background theories, but to present their own positions instead.

The rest of this chapter provides a historical context for the chapters that follow. We discuss four recurring themes of the book that cross-cut the section boundaries: constraints on development, the complexity of conceptual systems, the role of theory, and communication and social interaction. For each theme, we summarize first the classic views most befitting it, then the current contributions. The final section presents some issues for future research.

Constraints on development

The notion of constraints on semantic structures stems in part from Chomsky's arguments concerning the acquisition of syntax. Chomsky stressed the significance of language development (in particular, syntactic development) as a window onto the human mind. As a starting point, he made three assumptions concerning language and the learning process. First, grammars are systems of complex rules that determine which utterances are acceptable. The sentences we speak cannot have been memorized (see Miller, 1967, pp. 79–80, for a stunning demonstration of the vast number of sentences that would have to be memorized in order to store just a small sample of the infinitely many grammatical sentences of English); rather, they are creative, generative constructions. Second, the information a child receives is "impoverished" both in practice (because of our human tendency to make errors, including slips of the tongue and false starts) and in principle (because we receive only incomplete, indirect evidence about the structure of language; "the stimulus does not contain the elements that constitute our knowledge" [Chomsky, 1980, p. 35]). It would seem, then, that children could not induce the structure of the language from the finite sentences they hear around them using only general learning principles (for the role of parental speech input, see also Furrow & Nelson, 1986; Gleitman, Newport, & Gleitman, 1984). Third, despite the complexity of the task and the fragmentary nature of the input, the process of learning language is fairly uniform across speakers and nearly complete at an astonishingly early age. Indeed, all normal children learn the basics by age 4, and in many parts of the world children learn two or three languages simultaneously. Chomsky notes "the vast qualitative difference between the impoverished and unstructured environment, on the one hand, and the highly specific and intricate structures that uniformly develop, on the other" (1980, p. 34; see also Chomsky, 1975, 1988, for reviews). Taken together, these assumptions illustrate how impressive the accomplishment of language learning is and raise the question of how it is even remotely possible.

Chomsky's view is that there are highly abstract innate structures that constrain the acquisition of syntax. Children have an inborn outline of what language will be like (a "Language Acquisition Device"), and this guides them in learning its delicately complex structures. Language develops, just like any other organ or system in the body, such as the liver or the visual system. According to Chomsky, "in certain fundamental respects we do not really learn language; rather, grammar grows in the mind" (1980, p. 134). Thus, the human genetic endowment is said to impose limits on developmental processes in language (as well as other cognitive faculties).

According to Chomsky, nonnativist approaches to language acquisition are fundamentally misguided in their appeal to domain-general learning mechanisms such as "conditioning" or "assimilation" and "accommodation." Such general mechanisms endow the young child with too little knowledge of linguistic structures. Chomsky appeals to the "argument from poverty of the stimulus" to propose that children must have some idea of what to look for when learning their native tongue:

> Were it not for this highly specific innate endowment, each individual would grow into some kind of an amoeboid creature, merely reflecting external contingencies, one individual quite unlike another, each utterly impoverished and lacking the intricate special structures that make possible a human existence and that differentiate one species from another. (1980, pp. 33–34)

Gleitman and Wanner (1982) point out that all explanations of language learning assume some native ability. Even extreme empiricists such as Bloomfield (1933) and Skinner (1957) presume that children are born with the capacity to note similarity, form analogies, and generalize information. The disagreement lies in how richly specified and domain-specific the innate knowledge is.

Approaches that are relatively nonnativistic are also notable in that they do not admit of modularity, or the existence of "separate systems [of the mind each] with their own properties" (Chomsky, 1988,

p. 161; see also Fodor, 1975, 1983). Just as modularity is assumed for different physical systems (e.g., visual vs. circulatory system), Chomsky suggests that it is reasonable to assume modularity for different mental systems as well. Although modular systems interact with other forms of knowledge (Sadock, 1983), they are assumed to operate each according to its own set of rules. Modularity implies nativism: "The belief that various systems of mind are organized along quite different principles leads to the natural conclusion that these systems are intrinsically determined, not simply the result of common mechanisms of learning or growth" (Chomsky, 1975, pp. 40–41). Conversely, a nonnativistic approach implies lack of modularity.

Chomsky's analysis can be extended to semantic development, given that children learn word meanings as rapidly as they construct grammars. Extrapolating from the vocabulary of a 6-year-old, children are thought to add between five and nine new words to their lexicon *daily* between 18 months and 6 years of age (Carey, 1978; Dromi, 1987). Furthermore, word meanings are rarely given explicitly; they must be inferred (see Quine, 1960, for arguments concerning the indeterminacy of meaning).[3]

Just as children are predisposed with regard to the syntactic structures they will find, so too their conceptual and semantic systems are informed by preexisting expectations. Yet the precise form of these constraints, the degree to which they are specified innately, and their relation to conceptual and pragmatic constraints are not yet known and are among the topics discussed in this volume.

For instance, Eve Clark (Chapter 2) distinguishes conceptual constraints from lexical constraints, arguing that both are critical in acquiring not only conventionalized words but also direct, spontaneous lexical innovations by the child, such as *button-man* meaning a man who throws buttons. The lexical constraints include pragmatic principles: the conventionality assumption ("for certain meanings there is a form that speakers expect to be used in the language community") and the contrast assumption ("every two forms contrast in meaning"). The lexical constraints also include constraints on lexical meanings: the single-level assumption ("words apply at a single level [of abstraction]") and the no-overlap assumption ("the meanings of any two words do not overlap"). Clark argues that a full understanding of lexical acquisition requires an incorporation of conceptual universals as well as language-specific conventions of the surrounding society. The chapter is important for its incorporation of three levels of analysis: conceptual, lexical, and pragmatic. Clark suggests that conceptual categories provide one important starting point for children's hypotheses about what words mean, whereas pragmatic principles help refine and shape children's early hypotheses.

Ellen Markman (Chapter 3) proposes three constraints on word meaning: the whole-object assumption ("[a label] refers to the object as a whole, and not to its parts, or substance, or color, etc."), the taxonomic assumption ("[a label] refers to other objects of the same kind or same taxonomic category, and not to objects that are thematically related"), and the mutual exclusivity assumption ("each object will have only one label"). She points out that these constraints, although reasonable first-order approximations of the system to be learned, will eventually come into conflict and proposes a model for the resolution of conflicting interpretations by young children. These views are supported by a series of elegant experimental studies of word learning in young children. Markman is agnostic as to whether the constraints are specifically linguistic and suggests interesting ways that they may reflect more general cognitive predispositions.

Sandra Waxman (Chapter 4) argues for "implicit biases" that guide the process of word learning and proposes an interplay between conceptual level and linguistic form. Drawing on cross-cultural studies of ethnobiology, linguistic analyses, and developmental work, she argues that basic-level categories (e.g., *dog, grape*) are named consistently across cultures. Languages exert their effects at nonbasic levels, both superordinate and subordinate. Whereas novel nouns are presumed to focus attention on taxonomic relations at the superordinate level, novel adjectives are presumed to mark subordinate-level distinctions. Thus, semantic constraints cannot be considered apart from linguistic form.

For the most part, constraint theorists have focused on nouns, although Clark, Markman, and Waxman discuss the implications that constraints have for the learning of other parts of speech. Shatz and Wilcox (Chapter 9) take the critical step of applying a constraints approach to a "complex and irregular system," the English modal system (including, e.g., *should, might, hafta*). They argue that the convergence of constraints may operate in other complex systems as well. They also propose broadening the notion of constraint to include any "factors that channel or direct the process of acquisition," including input.

Although informed by Chomsky's approach, the chapters dealing with constraints make important departures as well. Semantic constraints are not assumed to be innately specified. (Indeed, on some views constraints may be the product of development; see Roberts & Goodman, 1985.) Perhaps most importantly, the present chapters examine closely the interplay between semantic biases and other factors, including world knowledge (Waxman), the language community (Clark; Shatz & Wilcox; Waxman), and general cognitive predispositions (Markman).

The complexity of conceptual systems

A second major theme is that language maps onto complex conceptual systems and that understanding these complex systems gets at the heart of the acquisition process. It is in part because of this complexity that Chomsky was motivated to propose constraints on acquisition. However, few thinkers have been as deeply fascinated with the nature of conceptual systems as the Swiss epistemologist Jean Piaget. We first provide an overview of his position regarding language–thought relations, then turn to a brief summary of some of the chapters addressing this theme.

Like Chomsky, Piaget saw language as a window onto the mind. However, whereas Chomsky was intrigued with linguistic structures underlying language acquisition and use, Piaget focused on cognitive underpinnings reflected in language. Specifically, he considered "the role of language in the formation of intelligence generally and of logical operations in particular" (1968, p. 88). His work is notable for its portrayal of the rich conceptual knowledge that underlies adult language comprehension. Knowledge is not merely a passive accumulation of associations or isolated facts. Rather, knowledge is actively structured by the individual. It is "a specific form of biological adaptation of a complex organism to a complex environment" (Flavell, 1985, p. 4). By adulthood, the normal human can engage in sophisticated hypothesis generation and hypothesis testing, can consider the logical relations among propositions as distinct from their content, can reason about time and space from multiple perspectives, and can consider the hypothetical. According to Piaget, these thought processes can be modeled formally. Although the particular logical systems Piaget proposed have been criticized by some as models of human thought (Brainerd, 1978; Flavell, 1985; Keats, Collis, & Halford, 1978), at the very least his work reminds us of the richness of adult conceptual understandings.

Piaget (1968) identified three points in development at which language might play an important role. He argued that the role of language is rather modest in all three cases.[4] The first point concerns the transition from sensorimotor intelligence (based solely in action, immediate perception, and the here and now) to representational intelligence (evident with the onset of language and the ability to evoke absent situations from memory or imagine future events). Whereas others before him attributed this change in thought to the onset of language, Piaget argued that language alone is not responsible for this transformation. Rather, other forms of the emergent semiotic function, such as motivated symbols found in imaginative play, deferred imitation of absent models, and images deriving from internalized actions are said to be equally responsible for (or indices of) changes in thought. Unlike Chomsky, who insists on the uniqueness and integrity of the language faculty (i.e., the biological abilities that underlie language), Piaget argued that language is responsible for changes in thought only as it is part of the semiotic function more generally. He also argued that language cannot be considered a mechanism of intellectual change, because the onset of intelligent thought in the form of sensorimotor schemes developmentally precedes the onset of language.

The second point of conceptual development that Piaget considered was the transition between preoperational and concrete operational thinking. He proposed that a hierarchical "logic of classes" emerges around age 7 to 8 in which children are able to relate subordinate and superordinate classes using necessary and sufficient criteria and are also able to form class intersections within matrices. At the same time children are thought to develop a "logic of relations" in which objects can be ordered by increasing magnitude. Again, where others have assumed that particular linguistic advances in predication, negation, and inflection (e.g., comparative endings) precipitate changes in categorical and ordinal reasoning, Piaget argued against this view. Among several pieces of evidence, he pointed out that children fail to demonstrate the logic of classes and relations until age 7 or 8. This delay suggested that language forms are assimilated to children's level of thinking. In essence, language at most serves as simply one more form of experience within which contradictions to one's constructions are made evident.

In addition to the shifts from sensorimotor intelligence to pre-operations and from preoperations to concrete operations, the third point of development at which language might seem to affect thought was the shift from concrete operational thought to formal operational thought. Piaget (1968, p. 95) conceded that language plays a role in the formation of propositional concepts such as implication (*if . . . then . . .*) and disjunction (*either . . . or . . .*) but argued that the appropriate linguistic forms are not themselves sufficient for prompting conceptual change. In this case, the properties of formal operations include not only the hypotheticodeductive use of propositions in inferential chains, but also 16 possible combinations of the component clauses of these propositions, the potential to organize propositions into a hierarchical lattice, and the potential to relate propositions by means of the mathematical group operations, including four transformations: identity, negation, reciprocal, and correlative (INRC). Piaget argued that these properties do not arise from language.

Piaget (1968) summarized his view on the relation between thought and language as follows:

> Language is thus a necessary but not a sufficient condition for the construction of logical operations. It is necessary because without the system of symbolic expression which constitutes language the operations would remain at the stage of successive actions without ever being integrated into simultaneous systems or simultaneously encompassing a set of interdependent transformations. Without language the operations would remain personal and would consequently not be regulated by interpersonal exchange and cooperation. It is in this dual sense of symbolic condensation and social regulation that language is indispensable to the elaboration of thought. Thus language and thought are linked in a genetic circle where each necessarily leans on the other in an interdependent formation and continuous reciprocal action. In the last analysis, both depend on intelligence itself, which antedates language and is independent of it. (p. 98)

Note that language is necessary for logical operations only in the sense that both language and logical operations depend on nonlinguistic intelligence.

Piaget also discussed the role of language throughout development (i.e., not just at transitional points) and argued that semantic understanding derives largely from the child's preexisting conceptual understanding (Inhelder & Piaget, 1964). When children are learning category terms (such as *cat*), quantification terms (such as *some*), relational terms (such as *brother*), and so forth, their levels of comprehension and production depend critically on their level of cognitive growth. In short, adequate semantic development requires the appropriate conceptual structures. Similar arguments are made concerning words expressing number, time, space, and causality. Thus, although Piaget believed that language and thought must interrelate in order for developmental change to take place, he also argued that language is but a reflection of thought at any single point in development. Overall, Piaget's position is referred to as *cognitive determinism,* in which the intellectual unfolding of the child's mind sets the pace for her linguistic developments (see Johnston, 1985, for a survey of several examples of cognition guiding and constraining the acquisition of English, e.g., with locative prepositions and dimensional adjectives).

Several of the chapters in this volume take up themes suggested by Piaget, though without endorsing his claims for cognitive determinism (see Gentner & Rattermann, Chapter 7, and Shatz & Wilcox, Chapter 9, in addition to those discussed later). One legacy is a recognition of the intricate layering of conceptual systems. Katherine Nelson (Chapter 8) points out that traditionally theorists have relied too heavily on linguistic, rather than psychological, models of word meaning. She suggests that the psychological problem is much richer than generally acknowledged: Words are parts of systems, idiolect differences abound, meanings change over time, meanings vary across contexts, and meanings are social constructions requiring interactions with others. Moreover, even when one considers nouns, words cannot be reduced to simple labels for objects. The case in point that Nelson pursues is the language of time (including *nighttime, tomorrow, right now, then*). Despite her attention to conceptual complexity, she rejects a straightforward Piagetian claim: "We have no firm basis at the present time for expecting general cognitive constraints on the expression of temporal relations." Rather, she argues for mutual influences among language, world knowledge, and the sociocultural milieu. Here the approach is Vygotskian in flavor (as discussed later).

An important testing ground for Piagetian theory is the acquisition of logical terms. Piaget's interest in logic stems from his broader interest in intellectual development and the role of language in explaining development from one level of thought to another (Inhelder & Piaget, 1964; Piagct, 1968). Thus, the language of logic is of critical interest and is discussed in two of the present chapters. James Byrnes (Chapter 10) focuses on the acquisition of two critical expressions of English, *if* and *because,* to detail the conceptual and linguistic requirements underlying their appropriate use. He argues that both the conceptual and the linguistic requirements are formidable and exert powerful influences on the course of acquisition. Given this analysis, it is striking that children are fairly conversant with these terms by 8 years of age. Byrnes ends with three specific proposals concerning the interaction of language and thought during the acquisition of complex systems: one derived from Karmiloff-Smith's (1986) proposal regarding the systematization of representations over time, one derived from a means–end approach to problem solving, and one derived from the metaphor of linguistic "bootstrapping."

Ellin Scholnick and William Hall (Chapter 11) identify two areas in which language–thought relations promise to be critical: logic (with particular focus on *if*) and metacognition. They provide precise hypotheses for the role of language as a supportive context and modulator and for the role of nonlinguistic cognitive contributions in providing a framework for and enriching linguistic expressions. As does Byrnes, they argue that language–thought relations are clearly a two-way street, and discerning these relations requires a precise knowledge of the systems under study. As Scholnick and Hall point out:

> One can find any of the possible models of language and thought relations from no overlap to complete identity, depending on the domain chosen. Similarly, whether language is the producer, by-product, or equal partner of thought in development may depend on the content area studied and the actual role that each process is thought to play.

The chapter provides an unusually rich convergence of conceptual analysis, linguistic analysis, and evidence from the conversational contexts in which children hear the terms being acquired. The relative contributions of language and thought are traced as a function of all three factors. Although it may not be surprising that complex systems must be explained with complex models, there have been too few attempts to construct detailed models of the interaction between language, thought, and context. The work of Byrnes, as well as Scholnick and Hall, is notable for its progress on this score.

The role of theory

The third theme is that theories guide the acquisition of concepts (and, correspondingly, language). Here we refer to "naïve theories," which are neither as formal nor as explicit as the constructs used by experts. This is a modern theme growing out of the interest of cognitive scientists in expertise and its developmental analogs (see McCloskey, Caramazza, & Green, 1980; Murphy & Medin, 1985; Neisser, 1987; Wellman, 1990). Despite the recent emergence of the metaphor of "child as theoretician," similar notions can be found in Piaget's respect for the complexity of conceptual systems (theories, after all, are needed to organize complex systems of beliefs, although Piaget does not speak of cognition in this way) and particularly in Whorf's discussion of habitual thought and world view.

Both Sapir (1929) and Whorf (1956) observe that languages – especially grammatical categories – construct implicit theories of the world. As they point out, there is no single, universal, genetically endowed framework for viewing the world. Rather, an individual's organization of knowledge reflects implicit assumptions about ontology, causality, and domains (Wellman, 1990). These assumptions are interconnected, interdependent, and to some extent coherent. It is in this sense that our assumptions of what kinds of things there are is "theory-laden" (Carey, 1985; Murphy & Medin, 1985). Whorf speaks of a "pattern-system" that is remarkably like what these days would be called a "naïve theory."

For the purposes of understanding the acquisition of semantic and conceptual systems, we can ask at what point in development theories are present in an individual, and whether theories are integral to word meanings. Frank Keil (Chapter 6) and Susan Gelman and John Coley (Chapter 5) take up these questions directly. Gelman and Coley argue that words are theory-laden, even for small children, and that language (in particular, naming) can help restructure concepts from a very young age. They review a range of studies showing that children as young as age 2 seem to expect categories to incorporate deep, nonobvious similarities, including internal structure and hidden essences.

Keil argues that relations among concepts can have important consequences for word meanings. For example, he discusses important conceptual differences between nominal kinds (e.g., *circle, odd number* – groupings defined by a single, well-specified criterion), natural kinds (e.g., *lion, gold* – "groups of entities that [cohere in nature and] are governed by a common set of laws" [Keil, 1989, p. 25]), and artifact concepts (e.g., *hammer, table* – groupings of human-made objects that are created intentionally). Conceptually, these three kinds of concepts differ in the importance of essences and causality (with natural kinds being most causally coherent and tied to essences). Correspondingly, Keil argues for differing routes of acquisition for the words that encode these concepts. This is a critical move, since in the past it has typically been assumed that acquisition works in the same way for all word meanings. Keil's framework not only argues that acquisition differs for different kinds of words (depending on the underlying conceptual structure), but also provides detailed suggestions about where to look for those differences. For example, causality should figure centrally in *semantic* representations of some words, given its importance in conceptual organization and theories. This work demonstrates that a close analysis of conceptual development has direct implications for the acquisition of word meanings.

For Keil, as well as Gelman and Coley, one strength of theories is that they enable us to bypass or overlook surface appearances or misleading perceptual cues. Causal beliefs, nonobvious commonalities, internal mechanisms become critical. For Gelman and Coley, language is an organizer of information that helps children in this regard.

Dedre Gentner and Mary Jo Rattermann (Chapter 7) provide a counterargument to the suggestion that young children bypass similarity. They suggest that there is much less evidence for theory-laden representations in young children. In particular, they provide evidence and arguments that similarity is a powerful organizer of language and thought in earliest childhood. In a broad range of cases, there is a developmental transition from relatively more reliance on perceptual similarity to relatively less. Theories are seen more as a consequence of development than as initiators or predispositions. When children hold theories is a lively and thorny issue; the rather different conclusions among the present chapters promise to give rise to fruitful discussions in the future.

The role of theory revisited: The importance of language

Two further claims by Whorf, informed by Sapir's writings and teachings, are particularly controversial and worth reviewing in this context. *Linguistic relativity* states that "structural differences between language systems will, in general, be paralleled by non-linguistic cognitive differences, of an unspecified sort, in the native speakers of the two languages" (Brown, 1976, p. 128); *linguistic determinism* states that "the structure of anyone's native language strongly influences or fully determines the world-view he will acquire as he learns the language" (Brown, 1976, p. 128). Whorf's focus was on grammatical categories in particular (e.g., plurality, gender, tense, aspect), as distinct from individual words or phrases. According to Whorf, grammatical patterns are "interpretations of experience." They orient the segmentation of sensory reality in particular ways. Thus, language has a distinct causal force in shaping conceptual systems:

> The forms of a person's thoughts are controlled by inexorable laws of pattern of which he is unconscious. These patterns are the unperceived intricate systemizations of his own language. . . . And every language is a vast pattern-system, different from others, in which are culturally ordained the forms and categories by which the personality not only communicates, but also analyzes nature. (p. 252)

For example, Whorf (1956, pp. 140–142; cf. Quine, 1960) suggested that there is no inherent or natural distinction between discrete objects with discernible boundaries or extensions (e.g., rocks) and continuous quantities without discernible boundaries (e.g., water); rather, the distinction is a product of the grammatical structure of English. In English, count nouns referring to discrete objects and mass nouns referring to continuous quantities have distinct grammatical properties. Only count nouns can be pluralized and preceded by articles. Moreover, there is a strong tendency to create countable, discrete quantities out of continuous masses using grammatical forms such as *a cup of* or *a stick of*. The consequence of this grammatical structure is that native speakers of English dichotomize the world into discrete and continuous quantities, whereas speakers of Hopi (in which all nouns are count nouns) do not.

For Whorf (1956), linguistic determinism extends well beyond our thinking about discrete versus continuous quantities to include our thinking about such fundamental concepts as time and space.[5] To illustrate, he contrasted the ways in which native speakers of "Standard Average European" languages such as English and French and native speakers of Hopi conceive of time. Standard Average European speakers conceive of time as a linear row of independent, discrete, countable units. Whorf hypothesized that this conception arose from Standard Average European linguistic constructions concerning time; for example, "10 days" is analogous to "10 people," in that each day is distinct from the one before it. Temporal counts, however, are plural in only an imaginary sense, because we cannot simultaneously perceive 10 days in the same way that we can perceive 10 people in a single spatial array. Standard Average European speakers conceive of time by means of a spatial metaphor made possible by linguistic structure. This metaphorical conception in turn affects habitual behavior, including the construction of calendars, clocks, and appointment books, as well as ordinary folk beliefs such as "Tomorrow is another day."

In contrast, Whorf argued, Hopi speakers lack such a conception of time, due in part to the grammatical unacceptability of constructions such as "10 days." (But see Hill, 1988, for disputes concerning Whorf's linguistic analyses of both English and Hopi.) In particular, Hopi linguistic patterning does not permit the construction of the Standard Average European spatial metaphor of time as a row of discrete temporal units. The Hopi conception of time is more a continuous stream of experience. Expressions for time are such that "10 days" are not analogous to 10 distinct entities paying a visit (as Standard Average European speakers think of time), but rather are analogous to 10 successive visits from the *same* entity (Whorf, 1956, p. 148). Accordingly, expressions in Hopi treat the present in terms of *preparation* for future "visits" from a day, wherein future experience accumulates and is dependent on prior experience. Whorf argues that the lack of an obsession with timekeeping instruments in the Hopi reflects this conception of time. In essence, Hopi speakers favor expressions such as "Well begun is half done" as opposed to "Tomorrow is another day" (p. 148). In short, Whorf argues powerfully for the primacy of grammatical patterning in conceptual systems.

Despite the appeal of Whorf's position to many scholars, direct empirical evidence for this position has been disappointing (e.g., Au, 1983; Brown, 1976; Carroll & Casagrande, 1958; Heider, 1972; see Au, 1988, for a review, but see Lakoff, 1987, for a more optimistic appraisal). Perhaps in part the domains that have been selected for analysis are not the right ones to reveal these relations (e.g., color terms have been extensively studied, yet color perception is presumably hard-wired into our perceptual system; see Bornstein, 1975; but see also Kay & Kempton, 1984; Lucy & Shweder, 1979). Whorf, like Boas and Sapir before him, was interested mainly in grammatical categories (obligatory, nonconscious, highly structured, and habitual) and habitual verbal behavior – he was not concerned with just any variation in language. As Lucy (1985) points out, the linguistic patterns that contribute to cognitive effects may be subtle and integrated across language systems; to quote Whorf, "A 'fashion' [of speaking] may include lexical, morphological, syntactic, and otherwise systematically diverse means coordinated in a certain frame of consistency" (1956, p. 158; see also Hymes, 1974). It has also been suggested that Whorf's is not a testable hypothesis to begin with, but rather an axiom of a framework for studying variability in linguistic and cultural patterning (Carroll, 1956, pp. 29–30; Mannheim, 1987).

None of the chapters in this book argue strongly for linguistic determinism as enunciated by Brown. Nonetheless, Whorf's influence can be seen in somewhat different form. Some of the linguistic constraints spelled out by Markman and Waxman may reflect a weak form of linguistic determinism – that is, by learning language children may become more attentive to taxonomic (e.g., *dog–cat*) as opposed to thematic (e.g., *dog–bone*) relations. Similarly, Gelman and Coley suggest that labels can redirect and reorganize children's classifications, allowing even young language learners to incorporate category anomalies (e.g., accepting a dodo as a bird). Furthermore, Gentner and Rattermann provide provocative evidence that relational labels (e.g., *Daddy, Mommy,* and *Baby*) can help children focus on relational similarity when mapping from one array of objects to another. Similarly, they suggest that children may more readily extract common relations between two events when one of them is described in a manner precisely designed to foster a metaphorical interpretation. Finally, Nelson suggests that language may make certain conceptual distinctions salient to the child (e.g., the tense system of English may highlight the distinction between past, present, and future) and may make possible the "construction of abstract concepts and complex representations that cannot be acquired solely from unmediated direct experience because they are culturally constituted through language" (e.g., *Saturday, hours*). In none of these cases do we have direct evidence for linguistic relativity. Nonetheless, all of these examples suggest that language may, at times, unconsciously pattern the child's view of reality.

Communication and social interaction

Critical to any complete theory of language and conceptual development is the role of social interaction. From those who take a functionalist approach to language learning in children (e.g., Bates & MacWhinney, 1982) to artificial intelligence researchers attempting to build a language-learning machine, the role of "input" or social exchanges takes on critical importance. The views of Soviet psychologist Lev Vygotsky are a starting point for any such theory.

Vygotsky's views on language acquisition are often contrasted with those of Piaget, although they share some important components. Both theorists argued that word meanings change with development and reflect underlying changes in thought (Vygotsky, 1962, p. 124); that significant portions of a preschooler's utterances (such as collective monologues) are egocentric and that egocentric speech sharply decreases in frequency between the ages of 3 and 7 (Vygotsky, 1962, p. 134); that younger children engage in "word magic," considering an object's label to be an inherent property of the object rather than a matter of convention (Vygotsky, 1962, p. 129); and that children often use linguistic constructions (such as *because*) in appropriate ways long before they grasp the conceptual relations such constructions typically convey (e.g., causality). In short, both Piaget and Vygotsky (as well as Whorf) believed that "grammar precedes logic" (Vygotsky, 1962, p. 127).

Also like Piaget (and Chomsky, though not Whorf), Vygotsky assumed that thought and language are distinct representational systems (Vygotsky, 1962). He based this assumption on examples of nonverbal thought (e.g., the problem-solving skills of apes and preverbal human infants) as well as nonsymbolic vocalizations (e.g., infant babbling). Vygotsky concluded that thought and language have distinct origins and originally follow independent tracks of development. However, at approximately age 2, these tracks seem to intersect for the first time wherein "thought becomes verbal and speech rational" (p. 44); that is, children discover the symbolic function of language as evident in their understanding that every object has a name. Thought and language can be conceptualized as two intersecting circles; their overlap is *verbal thought*. Thus, thought can exist nonverbally, and speech can exist without representational content (e.g., rote learning of a poem).[6]

What distinguishes Vygotsky most clearly from Piaget is his attention to social systems and their import for language and cognitive development. Piaget assumed that speech gradually becomes socialized with development. On his view, egocentric speech *precedes* socialized speech and reflects difficulties extending beyond the individual. In contrast, for Vygotsky egocentric speech was already always socialized. He assumed that speech is social from the start: "The primary function of speech, in both children and adults, is communication, social contact. The earliest speech of the child is therefore essentially social" (pp. 34–35). In children social speech can take two forms: egocentric and communicative.

Egocentric speech becomes progressively internalized, analogous to the progression from counting on fingers to mental counting. It is a transitional state that eventually gives rise to inner speech, or "speech for oneself," which serves as the medium of verbal thought: "In our conception, the true direction of the development of thinking is not from the individual to the social, but from the social to the individual" (p. 36).

Vygotsky found evidence for the social nature of egocentric speech in his naturalistic studies. Egocentric speech actually *declined* when children were placed in a group with other children who spoke a different language or who were deaf and nonspeaking (see Diaz & Berk, in press, for modern perspectives on private speech).

In Part IV, Maureen Callanan (Chapter 12) examines social interaction by studying how parents and children collaborate to help children construct and understand category hierarchies (e.g., that *jets* are *kinds of airplanes* or that *airplanes* are *kinds of vehicles*). She argues for an approach that combines Piagetian and Vygotskian views. Critical to this endeavor is an understanding of the role that parental input data can play in building theories of development.

Callanan distinguishes four different functions, two for the researcher and two for the child. For the researcher, parental input makes it possible to identify mismatches between parent and child in order to rule out parental teaching as a competing hypothesis of developmental change, and it fosters the identification of cultural attitudes regarding the parents' role in development (see also Shatz, in press). For the child, parental input serves as data that foster development and provides "scaffolding" for the child's construction of appropriate linguistic forms (see Bruner, 1983; Wertsch, 1985). Identifying patterns in the input does not automatically imply that acquisition entails more nurture than nature; rather, by examining the input one can gain a clearer understanding of the child's contribution as well as the causal links between input and acquisition.

Whereas Callanan focuses on adult–child communication, Lucia French, Marylou Boynton, and Rosemary Hodges (Chapter 13) take up the question of how peers learn to communicate with one another. Or as they put it, "How . . . do conversationally inept 2-year-olds manage to talk with one another?" This question is critical for disentangling the roles of parent, child, and context. With a mix of naturalistic and controlled observations, they provide a rich data base demonstrating the beneficial role of shared knowledge and shared physical context. This work implies that the development of both language and thought must be considered within the contexts of their use.

Questions and conclusions

At times clichés express basic truths, and such is the case here: The chapters in this volume raise as many questions as they answer. The questions that emerge, however, are focused and provocative. For example, from the studies of constraints, we can ask at what age particular constraints emerge, whether there is a preferred hierarchy of application when constraints conflict, and under which conditions the various constraints admit of exceptions. French, Boynton, and Hodges's study of early peer conversations raises the issue of what defines a "cognitive context," for the child as well as for the adult. And Callanan's study of parental input inspires us to ask about the relation between parents' theories of language and their ways of speaking with their children. In short, we are not left wondering simply whether language or thought is primary – itself an unanswerable puzzle (analogous to asking how the human body works). Rather, this research divides the larger enterprise into significant domains (analogous to asking how the human circulatory system works).

Of course, successful answers depend on successful questions – that is, they depend on parsing the problem correctly. Following Carey (1982), we believe that the study of language and thought requires a careful taxonomy of lexical distinctions, with an eye toward those that will yield the deepest implications for semantic development. The point is that not all words are susceptible to the same sort of semantic analysis, and capturing the appropriate distinction is critical to understanding the developmental course. Carey suggested distinctions between primitives and complex concepts; between natural kind terms and nominal terms; between open-class (content) words and closed-class (functor) words; between nouns and verbs.

Some of Carey's dichotomies are discussed in the present chapters (e.g., Keil as well as Gelman and Coley explore the distinction between natural kinds and nominal or artifact kinds). Additional contrasts are also suggested. Waxman distinguishes among basic, superordinate, and subordinate levels in a hierarchy, as well as between nouns and adjectives. Nelson contrasts implicit and explicit concepts (perhaps the Vygotskian distinction between spontaneous and scientific concepts) – which cross-cuts the distinctions above by focusing on process. Shatz and Wilcox implicitly propose a distinction between words that enter into complex and irregular systems and those that do not. A challenge for future researchers is to discover the nature of these distinctions and their implications for development.

A further challenge for researchers is to make use of evidence that will best answer the questions of interest, even when such evidence is difficult to come by. As one example, our understanding of constraints will be enriched by longitudinal work including younger children just beginning to break into the language system (especially those undergoing the naming explosion that Markman highlights in her chapter). Another striking example is the need for cross-linguistic data to address questions of universality and linguistic relativity. Slobin (1973, 1985) has convincingly argued that cross-linguistic evidence is perhaps our most powerful tool for examining grammatical and morphological development. Only such work is capable of sorting out what is "natural" or developmentally primitive from what is language-specific. We would urge researchers also to consider this tool seriously when studying semantic and conceptual development. Waxman as well as Shatz and Wilcox do so specifically, with provocative cross-linguistic results. Nelson's analysis of the language of time hints at potentially critical cross-linguistic effects. The constructions studied by Scholnick and Hall and by Byrnes are precisely the kinds of constructions that vary both formally and conceptually across languages and would be fascinating to study in languages other than English. A serious cross-linguistic effort would also make it possible to examine some of Whorf's intriguing, but untested notions directly. For example, does the child's notion of "individuation" vary conceptually depending on one's grammatical system (see also Quine, 1960), or are there universal commonalities? Currently there are a few programs of research examining semantic and conceptual development from a cross-linguistic perspective (e.g., Bowerman, 1985, 1987; Gentner, 1982; Gopnik & Choi, in press); we look forward to seeing more.

In sum, the perspectives set forth in this volume vary widely: The units of analysis range from the single word to the interactional (and cultural) context; the kinds of meanings range from semantic universals to language-specific nuances; the theoretical sympathies range from Chomskian to Vygotskian. Nonetheless, all of the contributors firmly agree that language–thought relations are bidirectional and that both conceptual complexity and linguistic transparency influence learning. The message that we hear repeatedly is that more focused hypotheses are needed, ones that are fully sensitive to the complexity of both language and thought and that articulate the intricate workings of their interrelations. We believe the chapters in this volume provide excellent models of the way such work can proceed fruitfully.

Notes

1. Carey (1982), however, points out that developmental primitives may not coincide with definitional or computational primitives.
2. We could list many other important theorists here, including Bloomfield, Sapir, Quine, Bruner, and Fodor. Instead, we have selected a representative sample of the broad range of positions that sparked and informed current research.
3. Although both Quine and Chomsky argue that one cannot directly infer a representation from the external stimulus (one can neither infer a

grammar from the input sentences nor infer meaning from pointing to an object and labeling it ["ostensive definition"]), Quine's "indeterminacy of meaning" is clearly distinct from Chomsky's "poverty of the stimulus." The latter assumes that the evidence for the mental structure is not even present in the input; the former assumes that the evidence is present – along with more information, besides. Whereas the poverty of the stimulus *requires* innate structures to account for knowledge, indeterminacy of meaning does not.

4. Whereas Chomsky is concerned with language as cognitive grammar, Piaget is concerned with language as talk.
5. Whorf distinguishes between the "apprehension of space" (or spatial perception), which he proposes is the same regardless of language, and the "concept of space," which is variable depending on the language one speaks (Whorf, 1956, pp. 158–159).
6. In contrast, note that in the Boas–Sapir–Whorf tradition, routinized behaviors are of special significance in determining *patterns* of thought.

References

Au, T. K. (1983). Chinese and English counterfactuals: The Sapir–Whorf hypothesis revisited. *Cognition, 15,* 155–187.
Au, T. K. (1988). Language and cognition. In R. L. Schiefelbusch & L. L. Lloyd (Eds.), *Language perspectives: Acquisition, retardation, and intervention* (2nd ed., pp. 125–146). Austin, TX: Pro-Ed.
Bates, E., & MacWhinney, B. (1982). Functionalist approaches to grammar. In E. Wanner & L. R. Gleitman (Eds.), *Language acquisition: The state of the art* (pp. 173–218). Cambridge University Press.
Bloomfield, L. (1933). *Language.* New York: Holt.
Bornstein, M. H. (1975). Qualities of color vision in infancy. *Journal of Experimental Child Psychology, 19,* 401–419.
Bowerman, M. (1985). What shapes children's grammars? In D. I. Slobin (Ed.), *The crosslinguistic study of language acquisition* (Vol. 2, pp. 1257–1319). Hillsdale, NJ: Erlbaum.
Bowerman, M. (1987, October). *Mapping thematic roles onto syntactic functions: Are children helped by innate "linking rules"?* Colloquium presented at the University of Michigan, Program in Linguistics, Ann Arbor.
Brainerd, C. J. (1978). *Piaget's theory of intelligence.* Englewood Cliffs, NJ: Prentice-Hall.
Brown, R. (1976). Reference: In memorial tribute to Eric Lenneberg. *Cognition, 4,* 125–153.
Bruner, J. (1983). *Child's talk.* New York: Norton.
Carey, S. (1978). The child as word learner. In M. Halle, J. Bresnan, & G. A. Miller (Eds.), *Linguistic theory and psychological reality* (pp. 264–293). Cambridge, MA: MIT Press.
Carey, S. (1982). Semantic development: The state of the art. In E. Wanner & L. R. Gleitman (Eds.), *Language acquisition: The state of the art* (pp. 347–389). Cambridge University Press.
Carey, S. (1985). *Conceptual change in childhood.* Cambridge, MA: MIT Press.
Carroll, J. B. (1956). Introduction. In J. B. Carroll (Ed.), *Language, thought,*

and reality: Selected writings of Benjamin Lee Whorf (pp. 1–34). Cambridge, MA: MIT Press.

Carroll, J. B., & Casagrande, J. B. (1958). The function of language classifications in behavior. In E. E. Maccoby, T. M. Newcomb, & E. L. Hartley (Eds.), *Readings in social psychology* (pp. 18–31). New York: Holt, Rinehart, & Winston.

Chomsky, N. (1975). *Reflections on language.* New York: Random House.

Chomsky, N. (1980). *Rules and representations.* New York: Columbia University Press.

Chomsky, N. (1988). *Language and problems of knowledge.* Cambridge, MA: MIT Press.

Diaz, R. M., & Berk, L. E. (Eds.). (in press). *Private speech: From social interaction to self-regulation.* Hillsdale, NJ: Erlbaum.

Dromi, E. (1987). *Early lexical development.* Cambridge University Press.

Flavell, J. H. (1985). *Cognitive development* (2nd ed.). Englewood Cliffs, NJ: Prentice-Hall.

Fodor, J. A. (1975). *The language of thought.* New York: Crowell.

Fodor, J. A. (1983). *The modularity of mind.* Cambridge, MA: MIT Press.

Furrow, D., & Nelson, K. (1986). A further look at the motherese hypothesis: A reply to Gleitman, Newport, & Gleitman. *Journal of Child Language, 13,* 163–176.

Gentner, D. (1982). Why nouns are learned before verbs: Linguistic relativity versus natural partitioning. In S. A. Kuczaj (Ed.), *Language development: Vol. 2. Language, thought, and culture* (pp. 301–334). Hillsdale, NJ: Erlbaum.

Gleitman, L., Newport, E., & Gleitman, H. (1984). The current status of the motherese hypothesis. *Journal of Child Language, 11,* 43–79.

Gleitman, L. R., & Wanner, E. (1982). Language acquisition: The state of the state of the art. In E. Wanner & L. R. Gleitman (Eds.), *Language acquisition: The state of the art* (pp. 3–48). Cambridge University Press.

Gopnik, A., & Choi, S. (in press). Do linguistic differences lead to cognitive differences? A cross-linguistic study of semantic and cognitive development. *First Language.*

Harsanyi, J. C. (1960). Explanation and comparative dynamics in social science. *Behavioral Science, 5,* 135–145.

Heider, E. R. (1972). Universals in color naming and memory. *Journal of Experimental Psychology, 93,* 10–20.

Hill, J. H. (1988). Language, culture, and world view. In F. J. Newmeyer (Ed.), *Linguistics: The Cambridge Survey: Vol. 4. Language: The socio-cultural context* (pp. 14–36). Cambridge University Press.

Hymes, D. (1974). Ways of speaking. In R. Bauman & J. Sherzer (Eds.), *Explorations in the ethnography of speaking* (pp. 433–451). Cambridge University Press.

Inhelder, B., & Piaget, J. (1964). *The early growth of logic in the child.* New York: Harper & Row.

Johnston, J. R. (1985). Cognitive prerequisites: The evidence from children learning English. In D. I. Slobin (Ed.), *The crosslinguistic study of language acquisition: Vol. 2. Theoretical issues* (pp. 961–1004). Hillsdale, NJ: Erlbaum.

Karmiloff-Smith, A. (1986). From meta-processes to conscious access: Evidence from children's metalinguistic and repair data. *Cognition, 23,* 95–147.

26   J. P. Byrnes and S. A. Gelman

Kay, P., & Kempton, W. (1984). What is the Sapir–Whorf hypothesis? *American Anthropologist, 86,* 65–79.
Keats, J. A., Collis, K. F., & Halford, G. S. (Eds.) (1978). *Cognitive development: Research based on a neo-Piagetian approach.* New York: Wiley.
Keil, F. C. (1989). *Concepts, kinds, and cognitive development.* Cambridge, MA: MIT Press.
Lakoff, G. (1987). *Women, fire, and dangerous things.* Chicago: University of Chicago Press.
Lucy, J. A. (1985). Whorf's view of the linguistic mediation of thought. In E. Mertz & R. J. Parmentier (Eds.), *Semiotic mediation* (pp. 73–97). New York: Academic Press.
Lucy, J. A., & Shweder, R. A. (1979). Whorf and his critics: Linguistic and nonlinguistic influences on color memory. *American Anthropologist, 81,* 581–607.
Mannheim, B. (1987, February). *Axiomatic relativism, anti-relativism.* Lecture to the Seminar on Group Dynamics, Institute for Social Research, University of Michigan, Ann Arbor.
McCloskey, M., Caramazza, A., & Green, B. (1980). Curvilinear motion in the absence of external forces: Naive beliefs about the motion of objects. *Science, 210,* 1139–1141.
Miller, G. A. (1967). *The psychology of communication.* Baltimore: Penguin Books.
Murphy, G. L., & Medin, D. L. (1985). The role of theories in conceptual coherence. *Psychological Review, 92,* 289–316.
Neisser, U. (1987). Introduction: The ecological and intellectual bases of categorization. In U. Neisser (Ed.), *Concepts and conceptual development: Ecological and intellectual factors in categorization* (pp. 1–10). Cambridge University Press.
Piaget, J. (1968). *Six psychological studies.* New York: Vintage Books.
Quine, W. V. O. (1960). *Word and object.* Cambridge, MA: MIT Press.
Roberts, R. J., Jr., & Goodman, G. S. (1985, April). *Reverse developmental trends: Development as the acquisition of constraints.* Paper presented at the biennial meeting of the Society for Research in Child Development, Toronto.
Sadock, J. M. (1983). The necessary overlapping of grammatical components. In J. F. Richardson, M. Marks, & A. Chukerman (Eds.), *Papers from the parasession on the interplay of phonology, morphology, and syntax* (pp. 198–221). Chicago: Chicago Linguistic Society.
Sapir, E. (1929). The status of linguistics as a science. *Language, 5,* 207–214.
Shatz, M. (in press). Using cross-cultural research to inform us about the role of language in development: Comparisons of Japanese, Korean, and English, and of German, American English, and British English. In M. Bornstein (Ed.), *Cultural approaches to parenting.* Hillsdale, NJ: Erlbaum.
Skinner, B. F. (1957). *Verbal behavior.* New York: Appleton-Century-Crofts.
Slobin, D. I. (1973). Cognitive prerequisites for the development of grammar. In C. A. Ferguson & D. I. Slobin (Eds.), *Studies of child language development* (pp. 175–208). New York: Holt, Rinehart, & Winston.
Slobin, D. I. (1985). Crosslinguistic evidence for the language-making capacity. In D. I. Slobin (Ed.), *The crosslinguistic study of language acquisition: Vol. 2. Theoretical issues* (pp. 1157–1256). Hillsdale, NJ: Erlbaum.
Vygotsky, L. (1962). *Thought and language.* Cambridge, MA: MIT Press.

Wellman, H. M. (1990). *The child's theory of mind.* Cambridge, MA: MIT Press.
Wertsch, J. V. (1985). *Culture, communication, and cognition.* Cambridge University Press.
Whorf, B. L. (1956). *Language, thought, and reality.* Cambridge, MA: MIT Press.

II. Relations between word learning and categorization

2. Acquisitional principles in lexical development

EVE V. CLARK

Languages depend for their content on words, and learning words makes up a large proportion of what children do as they acquire language. By one calculation, children learn on average nine new words a day between age 1 and age 6. And beyond age 6, by other estimates, they continue to add some six words a day to their vocabulary (see Carey, 1978; Liberman, 1989; Templin, 1957). But learning a word – its form and meaning – is no small task. It requires that one be able to identify the form of the word, its beginning and end, so that it can be picked out from the stream of speech and produced, eventually, in a form recognizable to others. And it requires that one learn what it means. This includes learning what *parts* of words mean, since knowing this offers children a way of expanding their current vocabulary much as adults do. When the occasion demands, children can construct new words out of known parts that they combine to convey novel meanings. They can also analyze known parts as they try to interpret new words.

But an unfamiliar word heard on a particular occasion could pick out an event or an object, a state or a relation, or a part of any of these. How does one narrow down the possibilities on each occasion in order to arrive at the conventional meaning? Children are aided in this task, I propose, by their reliance on various principles that help guide their acquisition of words. Two of these principles are general pragmatic principles that guide language use for adults as well as children. These two principles – conventionality and contrast – hold for adults and children alike. Moreover, their consequences for the lexicon play an important role in acquisition both

The preparation of this chapter and the research reported here were supported in part by the National Institute of Child Health & Human Development (NICHHD 5 R01 HD18908) and in part by the Sloan Foundation.

31

by constraining the options children consider for unfamiliar words and by offering a means for getting rid of unwanted overregularizations (see E. V. Clark, 1987, 1988, 1989, 1990). Children also rely on general principles that help them analyze the internal structure of form and meaning in words. They opt for simple forms over more complex ones, and they opt for transparent meanings over less transparent ones. These principles, though, appear to be discarded once children have mastered the repertoire of options in word formation. Finally, children attend to the productivity of the options used in adult speech and make use of this, much as adults do, in choosing among different forms. These principles, together, help constrain what children do in various ways as they assign meanings to forms and thereby transform the massive task of acquiring a vocabulary into a feasible endeavor.

Children produce their earliest recognizable words near the beginning of their second year. The first 50 or so fall into several domains – with one or two words each for people, animals, clothes, food, toys, greetings, and changes of place or state. Typical examples at the 50-word stage include some terms for greetings and routines: *hi, bye-bye, night-night, upsy-daisy*; for people: *mama, dada, baby* (self-reference); for animals: *doggie, cat/kitty, horsie, birdie*; for vehicles: *car, truck, bus*; for toys, clothes, and other small objects: *cup, bottle, spoon, shoe, sock, light* (light switch); and for certain changes in space or in state: *up, off, shut, wet, hurt* (see E. V. Clark, 1979a; Goldin-Meadow, Seligman, & Gelman, 1976; Nelson, 1973). As children add to their vocabulary, they gradually add new words to each domain and also add additional domains (see Dromi & Fishelzon, 1986, and, for a meticulous diary study, Dromi, 1987).

In this chapter, I begin by considering the principles of conventionality and contrast along with their consequences for the acquisition of the established vocabulary as well as of the building blocks for constructing innovative words. I then turn to several other principles that also affect children's acquisition of words and word structure. These are concerned with how transparent the meanings of unfamiliar words are; with how simple the forms of new words are; and with how productive in the speech community particular patterns are for constructing new meaning–form combinations. Transparency, simplicity, and productivity all at times interact with contrast and conventionality. Together these principles help guide children's acquisition of a vocabulary.

Conventionality and contrast

The two major pragmatic principles just introduced, conventionality and contrast, govern the lexicon, and do so not only for young children, but also for adult speakers in their everyday usage. Conventionality essentially assumes that words have conventional meanings. That is, unless speakers have some meaning in mind for which no conventional expression is already available, they will rely on established words to express their intended meanings. This principle can be stated as follows: For certain meanings there is a form that speakers expect to be used in the language community.

Conventionality here is to be taken in the sense discussed by Lewis (1969). A convention is essentially an agreement between two or more people about how something should be done – whether it is how to set up a mountain campsite, which side of the road to drive on, or which word to use to express a particular meaning. The utility of conventions in language comes from the mutual understanding they engender and from the consistency they offer over time. For example, *chair* designates chairs for all speakers who use this term in English-speaking communities, and the conventional meaning associated with *chair* remains consistent from one occasion to the next. (Meanings may change over time, of course, but such change must be sanctioned by the speech community or some subset of it.) Mutual understanding among speakers and consistency over time would appear to be necessary design features for a language to work as a communication system. Without conventionality, it is unclear that speakers and addressees could arrive at mutually agreed on interpretations of what the speakers were attempting to communicate. With conventionality, the paths of communication are considerably smoothed.

Each speech community relies on its members' knowledge of the conventions peculiar to that community. But each speaker typically belongs to more than one community. A community may be large, as it is for speakers of standard American English, for example, or it may be much smaller, as in the community of bird watchers or the community of embroiderers. Speakers may belong to a large community and simultaneously be members of several smaller communities as well. In each, membership is marked by observance of the conventions on the part of all the members.

Conventionality works hand in hand with the principle of contrast, namely, that different forms in a language have different meanings. This can be stated as follows: Every two forms contrast in meaning. That is, different forms typically have different meanings, as has been recognized for a long time (see, e.g., Bréal, 1897; de Saussure, 1919/1968; Paul, 1898), although the reverse does not hold. Two different meanings may be and often are expressed by the same form.

Together, these two pragmatic principles place certain constraints on the options speakers make use of to convey their intended meanings to their addressees. If speakers already have available to them a term that conventionally carries the pertinent meaning, they must make use of it, and not of something else; otherwise, their addressees will not be able to understand what they mean. And equally, if speakers wish to convey some meaning for which there is no conventional term available, they can construct a new word for that meaning on that occasion, provided they do so in circumstances that allow their addressees to arrive at the intended meaning. Such an innovative term, of course, must contrast in meaning with conventional meanings already in the lexicon. So if the speaker violates this condition and coins a new verb, *to hospital* say, and uses it in a setting where the conventional verb *to hospitalize* is available to express just the meaning for which the novel verb is being used, the addressee will reason as follows:

(1)   The speaker used the verb *to hospital*.
(2)   The meaning of *to hospital* seems to be "put into a hospital";
(3)   but that meaning is conventionally carried by *to hospitalize*, which means precisely "put into a hospital".
(4)   Therefore, the speaker must have meant something different from (2);
(5)   but there is nothing that allows me to compute a meaning different from (2).
(6)   Therefore, I find *to hospital* unacceptable.

If instead the speaker coins *to hospital* with a meaning that contrasts with *to hospitalize* – let's say it is intended to mean "endow a hospital with funds to build new wards" – then the addressee can accept that verb, having computed its intended meaning, because its meaning contrasts with that of *to hospitalize*. The "contract" being observed here depends on the kinds of principles put forward by Grice (1975; see further Clark & Clark, 1979).

The meanings of available, conventional terms place constraints on the possible meanings of innovative terms. Innovations must contrast in meaning with established terms; otherwise, they are unacceptable. This consequence of conventionality and contrast together can be expressed as the principle of pre-emption by synonymy: "If a potential innovation would be precisely synonymous with a well-established term, the innovative term is normally pre-empted by the well-established one, and is therefore considered unacceptable" (Clark & Clark, 1979, p. 798). Adults avoid coining words with meanings already represented in the lexicon, and when they do coin new words, they make them contrast with available conventional terms. Children should follow the same course, but their knowledge of the conventional lexicon is very limited compared with the adult's, so their innovations may often coincide in meaning with established terms – terms that children have yet to acquire (E. V. Clark, 1981).

Children attend to conventionality from the start in their own production of language. They take as their targets words produced by the adults around them, even though their own renditions of adult terms are often unrecognizable. From early on, almost as soon as they begin to talk, they seem to deliberately elicit conventional words, at first by pointing or pointing and staring, later – around age 2 – by actively asking, "What's that?" That is, children appear to recognize very early that language is *conventional*, that the speakers around them have words for objects, events, states, and relations, and that a major task in acquisition is to map those conventional terms into the appropriate conceptual categories (see E. V. Clark, 1983; Slobin, 1985b).

Children also observe contrast from very early on. They actively reject apparent synonyms, they assume that unfamiliar words refer to unfamiliar objects or actions, and they coin words to fill gaps. This early observance of contrast could develop with children's recognition of intentions as part of rational behavior:

> To discover Contrast as a pragmatic principle, children would have first to see the underpinnings of rational behavior – that people do things intentionally, and they always have a reason for choosing one word, x, on a particular occasion, rather than another, y. From this it would follow that x could not be equivalent to y, and so must contrast with it in some way (see Clark & Clark 1979). (E. V. Clark, 1988, p. 324)

In the next section, we will look in more detail at how children apply conventionality and contrast in the acquisition of unfamiliar words.

Acquiring unfamiliar words to fill gaps

Every day, small children hear many unfamiliar words, and they have to do their best on each occasion to come up with some hypothesis about what the speaker intended, and so what that word on that occasion might have meant. In doing this, children are guided to some extent by what they already know. They categorize objects and events, states, and relations from soon after birth onwards. The information they take in about these categories and their interrelations serves as a basis for their hypotheses about word meanings. As they amass knowledge about forms, functions, and histories for different categories and their members, they store more and more information that may be put to use once they begin trying to map words onto such categories (see E. V. Clark, 1977a, 1979b, 1983; Clark & Clark, 1979). By the time children produce their first words, at age 1 or so, they have stored a large amount of information about all kinds of things and events around them. But their knowledge of the world is necessarily still limited, and this in turn limits the kinds of hypotheses they initially entertain about word meanings. As their general knowledge grows, so does the sophistication of their mappings from conceptual categories to word meanings.

Lexical structure, though, does not bear any simple relation to conceptual structure. Languages differ considerably in how many lexical items they may deploy in a specific domain, and where the boundaries between meanings lie. Speakers of English, for example, rely essentially on just one verb for talking about getting dressed, *to put on*, and are indifferent to whether one is talking about a garment on the upper or lower body, on the extremities (hands or feet), or on the head, or about ornaments like rings, earrings, or bracelets. But speakers of Japanese take account of all these distinctions in choosing which of several verbs to use in talking about dressing (see, e.g., Backhouse, 1981; Kameyama, 1983). Other languages differ in the particular lexical structure that has grown up over the years for a specific domain and may use more terms than English for different kinds of camels or rice, say, or fewer terms than English for colors. In effect, the words of a language offer ways of representing only selected parts of any one domain, and they may focus the speaker's attention on alternative dimensions of a single domain. Different languages may offer different patterns of lexicalization to their speakers (Talmy, 1985), and these differences are therefore reflected in the input children receive from speakers of specific languages that then shapes and helps organize the lexical meanings and lexical structure children are trying to acquire (Bowerman, 1985).

Languages do not offer speakers an exhaustive mapping of each detail of every object or event. Rather, they are selective in what receives lexical expression. The relation between a conceptual category and its linguistic label is at best an indirect one. Although the label "stands for" the category the speaker is picking out, the actual relation between category and label is conventional and therefore arbitrary, so it may differ from one language to the next (Slobin, 1979). At the same time, languages are consistent in the "modulations" speakers can add to syntactic word classes. For example, nouns typically carry information about number and gender, and verbs information about aspect, tense, number, gender, and person (see Bybee, 1985). The inflections used to mark such modulations in meaning also offer children clues to word class and hence, indirectly, to the type of category being designated (see Gleitman, 1990; Naigles, 1990).

The conceptual basis

Children start by attaching basic or unmodulated lexemes to categories, or instances of categories – in particular to objects and actions. Some early word uses appear to be context-bound, appearing to be produced at first in only one context, then gradually being extended to other similar contexts, and then to an adult-like range of objects, actions, or events (Barrett, 1986). Only some early words are context-bound. Others, the majority, are extended immediately to a wide range of potential referents. Most of the earliest words children produce are used to pick out kinds of objects (e.g., *dog, duck, ball*), actions (e.g., *up, off, do*), and events (e.g., *bye-bye, peekaboo, bedtime*). But what leads them to attach labels to objects and actions, say, rather than to properties or parts? In the case of objects, the labels they attach seem to pick out the *whole object* – not just a part or a property. Indeed, 18-month-olds who are given labels for parts assume that the labels in fact pick out the whole object rather than just the part. Three-year-olds make the same assumption when they are given the label for a part of an unfamiliar, unlabeled object: They take the part label to be a label for the whole object (see Markman & Wachtel, 1988; Mervis & Long, 1987).

The kinds of categories of whole objects 1- and 2-year-olds appear to favor are categories at the *basic* or *generic level* – the level of categorization most likely to have single lexemes as labels across languages (see Berlin, Breedlove, & Raven, 1973; Mervis, 1987; Rosch, 1973). Moreover, when children attach labels to neighboring categories, they appear to look for *equal detail* in the alternatives they are considering. So a child who uses the label *bird* for chickens will look for a category at the same level of specificity when trying to map *duck* and is therefore more likely to attach it to the category of ducks than just to mallards or just to widgeon, both subkinds of ducks and therefore presenting more detailed points of comparison (Shipley & Kuhn, 1983). This ensures that the majority of the categories children label at age 1 to 2 are drawn from the same level of categorization. This is important for what has been called the *taxonomic assumption*, the assumption that labels pick out categories of objects (instances that belong to the same category) rather than associated clusters of objects. That is, children assume that the word *dog* picks out dogs, and not dogs-and-bones or dogs-chasing-cats, and that a label like *swing* picks out swings and not swings-with-children-on-them or swings-and-slides (Markman & Hutchinson, 1984).

The whole-object, generic-level, equal-detail, and taxonomic assumptions place constraints on what children (and to some extent adults as well) will count as a category that can be labeled. These assumptions, of course, all pertain to the conceptual categories children are beginning to build up and organize into groups of various kinds, including, in some domains, hierarchically structured taxonomies. This conceptual organization in turn has implications for the assumptions children make about the kinds of things that can have words attached to them.

The assumptions considered so far, though, all pertain to categories of objects. Indeed, research in this area has been confined almost exclusively to object categories. What of events and actions? Can children make similar assumptions when mapping words onto these kinds of categories? And do they do so? Research with adults suggests that event categories are taxonomic and in some domains are probably organized hierarchically just as many object categories are. In addition, there appears to be a basic or generic level of categorization for events, again just as for object categories (see Abbot, Black, & Smith, 1985; John, 1985; Rifkin, 1985; Rosch, 1978; Tversky

& Hemenway, 1984). Events appear to consist of sequences of actions, so categories of events appear to be superordinate to actions, which probably form the basic level of categorization. But the analyses available so far of how event and action categories are represented and stored lack many details. What counts as a subtype of action versus a (basic-level) action? Are action categories organized around prototypes, with a family resemblance structure, as object categories are?

Action categories differ from object categories in several ways. First, terms for actions are always relational in meaning. They link one or more participants, and there is no action without the pertinent participants. (Few object categories are relational.) Second, action categories have much vaguer boundaries than object categories do. It is difficult to decide, for instance, where an act of opening a door begins and ends – when the person approaches the door? reaches out a hand? grasps the doorknob? turns the handle? pushes the door away from the jamb? And when does the act of opening end? Third, the actual physical sequence of moves may differ considerably from one occasion of "opening" to another. Imagine opening a door, a can of sardines, a jar of marmalade, a briefcase, a book, a box of chocolates . . . All these acts receive the same label in English: *open*. The same point holds for acts of dressing: One puts on socks, shoes, gloves, underclothes, shirts, jeans, hats, coats – all with very different actions, yet all with the same label: *put on*. This diversity could make action categories harder to identify initially, so children might take longer to attach labels to them. This suggestion receives some support from the fact that children appear to be slower to learn labels for actions than for objects (Gentner, 1978, 1982). And they often rely heavily on a small number of general-purpose verbs (usually *do, go, get,* and *put*) in their first year or more of talking about actions (Berman, 1978b; E. V. Clark, 1978a, b). Children appear to apply verbs first to their own actions and only later to the actions of others as well. They do this earlier for verbs that map onto action categories for characteristic movements (e.g., *walk*) than they do for verbs that encode change and may require added inferences about causes, goals, or the internal states of others (Huttenlocher, Smiley, & Charney, 1983). Finally, it has been proposed that children organize their categories of actions and causality around prototypical events with typical intransitive or typical transitive causative actions (see Balcom, 1987; Slobin 1981, 1985b). Overall, it seems reasonable

Table 2.1. *Constraints on conceptual categories*

OBJECT CATEGORIES

Whole-object assumption: A word applied to an instance of an unfamiliar category refers to the whole object, not just to a part or property.

Generic- (basic-)level Assumption: Words pick out generic-level categories– categories that are optimally distinct from each other but whose members share a maximum number of parts and properties.

Equal-detail Assumption: Words pick out equally detailed instances of categories, and hence categories at the same level of specificity.

Taxonomic assumption: Words for objects pick out members of taxonomic categories, not sets of objects that are thematically related to each other.

ACTION CATEGORIES

Whole-action assumption: A word for an unfamiliar action refers to the act that links the different participants in that event as a whole, where the participants are picked out by object labels.

Generic- (basic-)level assumption (same as for objects)

Equal-detail assumption (same as for objects)

to assume that, here too, children rely on some limiting assumptions in setting up categories of actions that may carry labels, but actions and events have received less scrutiny than categories of objects.

Such assumptions play an important role in how children organize conceptual categories of objects, actions, and events (Table 2.1). Some assumptions apply only to object categories and others only to action categories. Others probably apply to both. Conceptual organization is important here because it offers the basis for children's hypotheses about the meanings of words they associate with contexts or occasions pertinent to specific categories. This holds just as much for their preliminary mappings of words for objects like *horse, ball,* and *milk,* as for actions like *come, get up,* and *open* and for events like *breakfast, bedtime,* and *bath.* It also seems to hold for their earliest hypotheses about relations in space such as containment and support; about orientation – on top of, beside, or in front of objects; about dimensionality – height, length, size; and about deixis – objects, places, or motion related to the position of the speaker (see E. V. Clark, 1979b). But the conventional meanings of words in a language are also shaped by what other words are available in a specific domain as well as by the words in the language at large.

Applying contrast

When children make use of contrast in adding a new word to their vocabularies, they do so by taking account of word meanings they already know in the pertinent domain and by then adding the unfamiliar word to that domain in relation to some object, event, or property not yet labeled. That is, on hearing an unfamiliar word in relation to some domain, the child-addressee must reason as follows:

(1)   The speaker is talking about domain X
(2)   and used the unfamiliar term *p*.
(3)   On this occasion, domain X contains one unfamiliar member.
(4)   Since the speaker didn't use *l* [or *m, n,* or *o,* all terms already known to the child in X],
(5)   the speaker must intend to indicate something other than referents of *l, m, n, o;*
(6)   so the speaker must intend *p* to pick out that unfamiliar object in domain X for which I don't yet have a word.
(7)   The term *p* therefore contrasts with the terms *l, m, n, o* that I already know in domain X.

Notice that in accepting the speaker's term *p*, the child does not necessarily have to assume that it is conventional, but that, probably, is the general assumption children make about unfamiliar terms offered for unfamiliar objects, events, relations, or properties under such circumstances. Often, of course, children may be unable to decide which kind the unfamiliar expression picks out on that occasion, and they may have to wait for another use before specifying its meaning somewhat. But parts of speech often offer clues (noun, verb, adjective), and so help narrow down the ways in which the new word contrasts with any already known. In addition, many unfamiliar words – perhaps most of them – are introduced to very young children in context, when the child and the adult speaker are in the presence of the kind of object, event, relation, or property that is being talked about and labeled.

Children then make use of the knowledge they already have about conceptual categories and how those are related or can be related to one another, plus their assumptions about the possible relations between categories and words, *and* their assumptions about words and how those are related to each other, in formulating hypotheses about possible meanings. Two of their major assumptions are pragmatic, conventionality and contrast. These apply not only to words

Table 2.2. *Constraints on lexical development*

PRAGMATIC PRINCIPLES
Conventionality assumption: For certain meanings there is a form that speakers expect to be used in the language community.
Contrast assumption: Every two forms contrast in meaning.
LEXICAL MEANINGS
Single-level assumption: Words apply at a single level.
No-overlap assumption: The meanings of any two words do not overlap.

but also to other linguistic units. And they interact both with each other and with other assumptions specific to lexical structure. Two of the latter are what I have called the *single-level assumption* and the *no-overlap assumption* (E. V. Clark, 1987). These capture the fact that children act as if the words they produce at first all apply at the same level and never overlap in meaning. These two assumptions may stem in part from three facts about conceptual categories: (a) Many of the categories children have are at the generic or base level; (b) children act as if comparisons among categories require equally detailed alternatives; and (c) such alternatives at the basic level for objects do not overlap – for instance, the category 'dog' does not overlap with the category 'cat' or 'horse'.

Children apply the single-level and no-overlap assumptions too broadly at first, and only later narrow their scope to match adult usage. Adults apply the single-level assumption only to terms for categories *at the same level* within a hierarchy. And they apply the no-overlap assumption only within a single lexical domain, again for terms at the same level. Notice that the terms *animal* and *dog* overlap in meaning within the hierarchy of animals, and the terms *dog* and *pet* overlap in the hierarchy of pets. But *cat* and *dog* do not overlap (both terms designate kinds of animals), nor do *dog* and *goldfish* (both terms designate kinds of pets). Many terms, of course, can belong, or simply be assigned for some occasion, to more than one domain. And although some domains are organized as hierarchies, many are not, especially among terms for actions, events, properties, and relations (see Fillmore, 1978). These pragmatic and lexical assumptions are summarized in Table 2.2.

Evidence for contrast

Children's earliest word uses pick out distinct categories of objects or events. One-year-olds who produce *dog* and *up*, for example, do not apply these words interchangeably, and they act from the start as though they assume the two have different meanings. But contrast on its own allows for many kinds and degrees of overlap in meaning, whether among words at the same level or words at different levels. For instance, the terms *up* and *down*, at the same level, overlap in meaning in that both apply to "vertical displacement," and the terms *horse* and *animal*, at different levels, overlap in that a horse is a kind of animal. When contrast is combined with the single-level and no-overlap assumptions, the three together are equivalent to the assumption of mutual exclusivity. (This is why mutual exclusivity is not listed as a distinct assumption in Table 2.2; see E. V. Clark, 1987; Markman, 1984, 1987; Markman & Wachtel, 1988). Evidence for mutual exclusivity, therefore, is simultaneously evidence for contrast, although evidence for contrast is not necessarily evidence for mutual exclusivity. So when 2-year-olds give up the single-level assumption for a domain and, for instance, produce novel compound nouns to designate subkinds of a category, as in *chow-dog* and *Dalmatian-dog* (from a child who already knew the word *dog*), or assign unfamiliar labels as subordinate terms when they already know another label for instances of the categories apparently being talked about, they provide further evidence for contrast, but not for mutual exclusivity (see Clark, Gelman, & Lane, 1985; Gelman, Wilcox, & Clark, 1989; Taylor & Gelman, 1989; and Waxman, 1990).

When speakers use a word that is unfamiliar to children, children consistently assume that their interlocuters must therefore have intended to convey *some other meaning* that contrasts with the meanings of terms already known. This has been carefully demonstrated in several recent studies of children's acquisition of unfamiliar words. Dockrell (1981),[1] for example, observed that 3-year-olds found it easier to arrive at the intended reference of an unfamiliar noun than of an unfamiliar verb. (For the latter, they tended to seize on an object closely associated with the target action). Moreover, just as the principle of contrast would predict, they found it much harder to identify the referent of an unfamiliar noun when it "replaced" a known word than when it simply filled a gap. In a series of detailed case studies, Dockrell documented the course that 3- and 4-year-olds followed when presented with an unfamiliar animal term, a novel mode of locomotion, and a novel shape or color term. In the animal-term study, for example, Dockrell presented children with several familiar toy animals for which the children all had names (e.g., *cow, sheep, pig*) plus one that was unfamiliar (a tapir). Then, in asking the children to put each animal named away in a box, Dockrell introduced an unfamiliar noun (the "gombe") for the strange animal. The children readily inferred that the unfamiliar term picked out the unfamiliar animal and treated it from then on as another animal term. Despite greater difficulty in learning unfamiliar loco-motion terms, children acted in much the same way there too. In the color and shape study, Dockrell looked at the effects of linguistic information on children's inferences about what an unfamiliar term picked out. She found (a) that children this age did use linguistic information about which domain a term belonged to (here, shape or color), and (b) that they preferred to rely on information about shape over color as a basis for word meaning (see also Au, 1990; Au & Markman, 1987; Baldwin, 1989; Dockrell & Campbell, 1986).

Younger children also make use of contrast in similar tasks. Golin-koff and her colleagues (1985, in press) found that children aged 2,4 to 2,10 made systematic inferences about the referents of unfamiliar words when presented with objects for which they already had la-bels alongside objects for which they lacked labels. (Their ability to provide labels for the entire set of objects was pretested for all the children.) Two-year-olds selected known objects in response to known labels 94% of the time and chose novel objects in response to un-familiar labels 89% of the time. On a second trial, they continued to respond to familiar (86%) and unfamiliar (81%) labels appropri-ately. On a third trial, Golinkoff and her colleagues offered a *second* unfamiliar label and some as yet unnamed objects alongside both familiar and previously labeled novel objects to see whether the ear-lier use of the first unfamiliar label pre-empted use of a second label for the same objects. It did. The children continued to pick out re-ferents for familiar labels with a high rate of appropriateness (97%) and chose a second kind of unfamiliar object as the referent for the second unfamiliar label (72%). (In these trials, the children could choose on each occasion among familiar objects, unfamiliar objects that they had already labeled, and unfamiliar objects not yet la-beled.) These findings offer further support for the view that young children make use of the principle of contrast from an early age in assigning meanings to unfamiliar words and that they use it to help fill gaps in their vocabulary (see E. V. Clark, 1981, 1987).

What happens if children already have a label for an object, and there is no other object around to serve as a possible referent for an unfamiliar label? Contrast would predict that children would take such a label to designate something other than the whole object – a part, a property, or a subordinate, for example. This indeed seems to be what happens. Markman and Wachtel (1988) showed that 3-year-olds systematically assign novel words to unfamiliar objects, thus replicating the findings of Dockrell and Golinkoff et al. They then presented other 3-year-olds with unfamiliar labels for parts of familiar or unfamiliar objects, indicating to the children which part a word was intended to pick out and then testing the children's comprehension and production of the new term. These 3-year-olds did two things. First, when they already knew a label for the object (familiar objects), they treated the novel label as picking out a part, and second, when they had no label already available (unfamiliar objects), they used the part label to pick out the whole object. They acted in a similar fashion when offered an unfamiliar label for the substance familiar or unfamiliar objects were composed of. In other words, the children seemed to avoid assuming two distinct labels applied to the same category – a finding predicted by the principle of contrast in interaction with the single-level assumption (object labels all contrast at the same level of specificity) and the whole-object assumption (words pick out whole objects).

Knowledge of a familiar label, in other words, stops children from using a second label for members of the same category. But when presented with the option of assigning an unfamiliar label to pick out a part of a familiar object, or the substance it is made from, they do so readily. And when presented simply with a second label in the presence of familiar category instances with known labels, where the instances differ from each other (e.g., kinds of dogs), children as young as 2 infer that the second label picks out a subkind. This pre-emption or blocking of unfamiliar labels when a familiar label has already been acquired is a very general consequence of the principle of contrast. The kinds of pre-emptions existing in the lexicon, of course, change as children learn that terms can contrast across levels and need not always be considered at just one level. As children get older, they restrict the single-level assumption, giving it up entirely for many domains. As they do so, they find out that many terms *overlap* in meaning to some degree, so they also restrict the no-overlap assumption until it applies only within each level of a hierarchy. They also learn that terms can label properties (parts, substance) and relations as well as objects and events. (They must give up the whole-object assumption here too). And they remain highly attentive to the language the adults around them use – they adopt conventional expressions of all kinds, while at the same time analyzing the parts words can be broken into along with the meanings of those parts.

Here I have looked at children's acquisition of unfamiliar terms for objects. There has been much less research on their acquisition of terms for actions or events, so whether the inferences children make about how words map onto categories of actions are similar to those for categories of objects remains an empirical question. But children are often faced with the problem of having no ready words for things they wish to talk about. Under those circumstances, they have to find some other way to convey their meaning. One they have frequent recourse to is the coining of a new word. Contrast and conventionality play a central role here too, since innovative terms must contrast in meaning with known conventional terms. I therefore turn next to some of the principles children rely on as they themselves construct words to carry new meanings.

Coining words to fill gaps

Although the number of conventional words they know is limited, children do not restrict their conversations to topics where they have words already available. Rather, from the start they talk about what they are interested in. Since they have relatively few conventional means for doing this, they often have to stretch their resources. Here they can have recourse to several options. One is to overextend conventional words already acquired. Children may stretch a term like *horse* to pick out not only horses but also dogs, cats, sheep, cows, and a variety of other four-legged mammal-shaped entities. Or they may stretch a term like *door* to encompass the act of opening a door, turning on a tap, removing peel from an orange, pulling a chair out from the table, unbuttoning a coat, or turning on a light (see Anglin, 1977; Barrett, 1978, 1986; E. V. Clark, 1973a, 1983; Rescorla, 1980). Notice that such overextensions rely on the single-level and no-overlap assumptions along with the principle of contrast. By the age of 2 or $2\frac{1}{2}$, however, children typically switch from overextensions to extensive questioning ("What's that?") to elicit conventional labels.

A second option is for children to rely on general-purpose words. Deictic terms constitute one class of general-purpose terms. A word like *that* can pick out an unlimited number of objects or events provided the speaker makes clear in context what, precisely, is being picked out on each occasion (see E. V. Clark, 1978c; Clark & Sengul, 1978). Although deictic terms can be used to pick out objects and events, they are rather limited when it comes to picking out relations, properties, or specific actions. Here children often have recourse to other kinds of general-purpose terms. They may use a single preposition like *in* (or the indeterminate form *'n*) as a general locative marker, or a general-purpose verb like *do, go,* or *get* to cover all sorts of actions. Not surprisingly, such verbs are very frequent in 2-year-old speech (see Berman, 1978b; Clark, 1978a, b; Huttenlocher et al., 1983).

A third option, and one that children begin to use early on, is to form new words out of existing ones. They coin nouns for objects by combining two known words (e.g., *bubble-hair* 'curly hair', *baby-towel* 'face cloth'), or by adding a suffix to a known word (e.g., *spyer* 'a spy', *angriness* 'anger'); and they coin verbs by using the word for the object most closely associated with the action in question (e.g., *to oar* 'to row', *to sand* 'to make into small particles', as in grinding pepper). These innovative words fill gaps for children and allow them to talk about things for which they still lack conventional words. Sometimes the gaps they fill are also gaps for adults, and there, children's choices of innovative forms to carry innovative meanings may coincide with adult choices. At other times, children's choices are limited by what they know so far about word formation. But many of the gaps children fill are not gaps for adult speakers, so some child innovations are illegitimate in the sense that, for adults, they are pre-empted by conventional terms with just those meanings. And in fact, as soon as children learn the conventional terms, they rely on them and no longer produce illegitimate coinages (see E. V. Clark, 1981, 1982a; Clark & Clark, 1979; for the shift to conventional terms, see Clark, Neel-Gordon, & Johnson, 1991).

The kinds of lexical innovations children produce, beginning around age 2,0, have been attested for many different languages in diaries and reports of vocabulary development for at least a century, but only recently have researchers begun to study them systematically. Studies so far have concentrated largely on what children know about word structure and hence about word formation by looking both at their ability to "gloss" or give possible meanings for novel word forms they have never heard before, and their ability to coin words for novel categories, categories chosen precisely because there is no word for that kind in the language being studied. When children innovate, though, they appeal to more than conventionality and contrast. Their innovations reveal systematic reliance on several other acquisitional principles.

These principles are principles for the processing of word forms, both for the analysis of words into parts (base and affix) and the assigning of meaning to those parts, and for the construction of innovative words where children must choose appropriate forms to express particular meanings. The forms children produce must be *transparent in meaning* to them before they can use them to express new meanings. This leads to two general predictions. First, children will use familiar base forms or combinations of such base forms before affixes; and second, they will prefer forms that have more specialized meanings (when these are available) over general-purpose forms. Early on, children will also place a premium on forms that are *simple in shape* and so require the least possible adjustment when assigned a new meaning. Among the predictions based on simplicity are, first, that children will use base forms before base and affix combinations; second, that among affixes they will use suffixes before prefixes;[2] third, that they will use bare compounds before compounds with affixes. At some points, then, transparency and simplicity may coincide in their predictions; at others, they diverge, with one form being more transparent and the other simpler, so it is possible empirically to order them. Early on, simplicity seems to take priority. When two forms are both transparent in meaning, for example, 2-year-olds pick the one with the simplest form. Later, once children have mastered many of the forms available, simplicity appears to play little or no role in the choice among available forms. Instead, in choosing among forms, children become sensitive to the relative *productivity* of specific meaning–form combinations.

Overall, these principles represent an attempt to capture the procedures children rely on as they analyze and coin new words, much as Slobin's "operating principles" are designed to capture children's preferences in the acquisition of syntax (Slobin, 1973, 1985b).

Simplicity of form

This principle captures the fact that when children first coin words, they make the fewest changes possible in forming a new word from building blocks already familiar to them. It can be stated as follows: Simpler forms are easier to acquire than more complex forms, where simplicity is measured by the degree of change in a form. The less a word form changes, the simpler it is. That is, children rely on familiar elements – at around age 2, typically whole words – in forming new words. Only from 2 on do they begin to add affixes to their repertoires, and for some time after this, they may have only limited knowledge of affix meanings and of how to combine them with existing words.

This principle allows for specific predictions about which kinds of changes children find complex and hence omit, and which they find easy, during the earlier stages of language acquisition. My emphasis here is on production, because children typically understand affixes and combinations of base and affix some time before they begin to produce them for themselves in innovative word forms (see, e.g., Clark & Berman, 1987; Clark & Hecht, 1982). Simplicity predicts, for example, that the earliest innovative compounds English-speaking children produce will be simple (bare) Noun + Noun compounds (e.g., *snow-tree* 'fir-tree') rather than compounds that contain affixes (e.g., *boat-driver, running-pants*). Their reliance on affixes in compounds and on verb- as well as noun-bases should be later because these require more changes or adjustments to the base forms used. On the same grounds, this principle predicts that Hebrew-speaking children will also find it easiest to produce bare Noun + Noun compounds first, and only later compounds with a head noun in its bound form.[3] In addition, the greater the changes required in going from the free form of a noun to its bound form, the later the acquisition of that type should be.

Simplicity predicts that when children produce innovative compound nouns, they should do so first by combining known words without modifications or changes to the forms of those words. Notice that only innovative forms allow for a test of acquisitional principles like simplicity of form. Established compounds in a language

Table 2.3. *Spontaneous novel Noun–Noun compounds
in Germanic languages*

Language	Child form	Adult gloss
Dutch	koppie-tafel	'coffee + table' (= table for coffee)
	water-man	'water + man' (= man who distributes water)
	trem-boeken	'tram + books' (= [books of] tram tickets)
	sport-hond	'sport + dog' (= dog with long, low body)
English	fire-dog	(= dog found at the site of a fire)
	snow-tree	(= fir tree, without any snow on it)
	plant-man	(= gardener)
	plate-egg	(= fried egg)
German	Korbwagen	'basket + wagon' (= small woven-straw pram)
	Wieguhr	'cradle + clock' (= kitchen scales)
	Fensterhaus	'window + house' (= house made of transparent blocks)
	Felsenberge	'rock + mountains' (= mountains made of rock)
Icelandic	fiatabill	'Fiat + car' (= Fiat)
	kubbabill	'block + car' (= car made of blocks)
	flugvélmadur	'airplane + man' (= pilot)
Swedish	fingerdeg	'finger + dough' (= playdough with fingerprints on it)
	golvkäpp	'floor + stick' (= stick for hitting on the floor)
	simbil	'swim + car' (= car that travels in water)

could be learned as if they were whole words, without any analysis of their internal structure. In what follows, I therefore focus only on innovative words – novel word forms with a meaning assigned for that occasion. As predicted, one of the earliest word-formation devices English-speaking children use, from as young as age 2, is Noun + Noun compounding. They combine familiar words to express novel meanings, meanings that are not computable out of context (see Clark & Clark, 1979; H. Clark, 1983). Children acquiring other Germanic languages also make extensive early use of simple Noun + Noun compounds where the first noun is the modifier and the second the head. Some typical examples drawn from several Germanic languages are shown in Table 2.3. In English, children consistently use compound stress for such forms, placing primary stress on the first, modifier, noun, and tertiary stress on the second, head, noun. By 2 or 2½, English-speaking children consistently interpret unfamiliar novel compounds as having modifier–head order, with heavier stress on the modifier than the head, and they readily

Table 2.4. *Producing agentive compounds with verb bases in English*

Stage	Word form	Example
1	*Verb + Noun(head)	*wash-man, open-man*
2	*Verb + Noun(object) *Verb-ing + Noun(object) *Verb-er + Noun(object)	*hug-kid, break-bottle moving-box, throwing-ball cutter-grass, puller-wagon*
3	Noun(object) + Verb-er	*water-drinker, well-builder*

Source: Clark, Hecht, and Mulford (1986).

produce compounds for contrasting subcategories, for example, *pencil-car* versus *carrot-car* (for cars made out of a pencil and a carrot, respectively). Among nouns, the majority of early child innovations in English consist of Noun + Noun compounds, with an occasional Verb + Noun one (e.g., *dry-hair* 'hair-dryer'). Hebrew-speaking children, in a similar task, are just as consistent in appropriately interpreting the *first* noun in a Noun^Noun compound as the head, and the second noun as the modifier. That is, children as young as 2 are already sensitive to the ordering of heads and modifiers in many constructions of their first language (for English, see Clark et al., 1985; for Hebrew, Berman and Clark, 1989).

Moreover, simplicity predicts that plain compounds will be used before compounds with affixes and compounds with a modifier-head order consistent with other constructions will be acquired before compounds with a different modifier–head order. When English-speaking children begin to use verbs in their compounds and to combine their verb and noun bases with affixes, they go through several stages before arriving at such productive adult compound patterns as the one illustrated by *basket-weaver* or *spoon-holder* (Noun + Verb-er).

These stages are summarized in Table 2.4. Among the earliest verb-base compounds are forms that combine a bare verb as modifier with a bare, generic head noun like *-man*, as in *push-man* or *open-man*. These are consistent with spontaneous Noun + Noun compounds in having modifier–head order, but are ungrammatical in English for talking about the agent, the person who *V*s (where *V* is the verb). At a second stage (around age 3 to 4), children start to incorporate the noun for the object affected into such compounds and, still using a bare Verb + Noun combination, place the verb in initial position as the head, and the noun second as the modifier.

Someone who builds walls is called a *build-wall*, and someone who opens doors, an *open-door*. This order is consistent with the head–modifier order of English verb phrases (e.g., [*he*] *throws the ball*), but not with the head-last order of complex nouns. Further evidence that the verb base is the head in such compounds comes from the addition of suffixes, like *-ing* or *-er*, always to the verb base, as in a *building-wall* or a *mover-box* for a person who builds walls and moves boxes, respectively (see Clark et al., 1985; Clark, Hecht, & Mulford, 1986).

Finally, around age 5 (or sometimes later), English-speaking children place the head – the verb and its affix – in final position to produce compounds like *wagon-puller* (someone who pulls wagons). As predicted by simplicity, children produce bare compounds first, then add affixes to the head (here the verb–base), and only after that get the modifier–head order for compound nouns. The order of head and modifier in such compounds in English causes difficulty, presumably, because of the differences in order for verb phrases (head first) and compound nouns (head last). In languages where the head–modifier order is consistent across different constructions, as in Hebrew, children do not make any errors in the word order of compounds during acquisition (Clark & Berman, 1987).

Simplicity of form also predicts that children will initially rely on word forms that require no change when they coin new words. In Hebrew, this would allow them to form compounds from nouns that do not require a change, but predicts that they will make errors on head nouns that have a special bound form within compounds. This prediction was tested for Hebrew in a study of how children interpreted and produced novel compounds. The fewer the changes required in the forms of head nouns, the earlier children mastered those forms in production. When more morphological changes were required, the harder children found the compound type and the later it was acquired. The percentages of correctly produced head nouns of four different types are shown for children aged 3 through 9 in Table 2.5. Head nouns that require no change in form posed no problem, as predicted, even for the youngest children tested. Feminine nouns that merely require the addition of a final /-t/ were the next easiest form in production, followed by masculine plural nouns that require the substitution of one suffix for another: Plural /-im/ has to be changed to /-ey/ when bound. Finally, the hardest change for children (and the only one that caused adults any difficulty) was

Table 2.5. *Percentage of compounds produced correctly for each head noun type in Hebrew*

Age	Target morphological type			
	No change	Final /-t/	Final /-ey/	Stem change
3	90	62	0	0
4	100	85	56	4
5	100	90	94	10
7	100	100	94	76
9	100	100	100	95
Mean	98	87	69	33

Source: Clark and Berman (1987).

where the word stem itself has to be changed when bound, as in the shift from the free noun *shafan* 'rabbit' to its bound form, *shfanˆ*.

Children also tend to retain base forms without any shifts in stress or palatalization, and so make their own coinages particularly transparent. For example, they coin *magic-man* to talk about a magician and, even when asked, typically fail to recognize the word *magic* in *magician* – its form and hence its meaning are still opaque to them. This same preference for transparency in coinage appears in such spontaneous innovations as *longness* (for *length*) and *volcano-y* (for *volcanic*). In essence, stress shifts and the concomitant changes or neutralizations of vowel quality, as well as palatalization, make the internal structure of many established words opaque. As a result, children take many years to master these processes and use them in their own coinages (see Condry, 1979; Moscowitz, 1973; Myerson, 1978).

Children take some time to work out what the possible forms of their language are, and until they do, they make the fewest possible changes in forms as they construct new words. This places a premium on zero derivation (no change), and on combinations of existing words, as in compounding, with no other changes in the constituent forms. It also predicts that affixation in general should be acquired later than zero derivation or compounding. Observations of spontaneous innovations across a number of languages support this general prediction in that compounding and zero derivation emerge before affixal forms in languages that have all three (see Clark, 1991). Simplicity of form is directly affected by what children know about possible word forms: While their repertoire remains small, they should adhere more strongly to simplicity. But once they analyze a larger range of complex word forms into their constituent parts (bases and affixes), they should rely less and less on simplicity in their own production of forms designed to carry innovative meanings.

Transparency of meaning

This principle captures the observation that when children stretch their vocabularies by coining new words, they do so by making use only of familiar words and affixes. That is, they follow the maxim that known elements can be used or combined to express new meanings. This preference, like simplicity, predicts children's early reliance on compounding and on zero derivation.

Among children's earliest coinages, as we have already seen, are Noun + Noun compounds where children make no change in the shapes and hence the meanings of the constituent base forms. The novel meaning comes from use of the *combination* of familiar nouns in context on that occasion of speech. One domain where this is particularly evident is in children's early attempts to coin agentive nouns. Prior to making use of the suffix *-er*, children opt for compound nouns with a noun or verb modifier and a generic noun such as *-man* as the head, as in *button-man* (man who throws buttons) in lieu of *thrower* or *button-thrower*. Only around age 4 do they shift to using the agentive affix, *-er*, most of the time (Clark & Hecht, 1982).

As soon as children work out the meanings of affixes, of course, these in turn become transparent and can be added to the repertoire of word-formation options for use in coinages. So what is transparent to children depends on what word structures and which affixes they have already identified and analyzed. But in many languages, one may have shifts in part of speech, for example, without any affixation. As predicted, in languages that license it, children rely very early on zero derivation and retain noun or verb bases unchanged in their coinages. In this way, the meaning of the familiar noun or verb remains accessible or transparent as *part* of the innovative meaning being expressed. In English, children can use a noun as a verb, a verb as a noun, or an adjective as a verb, with no suffix needed to indicate the part of speech intended. (That is given by the syntax and the inflections).

Table 2.6. *Spontaneous denominal verbs
coined by 2-year-olds*

Child verb	Adult form/gloss
ax	= to chop
broom	= to hit with a broom
button	= to turn on/off
cello	= to play the cello
key	= to open with a key
needle	= to mend, sew
nipple	= to nurse (a baby)
oar	= to row
pliers	= to remove with pliers
sand	= to grind finely
scale	= to weigh
string	= to fasten with a string
water	= to dip into water

Source: E. V. Clark (1982a).

English-speaking children rely extensively on familiar nouns to supply innovative verbs for talking about activities associated with the objects denoted by the nouns. A typical selection of novel denominal verbs from English-speaking 2-year-olds is given in Table 2.6. These children also use adjectives as verbs, as in "I'm darking this picture" (said as the child scribbled in black pencil over a picture she had just drawn), or "I sharped this pencil" (said by a child who had just learned how to use a pencil sharpener). And, on rare occasions in English, they also use a verb as a noun, as in a *rub* for an eraser.

Although zero derivation is treated as transparent early on, it may be more transparent to the speaker than to the addressee, since the interpretation of such coinages depends critically on the mutual knowledge shared by speaker and addressee on the occasion of speech. But children probably often succeed by default here, because much of child-to-adult speech occurs in the here-and-now. As they get older, they presumably become more skilled in using such devices and so making sure on each occasion that their intended meaning is clear. Transparency, then, depends both on knowledge of the meanings of different options in word formation and on the Gricean contracts shared by speaker and addressee for how to arrive

at the meanings of lexical innovations – contracts that depend crucially on conventionality and contrast combined.

Like simplicity, transparency is dependent on how much children
already know about the meanings and forms in their language. As
children are exposed to larger and larger paradigms of derivational
and compositional patterns linking meanings and forms, they are
able to use a larger array of options that have become transparent
to them.

Productivity

This principle accounts for the choices children (and adults) make
when there are several possible forms that could be used in coining
a new word. It can be stated as follows: The word-formation devices
used most often by adults in innovations are the most productive
and so the ones to use for constructing new words. But this does
not really capture what is meant by *productive*. In traditional treatments, it is typically defined in terms of the frequency of a form
type within established paradigms, but these presumably reflect past
productivity and not necessarily what is currently productive. Another approach to productivity is to link it to normative usage in a
language, where the academy or some other established group makes
recommendations about which form should be used to express a
particular kind of meaning. Yet another approach is to sample the
preferences of contemporary speakers of the language. Of these three
possibilities, only the third seems to capture both what adult speakers do and what most influences children who have reached a stage
where they can choose among several transparent options in coining a new word (Clark & Berman, 1984). All three views of productivity assume that speakers must keep track of the relative frequency of different elements of word structure in order to choose
among them. But evidence from overregularization errors suggests
that such tracking tallies types, not tokens (Guillaume, 1927). Moreover, children also seem to keep tags on word frequency more generally, perhaps because they must represent form–meaning pairs in
memory, and so may have to keep track of forms and potential
meanings separately for some time until they work out how they
are linked for specific words.[4]

Productivity comes into play when children have to decide among
several forms that are equally transparent and so available to the

child. This happens when simplicity and transparency per se are no longer an issue. At this point, children show a strong preference for the most productive of the options available. And contemporary preferences among adult speakers predict best which choices children will make within specific domains of meaning. This is apparent, for example, in their choices of agentive suffixes in English and in their choices of agent and instrument patterns in Hebrew.

In Hebrew, children are faced with a number of options when it comes to coining words for the agents of actions. Among these are the zero-derivation *beynoni* forms (where the verb is used as an agentive noun), the CaCCaC pattern (used for professions in Classical and Mishnaic Hebrew), and the CaCCan pattern (used for attributes of agents in earlier periods of Hebrew).[5] Adult speakers nowadays favor the CaCCan pattern overwhelmingly when coining new agent nouns, even though this does not reflect the forms most often found in the conventional vocabulary. (More striking still, adults also favor the CaCCan pattern for instrument nouns – a contemporary preference that appears to have no historical basis at all.) And the preference adults exhibit here accounts for the choices made by 7- and 9-year-old speakers of Hebrew.

The most productive elements in a language may also be the most frequently used. But sheer frequency alone, as reflected in the conventional word stock, is not enough. The meaning of the form has to be appropriate for what is to be expressed. For example, the suffixes *-er* (to express agency) and *-ly* (to express manner) occur with roughly the same frequency in English, but children as young as 4 reject *-ly* as a suffix to express agency in a series of unfamiliar nonsense words. When the meaning of different forms is roughly the same, however, frequency marks the most productive option. For example, when English-speaking 4-year-olds were given a memory task involving the agentive suffixes *-er*, *-ist*, and *-ian*, they consistently misremembered the less productive *-ist* and *-ian* as *-er*, even when they had heard only *-ist*, say, as the ending on a whole set of new words. That is, the most productive of the agentive suffixes accounted for virtually all the intrusions in memory for less productive suffixes (Clark & Cohen, 1984; see also Sterling, 1983).

But even among suffixes that share, say, agentive meaning, there are still differences in meaning. For instance, *-ist* is favored over *-er* in the domain of music – for example, *pianist, flautist, cellist* – and children also become sensitive to such domain-based restrictions quite early: Witness the coinage of *drummist* by one 4-year-old. And *-ist* is also favored over *-er* in technological domains – for example, *physicist, chemist, biologist* – perhaps because of the prevalence of Greek and Latin roots in word formation there.

Languages differ in which options in word formation are productive, and some general options depend on the typology of the language. For example, Germanic languages in general favor compounding in word formation, whereas Romance languages favor suffixation. Within particular languages at any one time, one finds that specific patterns of word formation for verbs and nouns may be highly favored, while other options that also exist and have been productive in the past are barely used. In English, zero derivation in forming verbs from nouns is highly productive (and has been for several hundred years); compounding for forming new nouns is also productive, but some compounding patterns are much more productive than others (e.g., the Noun$_{(object)}$ + Verb-er type, as in *wall-builder*, compared with the Verb + Noun type, as in *push-chair*). In French, most word formation relies on suffixes, but some are favored over others. Agentive *-eur*, for example, is far more productive than *-ien*. Compounds can occur in French, but they tend to be used in only some semantic domains, such as instruments (e.g., the innovative *ouvre-armoire* from a 5-year-old, with the same Verb + Noun$_{(object)}$ pattern as in established words like *tire-bouchon* 'corkscrew'). In Hebrew, the overall preferences are for zero derivation, suffixing, and word patterns, rather than for compounding, which appears more in written than in spoken Hebrew.

In summary, in some languages certain types of word formation are preferred over others – suffixing versus compounding, for instance. And within languages, some options available for expressing particular kinds of meanings are typically more highly favored than others by adult speakers. So although productivity is reflected in part by frequency of usage, it is frequency of innovative words, and so it is not necessarily reflected in the conventional vocabulary of the language. Rather, the conventional vocabulary offers a record of what has been productive in the past for those terms deemed useful enough to be added to the permanent store of words speakers use. Productivity, unlike simplicity of form or transparency of meaning, is not "given up" as children master the options for word formation in their language. Instead, it remains a major factor in determining speakers' choices for adults as well as children (Berman, 1987; Clark & Berman, 1984).

Conceptual structure and language use

To what extent does the structure of thought – conceptual categories and conceptual organization – affect the course children follow as they acquire lexical structure in language? Many languages display striking parallels in their lexical structure, parallels that, one could argue, are a product of universals in conceptual structure. At the same time, the precise distinctions conveyed within a lexical domain may differ considerably from one language to another. And children clearly become sensitive to which distinctions are "mapped" lexically in their first language at an early age. This suggests that universals of conceptual structure *and* patterns of language use in the society around them affect the course children follow as they acquire lexical meaning.

One window onto children's underlying conceptual organization is the range of nonlinguistic strategies they make use of during the earliest stages of acquisition. These strategies essentially make up for their lack of lexical knowledge and offer consistent ways of dealing with recurrent situations in which someone addresses them and they assume they are expected to do something in response (see Shatz, 1978). For instance, children who do not yet understand prepositions like *in, on, under, above,* or *below,* or locative phrases like *at the top, at the bottom,* or *in front of* rely on their general knowledge of possible relations in space – given the kind of reference point (a container, a surface, an object with or without inherent orientational features) and the kind of object available for placing. This basic conceptual knowledge translates into a small number of highly consistent, ordered strategies for placing an object, x, in spatial proximity to a reference point. If the reference point is a container, x goes inside; if it is a surface, x goes on top; and relations in space also require contact: x must touch the reference point (E. V. Clark, 1973b, 1977a, 1980).

Reliance on underlying conceptual and perceptual categories is also apparent in children's earliest word uses. When they overextend a word, using *moon,* for example, to designate the moon, balls of various kinds, doorknobs, oranges, the letter O, and many other round objects, they appear to be using the strategy of picking the best word available for objects that share the property of being round and relatively small. The vast majority of overextensions observed in children under 2,0 or 2,6 involve *shape* (Anglin, 1977; E. V. Clark, 1973a). And many of these also appear to involve just those shapes that appear most commonly as the basis for classifier use in languages with classifiers (E. V. Clark, 1977b).[6] Strategies like these, relied on consistently by young children, suggest that all children build on similar conceptual and perceptual categories. They call on such categories and their organization whenever they are faced with situations where they lack lexical knowledge, and so must rely on something else in dealing with or responding to the situation.

Children's nonlinguistic strategies could serve a further purpose: They could also provide children with initial hypotheses about the meanings of unfamiliar words. That is, children could begin by mapping words onto preestablished conceptual categories. (These categories need not be identical to adult categories, but will presumably overlap with them.) This is in fact taken as the starting point for children, their opening wedge into language, by researchers such as Slobin (1973, 1985b). The cognitive categories provide a foundation on which children build as they look for how words, morphemes, and syntax can be used to convey meanings. Children's nonlinguistic strategies, in other words, offer information about the kind of nonlinguistic basis children rely on during the earliest stages of language learning.

Another source of information about the contributions of conceptual and perceptual categories to language is the universals observable in lexical structure. As Greenberg (1966) pointed out, complexity in thought tends to be reflected in complexity of expression. That is, one finds consistent patterns of morphemes being added to mark additional complexity. Added morphemes, for instance, mark plural as distinct from singular (*dog/dog***s**, *child/child***ren**), ordinal as distinct from cardinal (*three/third***, *twenty/twenti***eth**), negative as distinct from positive (*happy/***un***happy*, *patient/***im***patient*), state as distinct from change-of-state (*solid/solid***ify**, *red/red***den**), and state as distinct from cause-of-change-of-state (*legal/legal***ize**, *large/***en***large*); present time as distinct from past or future (*work/work***ed**, *work/***will** *work*), actual as distinct from hypothetical (*work/***might** *work*); categories as distinct from subcategories (*oak/***scrub** *oak*, *blue/***light** *blue*); and, among kin terms, one generation away as distinct from two (*mother/***grand***mother*), blood relative as distinct from spouse's relative (*father/fa-*

ther-**in-law**); and so on (see Clark & Clark, 1978). In each instance, the more complex of two notions is marked with an added morpheme. Note that one does not find the reverse – the less complex of two notions being distinguished with an added morpheme.

Languages may differ in how words map onto particular domains. The mapping depends in part on the number of words available for talking about dimensions like size, height, and age, say, or the number available for talking about the kinds of objects one can sit on (*stool, chair, armchair, sofa,* etc.) (see Lehrer, 1974). Languages also differ in how they "package" particular kinds of semantic information, whether it appears in a verb or in an adverbial, whether it combines with notions of cause, path, goal, object-affected, or not, and whether some languages favor one typological pattern over another, as in expressions for motion in space (see Talmy, 1985). Some languages, for instance, combine information about motion and manner in the verb (e.g., English *run, dawdle, walk, trot, race, saunter*) and express path by means of particles and prepositional phrases (e.g., *run* **out**, *saunter* **along the lane**, *trot* **round the house**). Others combine motion and path in the verb (e.g., French *entrer* 'go + in', *sortir* 'go + out', *monter* 'go + up', *descendre* 'go + down') and express manner with adverbs and phrases (e.g., *sortir* **vite** 'go out quickly', *monter* **à quatre pattes** 'climb up [while] crawling').

Languages also differ in how they group spatial configurations linguistically – whether they require contact and support (as for English *on*) or merely adjacency without contact or support (as in the nearest equivalent expressions in Korean, Japanese, or Chinese). Some languages also incorporate information about the perspective from which the spatial array of objects is viewed – whether the object being located projects beyond or remains internal to the reference point object, as in Cora (see Bowerman, 1989). Languages differ too in how they group the arguments of transitive and intransitive verbs. In nominate-accusative languages, the subjects of intransitive and transitive verbs are treated alike and, for instance, receive the same case marking. In ergative languages, the subjects of intransitive verbs are grouped with the objects of transitives and receive the same case marking; subjects of transitive verbs receive a different case. Differences across languages in how information about meaning is distributed tend to show considerable consistency in which patterns go together within a particular language and so contribute to both ease of processing and ease of acquisition (see Bartsch &

Vennemann, 1972; Bowerman, 1985; Clark & Clark, 1978; Greenberg, 1963).

Variations such as these in lexical structure are reflected in all the language children are exposed to. So the specific way speakers of a language structure each part of the lexicon should interact with any initial structure children impose as a result of their general nonlinguistic strategies. Children who always place things "in" containers should map such a relation to the word *in* in English, and soon set up a contrast between putting something *in* versus *on*, where the latter connotes contact and support. Children acquiring Spanish map this whole range of relations – containment or support with contact – onto *en*. And children learning Korean group together the putting of one thing "in" or "on" another and the putting of two things "together" (Korean *kki-ta*), but only when the objects are related by tight fit or attachment. So the verb *kki-ta* can be used for putting a ring "on" a finger, a hand "in" a glove, or attaching two Lego pieces to each other, but this verb cannot be used for loose-fit or no-fit actions – for putting an apple "in" a bowl, a blanket "on" a bed, or putting two tables together (Bowerman, 1989). Children exposed to English hear a distribution of spatial terms that tells them geometry is important (containment, support, contact, covering, and symmetry or asymmetry of motion), while children exposed to Korean hear that tightness of fit is important and that when that obtains, geometry can be ignored. If children relied solely on conceptual categories and relations, they should be relatively unaffected by such differences in the input languages they hear. But if their early hypotheses about spatial meanings are also shaped by the ways language is used around them, they should begin to show the effects of such differences in mapping fairly early. Preliminary work by Bowerman and Soonja Choi suggests that children become sensitive to some of these differences by the end of their second year (Bowerman, 1989).

Children begin, it would seem, by drawing on their conceptual categories and organization for their first hypotheses about meaning. But the meanings they discover are also shaped by the way the words are used in the speech around them. Lexical meanings, in other words, are a product of both thought and society, so in learning meanings, children are necessarily influenced both by their ongoing conceptual development and by how words are used in their speech community. The precise contributions of thought and society, and how the two interact in achieving lexical meanings, await careful empirical research on specific domains in the lexicon.

Conclusions

Lexical acquisition and the principles that guide it offer an important vantage point from which to view the process of acquisition as a whole. Words in the lexicon offer a domain for the study of phonological processes and syntactic structure in addition to the semantic content associated with each word. Because words offer such general information about each language, the acquisition of a vocabulary is central to the acquisition of language as a whole.

Each language is subject to several general pragmatic principles that govern various aspects of its use and allow for the smooth working of Gricean contracts between speakers and addressees. Conventionality and contrast together play a critical role for both adults and children, particularly in providing the rationale for deciding that an unfamiliar word must mean something different from words that are already familiar. This is crucial in making the task of learning a vocabulary feasible for young children. Without this assumption, they would have a hard time comparing each unfamiliar word against all uses of known words to check first that the new word was not synonymous with one already mastered. Only after that possibility was eliminated could they go on to work out its actual meaning (see E. V. Clark, 1988, 1990).

But examination of how children learn conventional words and their meanings fills in only part of the acquisition picture. It can tell us little about the meanings they have associated with affixes on conventional words, or whether they have even identified affixes as such. Nor can it tell us whether they realize that compounds are in fact made up of two or more other words that may have an independent existence in the lexicon. (Occasional coinages in utterances like "I'm spiderman-woman," from a 2-year-old, suggest an absence of analysis.) The other half of the picture is filled in by the study of lexical innovations – the coinages children rely on to fill gaps and to provide labels for objects and actions they wish to talk about but lack words for. The majority of their coinages are nonce words, produced only once on a particular occasion to convey a particular meaning. But such coinages show us which internal parts of words children have identified as having a consistent meaning and which elements can combine with which. They tell us what children know in general about word structure, knowledge that is essential to word formation.

The principles and assumptions discussed here are concerned primarily with *language use* and specifically with *lexical* structures and meanings. Other principles are also critical, in particular the assumptions that guide solutions to the "mapping problem" as children link words to conceptual categories (E. V. Clark, 1977a, 1979b; Slobin, 1979, 1985a). They must identify kinds of objects, properties (shape, texture, color), relations (location, orientation), actions, and events as potential referents for words. These categories appear to provide the basis for children's initial hypotheses about word meanings. But their hypotheses are then shaped and refined by how the relevant words are used in the language around them. So while conceptual categories provide a major starting point for children's hypotheses about word meanings, the working out of specific word meanings is also shaped by the society that uses the language. Principles of conceptual structure play an indispensable role in the early acquisition of lexical meanings and lexical structure. But lexical meanings must conform to the conventions of the language community, and when the conventions do not map precisely onto the conceptual categories children start with, society plays a decisive role in refining and shaping children's early hypotheses about meanings. To understand lexical development fully, we must take account of the joint influences of conceptual structure and language use. Together, these provide the starting point for acquisition.

Notes

1. Dockrell's studies followed up Carey and Bartlett's (1978) finding that children very quickly assigned a new potential color word to the color domain, in contrast to other color terms. Prior to both these studies, Lyamina (1960) found that it was easier to teach children aged 1,6 to 2,6 a new word when its referent was the one unfamiliar object among a collection of familiar ones than in other kinds of settings. That is, Lyamina exploited children's reliance on contrast directly.
2. The addition of a suffix leaves the beginning of the word unchanged, so it remains more easily recognized than when a prefix is added. In fact, children consistently learn suffixes before prefixes (Slobin, 1973), and languages typically have either more suffixes than prefixes or only suffixes (Hawkins & Gilligan, 1988). Prefixing languages without suffixes are rare. From the point of view of simplicity, a change at the end of a word should be easier because (a) in comprehension, it does not affect recognition of the word, and (b) in production, it should be easier

to produce a familiar sequence followed by a modification in the form of a suffix than the reverse, a modification first and then the familiar word.

3. In Hebrew, some nouns remain unchanged in form when they appear as the heads of compounds. Other nouns have a special "bound" form that must be used in compounds. The particular shape of a bound form depends largely on its phonological properties. Feminine nouns ending in a final stressed /-a/, for example, add a final /-t/ in the bound form, e.g., *simla* 'dress' goes to *simlat*ˆ. (The caret will be used to indicate that a head noun is bound.) Some bound forms require much more than the addition of a suffix, e.g., use of a different vowel pattern in the base form or substitution of one suffix for another (see Clark & Berman, 1987).

4. Keeping track of the frequency of word types as well, possibly, as tokens also appears to play a role in proposals about how children change their language during development by comparing their own output with more adultlike targets drawn from the representations children have stored for comprehension (see, e.g., the proposals in E. V. Clark, 1982b; Clark & Hecht, 1983; MacWhinney, 1978, 1985).

5. Hebrew is a Semitic language in which the root word is identified by the consonants it contains (typically three consonants, but ranging from two to as many as six in some words). Vowels are intercalated with the consonants to mark inflection (e.g., present vs. past tense in verbs) and to mark different derivational patterns in word formation. Some intercalated vowel patterns carry suffixes or prefixes with them (see Berman, 1978a; Clark & Berman, 1984).

6. In classifier languages, numerals are always accompanied by a classifier as well as the noun for the entity being counted, e.g., "3 + long-thing + stick" or "5 + flat-thing + rug." (Analogous expressions in English are "3 **head** of cattle" or "2 **slices** of toast.") See Carpenter (1991).

References

Abbot, V., Black, J. B., & Smith, E. E. (1985). The representation of scripts in memory. *Journal of Memory and Language, 24,* 179–199.

Anglin, J. M. (1977). *Word, object, and conceptual development.* New York: Norton.

Au, T. K. (1990). Children's use of information in word learning. *Journal of Child Language, 17,* 393–416.

Au, T. K., & Markman, E. M. (1987). Acquiring word meanings via linguistic contrast. *Cognitive Development, 58,* 1021–1034.

Backhouse, A. E. (1981). Japanese verbs of dress. *Journal of Linguistics, 17,* 17–29.

Balcom, P. A. (1987, July). *The emergence of syntax: The acquisition of transitivity.* Paper presented at the Fourth International Congress for the Study of Child Language, Lund, Sweden.

Baldwin, D. (1989). Priorities in children's expectations about object label reference: Form over color. *Child Development, 60,* 1291–1306.

Barrett, M. D. (1978). Lexical development and overextension in child language. *Journal of Child Language, 5,* 205–219.

Barrett, M. D. (1986). Early semantic representations and early word-usage. In S. A. Kuczaj II & M. D. Barrett (Eds.), *The development of word meaning: Progress in cognitive development research* (pp. 39–67). Berlin: Springer.

Bartsch, R., & Vennemann, T. (1972). *Semantic structures: A study in the relation between syntax and semantics.* Frankfurt: Athenäum.

Berlin, B., Breedlove, D. E., & Raven, P. H. (1973). General principles of classification and nomenclature in folk biology. *American Anthropologist, 75,* 214–242.

Berman, R. A. (1978a). *Modern Hebrew structure.* Tel-Aviv: University Publishing.

Berman, R. A. (1978b). Early verbs: Comments on how and why a child uses his first words. *International Journal of Psycholinguistics, 5,* 21–39.

Berman, R. A. (1987). Productivity in the lexicon: New-word formation in Modern Hebrew. *Folia Linguistica, 21,* 425–461.

Berman, R. A., & Clark, E. V. (1989). Learning to use compounds for contrast: Data from Hebrew. *First Language, 9,* 247–270.

Bowerman, M. (1985). What shapes children's grammars? In D. I. Slobin (Ed.), *The crosslinguistic study of language acquisition: Vol. 2. Theoretical issues* (pp. 1257–1319). Hillsdale, NJ: Erlbaum.

Bowerman, M. (1989). Learning a semantic system: What role do cognitive predispositions play? In M. L. Rice & R. L. Schiefelbusch (Eds.), *The teachability of language* (pp. 133–169). Baltimore: Brookes.

Bréal, M. (1897). *Essai de sémantique.* Paris: Hachette.

Bybee, J. L. (1985). *Morphology: A study of the relation between meaning and form.* (Typological studies in language, 9.) Amsterdam: Benjamins.

Carey, S. (1978). The child as word learner. In M. Halle, J. Bresnan, & G. A. Miller (Eds.), *Linguistic theory and psychological reality* (pp. 264–293). Cambridge, MA: MIT Press.

Carey, S., & Bartlett, E. J. (1978). Acquiring a single new word. *Papers and Reports on Child Language Development* [Stanford University], *15,* 17–29.

Carpenter, K. L. (1991). Later rather than sooner: Extralinguistic categories in the acquisition of Thai classifiers. *Journal of Child Language, 18,* 93–113.

Clark, E. V. (1973a). What's in a word? On the child's acquisition of semantics in his first language. In T. E. Moore (Ed.), *Cognitive development and the acquisition of language* (pp. 65–110). New York: Academic Press.

Clark, E. V. (1973b). Nonlinguistic strategies and the acquisition of word meanings. *Cognition, 2,* 161–182.

Clark, E. V. (1977a). Strategies and the mapping problem in first language acquisition. In J. Macnamara (Ed.), *Language learning and thought* (pp. 147–168). New York: Academic Press.

Clark, E. V. (1977b). Universal categories: On the semantics of classifiers and children's early word meanings. In A. Juilland (Ed.), *Linguistic studies presented in Joseph Greenberg* (pp. 449–462). Saratoga, CA: Anma Libri.

Clark, E. V. (1978a). Discovering what words can do. In D. Farkas, W. M. Jacobsen, & K. W. Todrys (Eds.), *Papers from the Parasession on the Lexicon* (pp. 34–57). Chicago: Chicago Linguistic Society.

Clark, E. V. (1978b). Strategies for communicating. *Child Development, 49,* 953–959.

Clark, E. V. (1978c). From gesture to word: On the natural history of deixis in language acquisition. In J. S. Bruner & A. Garton (Eds.), *Human growth and development: Wolfson College Lectures, 1976* (pp. 85–120). Oxford: Oxford University Press.

Clark, E. V. (1979a). Building a vocabulary. In P. Fletcher & M. Garman (Eds.), *Language acquisition* (pp. 149–160). Cambridge University Press.

Clark, E. V. (1979b). *The ontogenesis of meaning.* Wiesbaden: Athenaion.

Clark, E. V. (1980). Here's the *top:* Nonlinguistic strategies in the acquisition of orientational terms. *Child Development, 51,* 329–338.

Clark, E. V. (1981). Lexical innovations: How children learn to create new words. In W. Deutsch (Ed.), *The child's construction of language* (pp. 299–328). New York: Academic Press.

Clark, E. V. (1982a). The young word-maker: A case study of innovation in the child's lexicon. In E. Wanner & L. R. Gleitman (Eds.), *Language acquisition: The state of the art* (pp. 390–425). Cambridge University Press.

Clark, E. V. (1982b). Language change during language acquisition. In M. E. Lamb & A. L. Brown (Eds.), *Advances in developmental psychology* (Vol. 2, pp. 173–197). Hillsdale, NJ: Erlbaum.

Clark, E. V. (1983). Meanings and concepts. In J. H. Flavell & E. M. Markman (Eds.), *Handbook of child psychology: Vol. 3. Cognitive development* (pp. 787–840). New York: Wiley.

Clark, E. V. (1987). The Principle of Contrast: A constraint on language acquisition. In B. MacWhinney (Ed.), *Mechanisms of language acquisition: The 20th Annual Carnegie Symposium on Cognition* (pp. 1–33). Hillsdale, NJ: Erlbaum.

Clark, E. V. (1988). On the logic of Contrast. *Journal of Child Language, 15,* 317–335.

Clark, E. V. (1989, July). *Conventionality and Contrast: Pragmatic principles have lexical consequences.* Paper presented at the Conference on Lexical Structure, University of Arizona, Tucson.

Clark, E. V. (1990). On the pragmatics of Contrast. *Journal of Child Language, 17,* 417–431.

Clark, E. V. (1991). *Lexical development and word-formation in acquisition.* Unpublished manuscript.

Clark, E. V., & Berman, R. A. (1984). Structure and use in the acquisition of word formation. *Language, 60,* 547–590.

Clark, E. V., & Berman, R. A. (1987). Types of linguistic knowledge: Interpreting and producing compound nouns. *Journal of Child Language, 14,* 547–567.

Clark, E. V., & Clark, H. H. (1979). When nouns surface as verbs. *Language, 55,* 767–811.

Clark, E. V., & Cohen, S. R. (1984). Productivity and memory for newly formed words. *Journal of Child Language, 11,* 611–625.

Clark, E. V., Gelman, S. A., & Lane, N. M. (1985). Compound nouns and category structure in young children. *Child Development, 56,* 84–94.

Clark, E. V., & Hecht, B. F. (1982). Learning to coin agent and instrument nouns. *Cognition, 12,* 1–24.

Clark, E. V., & Hecht, B. F. (1983). Comprehension, production, and language acquisition. *Annual Review of Psychology, 34,* 325–349.

Clark, E. V., Hecht, B. F., & Mulford, R. C. (1986). Coining complex compounds in English: Affixes and word order in acquisition. *Linguistics, 24,* 7–29.

Clark, E. V., Neel-Gordon, A., & Johnson, S. (1991). *Convention and contrast in the acquisition of verb meanings.* Unpublished manuscript.

Clark, E. V., & Sengul, C. J. (1978). Strategies in the acquisition of deixis. *Journal of Child Language, 5,* 457–475.

Clark, H. H. (1983). Making sense of nonce-sense. In G. B. Flores d'Arcais

& R. J. Jarvella (Eds.), *The process of language understanding* (pp. 297–331). New York: Wiley.

Clark, H. H., & Clark, E. V. (1978). Universals, relativity, and language processing. In J. H. Greenberg (Ed.), *Universals of human language: Vol. 1. Method and theory* (pp. 225–277). Stanford, CA: Stanford University Press.

Condry, S. M. (1979). *A developmental study of processes of word derivation in elementary school children and their relation to reading.* Unpublished doctoral dissertation, Cornell University, Ithaca, NY.

de Saussure, F. (1968). *Cours de linguistique générale.* Paris: Payot. (Original work published 1919.)

Dockrell, J. E. (1981). *The child's acquisition of unfamiliar words: An experimental study.* Unpublished doctoral dissertation, University of Stirling, Stirling, Scotland.

Dockrell, J. E., & Campbell, R. N. (1986). Lexical acquisition strategies in the preschool child. In S. A. Kuczaj II & M. Barrett (Eds.), *The development of word meaning: Progress in cognitive development research* (pp. 121–154). Berlin: Springer.

Dromi, E. (1987). *Early lexical development.* Cambridge University Press.

Dromi, E., & Fishelzon, G. (1986). Similarity, specificity, and contrast: A study of early semantic categories. *Papers and Reports on Child Language Development* [Stanford University], *25,* 25–32.

Fillmore, C. J. (1978). On the organization of semantic information in the lexicon. In D. Farkas, W. M. Jacobsen, & K. Todrys (Eds.), *Papers from the Parasession on the Lexicon* (pp. 148–173). Chicago: Chicago Linguistic Society.

Gelman, S. A., Wilcox, S. A., & Clark, E. V. (1989). Conceptual and lexical hierarchies in young children. *Cognitive Development, 4,* 309–326.

Gentner, D. (1978). On relational meaning: The acquisition of verb meaning. *Child Development, 49,* 988–998.

Gentner, D. (1982). Why nouns are learned before verbs: Linguistic relativity vs. natural partitioning. In S. A. Kuczaj II (Ed.), *Language development: Vol. 2. Language, thought, and culture* (pp. 301–334). Hillsdale, NJ: Erlbaum.

Gleitman, L. R. (1990). The structural sources of verb meanings. *Language Acquisition, 1,* 3–55.

Goldin-Meadow, S., Seligman, M. E. P., & Gelman, R. (1976). Language in the two-year-old. *Cognition, 4,* 189–202.

Golinkoff, R. M., Hirsh-Pasek, K., Baduini, C., & Lavallee, A. (1985, October). *What's in a word? The young child's predisposition to use lexical contrast.* Paper presented at the Boston University Conference on Child Language, Boston.

Golinkoff, R. M., Hirsh-Pasek, K., Bailey, L. M., & Wenger, N. R. (in press). Young children and adults use lexical principles to learn new nouns. *Developmental Psychology.*

Greenberg, J. H. (1963). Some universals of grammar with particular reference to the order of meaningful elements. In J. H. Greenberg (Ed.), *Universals of language* (pp. 73–113). Cambridge, MA: MIT Press.

Greenberg J. H. (1966). *Language universals.* The Hague: Mouton.

Grice, H. P. (1975). Logic and conversation. In P. Cole & J. L. Morgan (Eds.), *Syntax and semantics: Vol. 3. Speech acts* (pp. 41–58). New York: Academic Press.

Guillaume, P. (1927). Le développement des éléments formels dans le langage de l'enfant. *Journal de Psychologie, 24,* 203–229.

Hawkins, J. A., & Gilligan, G. (1988). Prefixing and suffixing universals in relation to basic word order. In J. A. Hawkins (Ed.), Papers in universal grammar: Generative and typological approaches [Special issue]. *Lingua, 74* (2–3), 219–259.

Huttenlocher, J., Smiley, P., & Charney, R. (1983). Emergence of action categories in the child: Evidence from verb meanings. *Psychological Review, 90,* 72–93.

John, O. (1985). *Actions, verbs, and the role of context: Differences between categories of objects and those of actions and events.* Unpublished manuscript, University of Oregon and Oregon Research Institute, Eugene.

Kameyama, M. (1983). Acquiring clothing verbs in Japanese. *Papers and Reports on Child Language Development* [Stanford University], *22,* 66–73.

Lehrer, A. (1974). *Semantic fields and lexical structure* (North-Holland Linguistic Series 11). Amsterdam: North-Holland.

Lewis, D. K. (1969). *Convention: A philosophical study.* Cambridge, MA: Harvard University Press.

Liberman, M. (1989, June). *How many words do people know?* Invited address, 27th Annual Meeting of the Association of Computational Linguistics, University of British Columbia, Vancouver.

Lyamina, G. M. (1960). Razvitie ponimaniya rechi u deteĭ vtorogo goda zhinzni [Development of speech comprehension in children in the second year of life]. *Voprosy Psikhologia, 3,* 106–121.

MacWhinney, B. (1978). The acquisition of morphophonology. *Monographs of the Society for Research in Child Development, 43* (1–2), Serial No. 174.

MacWhinney, B. (1985). Hungarian language acquisition as an exemplification of a general model of grammatical development. In D. I. Slobin (Ed.), *The crosslinguistic study of language acquisition: Vol. 2. Theoretical issues* (pp. 1069–1155). Hillsdale, NJ: Erlbaum.

Markham, E. M. (1984). The acquisition and hierarchical organization of categories by children. In C. Sophian (Ed.), *Origins of cognitive skills: The 18th Annual Carnegie Symposium on Cognition* (pp. 371–406). Hillsdale, NJ: Erlbaum.

Markman, E. M. (1987). How children constrain the possible meanings of words. In U. Neisser (Ed.), *Concepts and conceptual development: Ecological and intellectual factors in categorization* (pp. 255–287). Cambridge University Press.

Markman, E. M., & Hutchinson, J. (1984). Children's sensitivity to constraints on word meaning: Taxonomic vs. thematic relations. *Cognitive Psychology, 8,* 561–577.

Markman, E. M., & Wachtel, G. F. (1988). Children's use of mutual exclusivity to constrain the meanings of words. *Cognitive Psychology, 20,* 121–157.

Mervis, C. B. (1987). Child-basic object categories and early lexical development. In U. Neisser (Ed.), *Concepts and conceptual development: Ecological and intellectual factors in categorization* (pp. 201–233). Cambridge University Press.

Mervis, C. B., & Long, L. M. (1987, April). *Words refer to whole objects: Young children's interpretation of the referent of a novel word.* Paper presented at the biennial meeting of the Society for Research in Child Development, Baltimore.

Moscowitz, B. A. (1973). On the status of vowel shift in English. In T. E. Moore (Ed.), *Cognitive development and the acquisition of language* (pp. 233–260). New York: Academic Press.

Myerson, R. F. (1978). Children's knowledge of selected aspects of *Sound Pattern of English*. In R. N. Campbell & P. T. Smith (Eds.), *Recent advances in the psychology of language: Formal and experimental approaches* (pp. 377–402). London: Plenum.

Naigles, L. G. (1990). Children use syntax to learn verb meanings. *Journal of Child Language, 17*, 357–374.

Nelson, K. (1973). Structure and strategy in learning to talk. *Monographs of the Society for Research in Child Development, 38* (1–2), Serial No. 149.

Paul, H. (1898). *Principien der Sprachgeschichte* (3rd ed.). Halle: Niemeyer.

Rescorla, L. (1980). Overextension in early language development. *Journal of Child Language 7*, 321–335.

Rifkin, A. (1985). Evidence for a basic-level in event taxonomies. *Memory and Cognition, 13*, 538–556.

Rosch, E. H. (1973). On the internal structure of perceptual and semantic categories. In T. E. Moore (Ed.), *Cognitive development and the acquisition of language* (pp. 111–144). New York: Academic Press.

Rosch, E. (1978). Principles of categorization. In E. Rosch & B. B. Lloyd (Eds.), *Cognition and categorization* (pp. 27–48). Hillsdale, NJ: Erlbaum.

Shatz, M. (1978). On the development of communicative understandings: An early strategy for interpreting and responding to messages. *Cognitive Psychology, 10*, 271–301.

Shipley, E. F., & Kuhn, I. F. (1983). A constraint on comparisons: Equally detailed alternatives. *Journal of Experimental Child Psychology, 35*, 195–222.

Slobin, D. I. (1973). Cognitive prerequisites for the acquisition of grammar. In C. A. Ferguson & D. I. Slobin (Eds.), *Studies of child language development* (pp. 175–208). New York: Holt, Rinehart & Winston.

Slobin, D. I. (1979, April). *The role of language in language acquisition*. Address to the meeting of the Eastern Psychological Association, Philadelphia.

Slobin, D. I. (1981). The origins of grammatical encoding of events. In W. Deutsch (Ed.), *The child's construction of language* (pp. 185–199). New York: Academic Press.

Slobin, D. I. (1985a, October). *Developmental paths between form and meaning: Crosslinguistic and diachronic perspectives*. Keynote address, 10th Annual Boston University Conference on Child Language, Boston.

Slobin, D. I. (Ed.). (1985b). *The crosslinguistic study of language acquisition* (2 vols.). Hillsdale, NJ: Erlbaum.

Sterling, C. M. (1983). The psychological productivity of inflectional and derivational morphemes. In D. Rogers & J. A. Sloboda (Eds.), *The acquisition of symbolic skills* (pp. 179–185). London: Plenum Press.

Talmy, L. (1985). Lexicalization patterns: Semantic structure in lexical forms. In T. Shopen (Ed.), *Language typology and syntactic description: Vol. 3. Grammatical categories and the lexicon* (pp. 57–149). Cambridge University Press.

Taylor, M., & Gelman, S. A. (1989). Incorporating new words into the lexicon: Preliminary evidence for language hierarchies in two-year-old children. *Child Development, 60*, 625–636.

Templin, M. (1957). *Certain language skills in children: Their development and interrelationship* (Institute of Child Welfare Monograph 26). Minneapolis: University of Minnesota Press.

Tversky, B., & Hemenway, K. (1984). Objects, parts, and categories. *Journal of Experimental Psychology: General, 113,* 169–193.

Waxman, S. R. (1990). Linguistic biases and the establishment of conceptual hierarchies: Evidence from preschool children. *Cognitive Development, 5,* 123–150.

3. The whole-object, taxonomic, and mutual exclusivity assumptions as initial constraints on word meanings

ELLEN M. MARKMAN

Starting at about 18 months of age, children become remarkably capable of learning the vocabulary of natural languages. Yet word learning presents a problem of induction that must somehow be solved by such very young children, with their limited information-processing abilities. In order for children to acquire language as rapidly as they do, they must have biases that enable them to rule out many alternative hypotheses for the meanings of a word and that lead them instead to focus on hypotheses that are reasonably likely to be correct (Markman, 1989; Markman & Hutchinson, 1984; Markman & Wachtel, 1988). A sophisticated, intelligent adult, let alone a 2-year-old, would never be able to settle on the meaning of a word by open-mindedly considering every possible hypothesis and waiting for evidence that would rule out all but one (Quine, 1960). It has been suggested that children use several assumptions to solve the inductive problem posed by word learning; among these are the whole-object assumption, the taxonomic assumption, and the assumption of mutual exclusivity. In this chapter, I will review some of the evidence that children rely on these assumptions to guide their initial hypotheses about what words mean and will try to reconcile this argument with some conflicting evidence about whether these constraints are available to young children just starting to acquire language.

The taxonomic and whole-object assumptions

When an adult points to an object and labels it, the novel term could refer to an object category, but it could also refer to a part of the

I thank the editors for their helpful comments on this manuscript. This work was supported in part by NIH Grant HD 20382.

object or to its substance, color, or weight, and so on. As just mentioned, it is very unlikely that children wait until enough evidence has accumulated to decide among the alternative hypotheses. Instead, one way children initially constrain word meanings is to assume that a novel label refers to the whole object and not to its parts, substance, or other properties.

Once children decide that a term refers to the whole object, they must still decide how to extend it to other objects. The term could refer to some external relation between two objects. Spatial and causal relations and possessor–possessed are some examples of common relations between objects that a term could in principle label. More generally, objects can be related through the variety of ways in which they participate in the same event or theme (e.g., cats eat mice; people read books; birds build nests). Many studies of classification by children demonstrate that children often find thematic relations particularly salient and interesting (for discussions see Markman, 1989; Markman & Callanan, 1983). The existence of a powerful thematic relation between two objects does not, however, make them the same kind of thing.

Thus, if children are attending to thematic relations between objects, how is it that they so readily learn labels for kinds of objects instead? To answer this question, Hutchinson and I (Markman & Hutchinson, 1984) proposed that children constrain the possible meanings of words in such a way that they rule out thematic meanings. That is, as a first hypothesis about what a novel label might mean, children do not consider thematic relations despite the fact that they consider such relations to be good ways of organizing the objects themselves. Thus, when children believe that they are learning a new *word*, they shift their attention from thematic to taxonomic organization.

In sum, it is argued that upon hearing a novel label, children honor the *whole-object* and *taxonomic* assumptions. This means that when children hear a novel label, they assume that the label refers to the object as a whole, and not to its parts, substance, or color, and so on, and that it refers to other objects of the same kind or same taxonomic category, and not to objects that are thematically related.

To narrow the hypotheses down to object categories, of course, leaves open the question of which of the numerous possible categories the label refers to. Objects can be categorized in many different ways and at many different levels – for example, basic, subordinate, or superordinate levels within a hierarchy. Which category children map the label onto is itself an interesting question, one that is addressed in this volume by Waxman (Chapter 4; see also Markman, 1989; Mervis, 1987; Waxman, 1990).

The whole-object and taxonomic assumptions predict that children should interpret novel labels as labels for objects of the same type rather than objects that are thematically related. To test this, Markman and Hutchinson (1984) compared how children organized objects when they were not provided with an object label versus when the objects were given a novel label.

One set of studies was conducted with 4- and 5-year-olds to test the hypothesis that hearing a new word would lead them to look for taxonomic relations rather than thematic relations. The children were assigned to one of two conditions. In one of the conditions, they were asked to find a picture that was the same as the target (e.g., "See this? Can you find another one?"). The other condition was the same except that a nonsense syllable was used to label the target picture (e.g., "See this dax? Can you find another dax?"). In both conditions, the children were first shown the target picture. They were then shown two other pictures and had to select one of them as being the same as the target. One of the pictures was related in a thematic way to the target, for example, as milk is to cow. The other picture was a member of the same superordinate category as the target, for example, as pig is to cow.

As is typical of children this age, when no word was provided, the children did not often make categorical choices. When they had to choose between another member of the same superordinate category and a thematically related object, they most often selected the thematically related object. As predicted, hearing a new word caused the children to seek taxonomic relations. Children who heard the target picture labeled with a unfamiliar word were much more likely than those hearing no label to select categorically.

Children are hypothesized to focus on categorical relationships because of the sheer presence of the word, and not because of any particular knowledge about the meaning of the word. The final study of Markman and Hutchinson (1984) was designed to provide evidence that children use abstract knowledge about words rather than specific known meanings to facilitate taxonomic responding. In this study, pictures of artificial objects were used instead of real objects. Children are not likely to translate unfamiliar names for these pictures into known words, because they do not know real names for them. If the presence of an unfamiliar word still causes children to shift from thematic to taxonomic responding when the materials are also unfamiliar, this would rule out translation as an explanation of the effect.

In this study, the experimenter first taught the children the taxonomic and thematic relations for the artificial objects before asking them to select the picture that was like the target. The results of this study with artificial objects replicated those of the study with known objects. As usual, when the children were simply asked to find another object like the target, they most often chose the thematic relation. When the target picture was labeled with an unfamiliar word, the children again were more likely to select categorically. This demonstrates that 4-year-old children place an abstract constraint on what single nouns might mean. For them, count nouns refer mainly to objects of the same kind rather than to objects that are united by thematic relations.

Markman and Hutchinson (1984) also demonstrated that children as young as 2 and 3 years place constraints on what unfamiliar words might mean. When presented with two basic-level objects, such as two different kinds of dogs, and a third object that was thematically related, such as dog food, very young children showed some tendency to select a dog and dog food. If, however, one of the dogs was labeled with an unfamiliar term, the children were now more likely to select two dogs (Markman & Hutchinson, 1984).

Hutchinson (1984) has provided evidence for the generality of the labeling effect. She raised the concern that the oddity task forces children to select another object to go with the target. Although children who hear a label select taxonomically under these conditions, they may not be so likely to generalize when they are not forced to. So Hutchinson (1984) used a procedure that was designed to resemble naturalistic conditions more closely. Children were taught a novel word for the target object, as before, but were free to select none, one, or two additional objects, one of which was related taxonomically, and one of which was related thematically, to the target. With the exception of the 3-year-old boys, Hutchinson replicated the Markman and Hutchinson (1984) results with this procedure. That, is 3-year-old girls and 4- and 5-year-old children will spontaneously extend a term to label taxonomically related objects, even when they are free not to.

Waxman and Gelman (1986) found that a label will induce 3-year-olds to classify taxonomically at the superordinate level, at least for superordinate categories for which the children do have a label. Moreover, they found that a novel label, actually a Japanese term, helped children organize objects taxonomically in a free classification task, instead of an oddity procedure. Waxman and Gelman compared the effectiveness of hearing a novel label with other means of highlighting the salience of categories. In some cases, children were shown typical instances of the category and told to think about them as a group. In other cases, they were given the common English superordinate term for the categories. Four-year-olds benefited from all of these manipulations. Three-year-olds, however, were helped by the use of labels, but not by seeing typical instances. Moreover, 3-year-olds did just as well when Japanese labels were provided for these familiar superordinate categories as when the known English labels were provided.

One limitation of all of the studies described so far that provide evidence for the taxonomic and whole-object assumptions is that there are not any very salient thematic relations available at the time the object is first labeled. An object is labeled and then other objects are provided such that the label could be extended to thematic or taxonomic relations, but salient thematic relations are not present at first. One question, then, is whether the taxonomic assumption is powerful enough to override children's preference for thematic relations if objects are engaged in dynamic, salient, thematic relations at the time of labeling. Backscheider and I tested this by providing a novel label at the time objects were shown engaging in a dynamic thematic relation (Backscheider & Markman, 1990). For example, children watched as a doll was repeatedly seated in a chair. Half of the children heard a label at that time, for example, "See the bif," and half heard "See this." All of the children were then given an array of objects that could be organized into taxonomic or thematic groups. Hearing a label caused the children to select objects of the same kind, although in the absence of a label they organized objects according to the thematic event that had been depicted. Thus, we again found that labeling increased the amount of taxonomic responding.

Baldwin (1989) pointed out another potential paradox in the literature on classification and early word learning. On classification tasks, young children often sort on the basis of color rather than common category (Melkman, Tversky, & Baratz, 1981; Suchman & Trabasso, 1966), yet children rarely overgeneralize words on the basis of color (Clark, 1973). Baldwin (1989) argued that children may be biased upon hearing a novel label to look for common form or taxonomic category rather than color. Using a procedure analogous to that of Markman and Hutchinson (1984), Baldwin found that labeling an object reduces children's tendency to sort on the basis of color and increases their tendency to sort on the basis of taxonomic category.

In a related study, Landau, Smith, and Jones (1988) compared which objects 2- and 3-year-old children and adults would classify together depending on whether the task was to extend a novel count noun to new instances or to put objects together in a nonlinguistic classification task. Objects could be sorted on the basis of shape, size, or texture. Here, too, there was a developmental difference, with 3-year-olds and adults sorting on the basis of shape more often than 2-year-olds. Of greatest interest for the whole-object assumption is that labeling an object increases young children's tendency to sort on the basis of overall shape. In the case of the objects that Landau et al. used (e.g., Us), sorting by shape might be tantamount to sorting by object type. If so, then these findings as well as those of Baldwin (1989) and Au (1989; Au & Markman, 1987) are consistent with the argument that children are biased to interpret novel labels as referring to the whole object.

Soja, Carey, and Spelke (1985) raised the question of what ontological type children will assume a word refers to. In particular, they asked whether children will treat a label as referring to a physical object or the object's substance. They also asked whether children's apparent adherence to the whole-object assumption could be accounted for by their attention to shape per se or to the physical object itself. In one condition, children heard, for example, "This is my blicket" in the presence of a novel physical object (e.g., a brass pyramid). They were then asked which was the blicket while shown another of the same kind of object but made of a different substance (e.g., a plastic pyramid) and some pieces of the same substance (e.g., pieces of brass). When the children heard a label in the presence of a solid object, they treated the label as a label for the object, not its substance, thus supporting the whole-object assumption. Soja et al. subsequently investigated how children would interpret a label when there was no solid object present. In this condition, the children saw a new nonsolid substance (e.g., skin lotion with gravel in it) arranged into a distinctive form and heard it labeled as before, for example, "This is my blicket." Here the choices were between another nonsolid substance formed into the original shape versus three small blobs of the original substance. Now children interpreted the novel label as referring to the substance itself, not the shape. In other words, shape is used only in extending a term to another like object, not as a property of a nonsolid substance.

Thus, this work reveals again that children will interpret a novel label as referring to the object as long as there is an object present. If instead children hear a label in the presence of a nonsolid substance, they will interpret the term as referring to the substance, not its shape. Here, then, is some evidence of how the whole-object assumption is overcome – if there is no candidate whole object to label, children are willing to violate the assumption and treat the novel term as referring to something else, substance in this case.

Bauer and Mandler (1989) set out to determine whether the labeling effect would hold up for even younger children. They asked whether labeling would increase 16- to 31-month-old children's tendency to sort taxonomically. Unexpectedly, even the youngest children sorted taxonomically from the start. That is, even with no labels children sorted taxonomically about 75% of the time. Labeling did not increase this already high level of performance. Bauer and Mandler (1989) thus convincingly demonstrated that quite young children are capable of sorting taxonomically. They also argued that there may not be any general preference to sort thematically. However, because of the already high rate of sorting taxonomically, they were unable to test whether children of this age adhere to the taxonomic assumption. That is, it is still important to know whether in those cases where children do show a thematic preference, hearing a label will cause them to shift to taxonomic sorting. This question was addressed by Backscheider and Markman (1990).

Backscheider and Markman (1990) discussed several possible reasons that Bauer and Mandler (1989) found such a high rate of taxonomic responding in their young children. First, Bauer and Mandler (1989) used a reinforcement procedure whereby they briefly pretrained children to select taxonomically and maintained this selective reinforcement of taxonomic choices throughout the testing procedure. Second, although they used thematic relations quite similar to those of Markman and Hutchinson (1984), these relations may not have been the most salient or interesting to younger children. In a control study, Bauer and Mandler reinforced children for thematic responding and found that, when reinforced, the children could select thematic options. But this is uninformative about the relative salience of the items. So Backscheider and I selected thematic items that were likely to be highly familiar even to 18-month-olds. Moreover, we did not differentially reinforce taxonomic responding. Our results replicated the original Markman and Hutchinson (1984) findings, even with 18- to 24-month-olds. In the absence of a label, very young children selected taxonomically only 32% of the time. In other words, they did reveal a thematic bias. In marked contrast, when an object was given a novel label, the children interpreted the novel label as referring to objects of the same taxonomic category 77% of the time. Thus, the taxonomic assumption is used by children by 18 months of age.

The whole-object and taxonomic assumptions and early language acquisition

In this section, I will consider what kind of developmental evidence would be required to support the claim that children need the whole-object and taxonomic assumptions to break into language in the first place – that they serve as the initial constraints on word learning. As Nelson (1988) has pointed out, even if we have evidence that these constraints are used by 3- and 4-year-olds, that does not demonstrate that they were needed in the first place. By 3 years of age, children know enough language that they could have induced these assumptions from the language they have learned and then used them as convenient heuristics, rather than as necessary limits on the hypothesis space. What kind of evidence would support the claim that such constraints are required for lexical acquisition to take place at all?

At first sight, one might think that we have to demonstrate that babies are aware of these assumptions before they produce or even comprehend their first word. If such assumptions are used to figure out word meanings in the first place, we should be able to find evidence that babies honor them before any language has been learned (Nelson, 1988). However, there is reason to believe that the whole-object and taxonomic assumptions could, in fact, be necessary for language acquisition, and yet still appear after some language has been acquired. The reason I make this claim is that some-where around 18 months of age, the character of children's language learning appears to change dramatically. At this point children start acquiring words at an extraordinarily fast pace – in some cases sev-eral new words each day. This *naming explosion* or *vocabulary spurt* may mark a qualitatively new way of acquiring language. For this fast rate of acquisition to take place, the learning must be con-strained. But before the onset of the naming explosion, "word" learning might occur through a more "brute force" paired-associate kind of learning. Children may well acquire the first 50 or so words in their vocabulary by some slow associative learning mechanism, but this would account for only a tiny fraction of their language. At some point the learning changes and becomes very rapid. This new fast form of learning may be made possible by the emergence, con-solidation, or learning of such constraints on word meaning.

The naming explosion. Bloom, Lifter, and Broughton (1985) have said that "one of the most consistent observations in child language is the often precipitous increase in vocabulary size and volubility sometime during the last half of the second year . . . a precipitous increase in the use of *object* words, in particular." The existence of fast word learning has been acknowledged by several investigators spanning quite different theoretical positions (Bloom et al., 1985; Corrigan, 1983; Dromi, 1987; Halliday, 1975; McShane, 1979; Nelson, 1973).

Here is a composite view of what happens developmentally both before and after the naming explosion. Some babies begin to speak at 8 months and others not until 18 months or older. Especially in early talkers there is a period of time when the rate of acquisition of terms is slow. A child might acquire one or two words a month, for example. These first words sometimes include object labels but might also include an assortment of words from other grammatical form classes, for example, *hi, bye-bye, more, up, all gone.* It is also during this period that some investigators report what appear to be potential counterexamples to the taxonomic constraint, where chil-dren interpret words in "complexive" thematic ways, in which, for example, a duck, a bathtub, and yellow things are all called *duck* (Bloom, 1973; Bowerman, 1987, Dromi, 1987; Rescorla, 1980). Yet in a careful study to be discussed later, Huttenlocher and Smiley (1987) failed to find complexive meanings even at these earliest stages. Some of the early words are used only in limited contexts (Bretherton et al., 1981). For at least some of the words that children acquire in this period, they hear hundreds of trials (e.g., *hi* and *bye-bye*). This period has been called *prelexical* (Nelson & Lucariello, 1985), *performative* (Snyder, Bates, & Bretherton, 1981), *nonreferential* (Snyder et al., 1981), and *associative* (Lock, 1980). In other words, some of the earliest uses of "words" by beginning language learners do not appear to be wordlike. Children may not be using the words to refer to objects in the world, but rather the word may be just another associate the child has to a given situation – a routinized, ritualized part of an activity and not genuine naming.

Very roughly around 18 months of age a shift occurs. Children begin to acquire words very rapidly – in the most carefully documented case a child learned 45 words in a week (Dromi, 1987). During this time, a large proportion of the new terms acquired are object labels (Bloom et al., 1985; Bridges, 1986; Dromi, 1987; Lock, 1980). In fact, this vocabulary spurt is often called the *naming* explosion to reflect the large preponderance of nouns that are learned. Moreover, complexive interpretations of words are no longer found (Dromi, 1987). All of these features of this phase of learning – the rapidity of learning, the fast learning of object labels per se, and the absence of thematic interpretations of terms – are just what would be expected for children who honor the taxonomic and whole-object assumptions (assumptions akin to the nominal insight postulated by McShane, 1979).

Thus, to return to the issue of whether the whole-object and taxonomic assumptions are in place by the time lexical acquisition begins, if we take the onset of the naming explosion as the beginning of genuine word learning, these constraints should be evident by then. As yet we do not know whether this developmental relationship will be found, but Backscheider and Markman's evidence that children honor the taxonomic assumption by 18 months of age is encouraging. Moreover, Huttenlocher and Smiley (1987) have evidence from children's very early word use that early language learners honor the taxonomic assumption.

Huttenlocher and Smiley (1987) examined the language use of children they followed from the time of their first word (around 13 months for most of the children) until the children were 2 or $2\frac{1}{2}$ years old. Their goal was to determine the basis on which children extend words beyond their original context and to test whether early on children extend words complexively. A complexive use of a word would be tantamount to what we referred to as a thematic use—extending the word to a spatial, temporal, or causal associate of an object, rather than to objects of like kind. Previous researchers have reported finding that children's early word meanings are sometimes complexive (Nelson, 1974; Snyder et al., 1981).

Huttenlocher and Smiley (1987) argued that some of the previously reported instances of apparent complexive extensions of words by children may actually have been nonreferential uses of language. For example, a child who says "cookie" while reaching toward a cookie jar is not necessarily labeling the jar "cookie." Instead, the child might know that cookies are kept in the jar, and since the child is in the one-word stage, about the only way to formulate a request for a cookie when no cookie is visible is to say "cookie." Huttenlocher and Smiley set forth criteria to differentiate between that and other communicative uses of language from genuine complexive extensions. They found that even from the onset of language production, children were not using words to refer to complexively (thematically) organized objects. Instead, early language learners generalized object labels in ways that fit the whole-object and taxonomic assumptions.

Baldwin and Markman (1989) looked at what might be considered a precursor of the taxonomic assumption, namely, does labeling an object for a baby cause the baby to pay more attention to that object than if it were not labeled? We argued that if infants are biased to attend more to objects when they hear them labeled, that could help them notice word–object pairings. To test this, a first study compared how long 10- to 14-month old infants looked at unfamiliar toys when a novel label was provided versus when no label was offered. As predicted, labeling the toys increased infants' attention to them.

A second study examined whether labeling increased infants' attention to objects over and above what pointing, a powerful non-linguistic method for directing infants' attention, can accomplish on its own. Infants ranging in age from 10 to 20 months were shown pairs of unfamiliar toys in two situations: (a) in a pointing-alone condition, in which the experimenter pointed a number of times at one of the toys, and (b) in a labeling and pointing condition, in which the experimenter labeled the target toy while pointing to it. While pointing occurred, the infants looked just as long at the target toy whether or not it was labeled. However, during a subsequent play period in which no labels were uttered, the infants gazed longer at the target toys that had been labeled than at those that had not. Thus, labeling can increase infants' attention to objects beyond the time the labeling actually occurs. This tendency of language to sustain infants' attention to objects may help them learn the mappings between words and objects. It could also serve as a precursor or component of the full-blown whole-object assumption.

To summarize, a number of studies using several different methods together demonstrate that children from 18 months of age on honor the whole-object and taxonomic assumptions. Although studies have not yet been conducted that would allow us to say with certainty whether these assumptions are what make it possible for the naming explosion to take place, 18 months of age is close enough to the average age of the vocabulary spurt to suggest that this is possible. Moreover, the work of Huttenlocher and Smiley (1987) suggests that the assumption guides children's language acquisition right from the start of production – by 13 months of age.

Mutual exclusivity assumption

The whole-object assumption leads children to treat novel terms as labels for whole objects – not for parts or substances of objects or for other properties. But children must, of course, learn terms that refer to parts, substances, and other properties. The *mutual exclusivity assumption,* to be discussed in this section, helps children override the whole-object assumption, thereby enabling them to acquire terms other than object labels.

In addition to using the whole-object and taxonomic assumptions, children constrain word meanings by assuming at first that words are mutually exclusive – that each object has only one label. Given the nature and function of category terms, they often tend to be mutually exclusive. A single object cannot be both a chair and a dresser or a chair and a table. A single object cannot be both a cow and a bird or a cow and a dog. Of course, there are exceptions: Categories can overlap, as in *dog* and *pet*, and they can be included, as in *poodle* and *dog*. Thus, mutual exclusivity is a reasonable, though not infallible, assumption to make. Sometimes children are led astray by assuming terms to be mutually exclusive. Adhering to this assumption helps explain why children find class inclusion difficult (because it violates mutual exclusivity) and why the part–whole relation of collections is simpler (because it maintains mutual exclusivity) (Markman, 1987, 1989).

The advantages are that by assuming mutual exclusivity, children avoid making redundant hypotheses about the meanings of category terms; they are provided with a simple indirect strategy for learning category labels; and they are aided in overcoming the limitations of the whole-object assumption.

While honoring the mutual exclusivity assumption, children nevertheless violate mutual exclusivity under some circumstances. To acquire class-inclusion relations, for example, children must override their initial tendency to assume that terms are mutually exclusive. With enough evidence to the contrary, or enough information about the referent of a term, children will allow multiple labels for the same object. The mutual exclusivity bias guides children's initial hypotheses about a word's meaning, and without evidence to the contrary, children will maintain this hypothesis. But mutual exclusivity can be overridden. Thus, violations of mutual exclusivity in children's lexicons are not necessarily evidence against this principle. Gathercole (1987), Merriman (1987), and Nelson (1988) have all pointed out cases in which mutual exclusivity has clearly been violated, and a complete theory of how these constraints guide children's word learning must account for the counterexamples to and violations of the principle. As an initial step toward gaining such an understanding, we hypothesize that children are biased to assume, especially at first, that terms are mutually exclusive but will relinquish that assumption when confronted with clear evidence to the contrary (see also Merriman & Bowman, 1989; Woodward & Markman, in press).

Clark (1983, 1987) postulates another, related principle to help account for semantic acquisition. She argues, following Bolinger (1977), that every word in a dictionary contrasts with every other word and that to acquire words children must assume that word meanings are contrastive. Mutual exclusivity is one kind of contrast, but many terms that contrast in meaning are not mutually exclusive. Terms at different levels of a class-inclusion hierarchy, such as *dog* and *animal*, contrast in meaning in Clark's sense, since obviously the meaning of *animal* is different from that of *dog*. Yet these terms violate mutual exclusivity. Mutual exclusivity is a more specific and stronger constraint than the principle of contrast. Some of the evidence that Clark (1987) cites for the principle of contrast is, in fact, evidence for mutual exclusivity as well. One problem with this evidence, as discussed in Markman and Wachtel (1988) and Markman (1989) is that it comes almost entirely from production data. There may be many reasons for the limitations on the production of beginning language learners that would prevent them from expending valuable resources on redundant information. Limitations on production may limit a child's productive lexicon without there being any need to invoke mutual exclusivity or lexical contrast. A lexical constraint, if it is operating, should be apparent in comprehension as well as production. In fact, the best evidence for contrast or mutual exclusivity would come from comprehension, not production. Experimental studies of children's comprehension of terms would provide the clearest test of whether children widely assume that terms are mutually exclusive. I now summarize several such studies.

The simplest situation where the principle of mutual exclusivity could be applied is one in which two objects are presented, one of which already has a known label and one of which does not. If a new label is then mentioned, children should (a) on the taxonomic assumption, look for an object as a first hypothesis about the meaning of the label; (b) on the mutual exclusivity assumption, reject the already labeled object; and (c) therefore, assume that the other object is being referred to by the novel label. In this way, the mutual exclusivity assumption could provide an indirect means of learning a new object label. That is, children could learn the referent of a term without anyone ever explicitly pointing it out. Three recent studies have found that young children can learn object labels by such indirect means (Golinkoff, Hirsch-Pasek, Baduini, & Lavallee, 1985; Hutchinson, 1986; Markman and Wachtel, 1988).

In Study 1 of Markman and Wachtel (1988), 3-year-olds were presented with six pairs of objects, one member of each pair being an object that the children could label (e.g., banana, cow, spoon) and one member being an object for which the children did not yet know the label (e.g., a lemon wedgepress, tongs).

There was a control condition in which each child was shown the six pairs of objects and asked by a puppet to "show me one." This was to ensure that if children select a novel object when they hear a novel label, it is due to the labeling per se and is not just a response bias to go with the novel object. In the novel-label condition, the procedure was identical except that the child was asked to "show me the *x*," where *x* was a nonsense term.

Children who heard a novel term applied in the presence of two objects, one of which was familiar and one of which was unfamiliar, had a striking tendency to select the novel object as the referent for the novel term. Yet in the control condition the children performed at chance level. Thus, the tendency to select an unfamiliar object as the referent for a novel label does in fact reflect children's adherence to the mutual exclusivity principle, because they do not have such a bias when no labels are provided.

In summary, in this simple situation, 3-year-old and even younger children (Golinkoff et al., 1985; Hutchinson, 1986) map an unfamiliar word to an unfamiliar object. We interpreted this as evidence that very young children use the principle of mutual exclusivity to figure out the meaning of a new word. Merriman and Bowman (1989) have argued, however, that children could map a novel label to a novel object without relying on mutual exclusivity. Suppose instead that children have a bias to fill lexical gaps. Upon seeing an object for which they do not yet have a label, they will be motivated to learn what it is called. Thus, when they hear a novel label, they will interpret it as referring to an as yet unnamed object rather than to an object with a known name. Children could succeed in mapping a novel label to a novel rather than a familiar object because they are motivated to find first labels for things and not because they reject second labels. It is very likely that children do have a bias to fill lexical gaps. Whether that bias alone could account for these young children's performance or whether children also rely on mutual exclusivity cannot be decided on the basis of current evidence.

Merriman and Bowman (1989) have documented several ways in which mutual exclusivity guides young children's interpretation of a novel term that are not subject to this alternative interpretation. Depending on the circumstances, when a second label is given to an already named object, mutual exclusivity leads children sometimes to reject the second label and sometimes to correct the old label by narrowing its extension to exclude the object just named. Further, mutual exclusivity motivates preschoolers to keep word extensions from overlapping and thus prevents labels from extending to objects already labeled.

In each of the cases described so far, with the exception of simply rejecting the second label, children could satisfy the mutual exclusivity assumption while simultaneously satisfying the whole-object assumption. The next study from Markman and Wachtel (1988) examined what happens when this is no longer possible, and the whole-object and mutual exclusivity assumptions may conflict.

Suppose that a novel word is used to describe a single object. According to the whole-object assumption, a child should first hypothesize that the new word refers to the object as an exemplar of a category of similar objects, and not to the object's parts, substance, and so on. Suppose, however, that the object described by the novel term is an object for which the child already has a label. In this case, in order to adhere to the principle of mutual exclusivity, the child would have to reject the novel term as a label for the object, but then may not have any clear alternative meaning for the term. That is, since there is no other object around to label, the simple novel label–novel object strategy cannot be used. Under these circumstances, children could decide to abandon mutual exclusivity and interpret the novel term as a second label for the object. Another possibility is that they could reject the term as a label for the object without coming up with an alternative meaning. Rejecting one meaning for the term, however, leaves children with a term that is not yet attached to any referent. This in itself may motivate them to try to find some meaning for the novel term. The mutual exclusivity principle does not explain how children select among potential meanings, but they might analyze the object for some interesting part or property and interpret the novel term as applying to it. Studies 2 through 6 of Markman and Wachtel demonstrated that 3- and 4-year-old children can use mutual exclusivity in this more difficult situation to learn terms for parts and for substances. When a novel label was mentioned in the presence of an object with a known label, children rejected the term as a second label for the object and interpreted it instead as a label for a part of the object or its substance.

Taken together, the studies of Markman and Wachtel suggest how the assumption of mutual exclusivity can help children acquire not only category terms, but other kinds of terms as well. First, at a minimum it enables children to reject one hypothesis or one class of hypotheses about a term's meaning. Namely, the new term should not be another object label. Second, the mutual exclusivity assumption has a motivational force. Having rejected one meaning of a term, children will be left with a word for which they have not yet figured out a meaning. This should then motivate them to find a potential meaning for the novel term, leading them to analyze the object for some other property to label. In this way, the mutual exclusivity assumption motivates children to learn terms for attributes, substances, and parts of objects. It also predicts that children should be much better able to learn color terms, shape terms, and so on, with objects that have already been labeled.

This function of mutual exclusivity helps to overcome a major limitation of the whole-object assumption that leads children to look for object labels. Although the whole-object assumption provides a critical first hypothesis about word meanings, children must eventually be able to learn terms for properties of objects and not just terms for objects alone. These two principles complement one another, then, with the whole-object assumption being applied first and the mutual exclusivity principle being applied in cases where children already know a label for an object, motivating them to learn terms other than object labels. One can envision how the mutual exclusivity principle can be used to constrain the meanings of terms successively. Suppose that a child already has words for apple and for red, and now someone refers to the apple as "round." By mutual exclusivity, the child can eliminate apple and red as the meaning of "round" and try to analyze the object for some other property to label.

In the studies reviewed so far, children heard objects labeled or were asked to interpret labels but were given very little additional information about the meaning of the novel terms. In another learning situation that has been studied, a new term is introduced by contrasting it with a well-known word from the same semantic domain. The rationale here is that hearing the known word should enable children to determine the relevant semantic domain (Carey & Bartlett, 1978; Dockrell, 1981; Heibeck & Markman, 1987). For example, a child who hears, "Bring me the oval one, not the square one" should infer that "oval" is a shape term because it was contrasted with "square." Some recent puzzling findings in this literature may be explained by assuming that children adhere to mutual exclusivity or, more precisely in this case, lexical contrast (Clark, 1987). At first, it appeared that children could use lexical contrast to learn novel terms in several different semantic fields, including color, material, and shape (Carey & Bartlett, 1978; Heibeck & Markman, 1987). However, Heibeck and Markman pointed out that in each of these cases, the objects that children saw were identical except for one salient dimension – the one being taught. They found that in these very simple situations in which the novel terms were taught, lexical contrast was not any more effective than simply saying, "Bring me the oval one, not that one." Because the objects differed on only one dimension, hearing the term contrasted with another member from the semantic domain was not needed.

To remedy this problem, Au and Markman (1987) used lexical contrast to teach children novel terms, where the objects that were depicted differed along several dimensions. In these cases, the semantic contrast would be needed to help the children narrow the domain. The results from the study were inconsistent, however. Contrasting a novel material term, for example, *acrylic,* with known material terms, for example, *wood* and *cloth,* did help children interpret novel terms as referring to the material of the object. However, contrasting a novel color term, for example, *mauve,* with known color terms, for example, *red* and *green,* did not help children learn that *mauve* is a color name. The children were just as likely to interpret *mauve* as a label for a novel material, whether or not it was contrasted with color terms.

Au and Laframboise (in press) proposed an explanation for this finding that assumes that children honor mutual exclusivity of terms within a semantic domain. Their argument is that color terms are readily stretched to cover nonfocal colors. For example, some children who viewed a mauve object called it purple. The reason that *mauve* was not interpreted as a color term, even when it was contrasted with known terms, is that the children may have believed they already had a term for that color, for example, *purple,* and thus resisted learning a second one. Au and Laframboise reasoned that one way around the problem of a child's preexisting color terms preempting the interpretation of a new term was to contrast the novel term with the child's color term for that color. Children would be told, for example, "Bring me the mauve one, not the purple one." Au and Laframboise compared how well children could learn a new color term when it was contrasted with their own term for that color versus a randomly selected color term. As before, when children were taught a novel color term by hearing it contrasted with a familiar, randomly selected color term, the contrast did not help them acquire the term. However, contrasting the novel term with the children's own term did help them learn the term.

In Markman and Wachtel's procedure, children were presented with a situation in which the substance or parts of an object were deliberately made very salient in order to help provide the children with an alternative hypothesis to a category label if they chose to reject the category label. Taylor and Gelman (1988) also provided young children with either first or second labels for objects, but they did not try to make any dimension particularly salient. They then determined whether the children were more likely to interpret the label as a category term, a property term, or a name for a particular toy. When children were taught a novel label for an unfamiliar object, they tended to honor the whole-object and taxonomic assumptions. The 2-year-old children often treated novel nouns as category terms – labels that refer to the originally labeled object and to others of the same kind. Labels for objects with known category names were treated differently, though it is hard to tell from this study whether the children were honoring mutual exclusivity. When the children heard a second label for an object, they tended to treat the term as referring only to that object. It could be that the children were treating the term as a proper name, which would be one way of avoiding having two category labels for the same object and thus preserving mutual exclusivity. Another possibility is that these young children were treating the term as a label for a subordinate category and hence were able to overcome mutual exclusivity in this case.

To distinguish between these possibilities, Taylor and Gelman (1989) again labeled well-known objects with novel nouns, but this time differentiated between proper-name interpretations and subordinate category interpretations of the second label. Some of the children did in fact interpret the second label as a proper name when the object was animate (e.g., a stuffed bear). Thus, 2-year-olds might resist a second category label when a proper name is a possible alternative, even when this violates the form-class information in the label. That is, even though children were taught a count noun, "This is a tiv," and not a proper name (e.g., "This is Tiv"), they still interpreted the novel term as a proper name. Yet more of the children were capable of learning the novel term as a subordinate term, which entails overcoming mutual exclusivity.

Ways in which children override the mutual exclusivity assumption

Gelman, Wilcox, and Clark (1989) also taught 3- through 5-year-olds second labels for objects but varied whether the second label was a simple label or a compound noun (such as oak-tree or taxi-car). They reasoned that the compound form might provide a linguistic clue that the objects were to be labeled at more than one hierarchical level. Under these circumstances the children made quite a few errors in learning the second label, and the majority (74% in Experiment 1 and 67% in Experiment 2) of the errors they made were treating the labels as mutually exclusive subsets. Hearing compound nouns as second labels helped the children learn two labels for the same object, especially at the subordinate level. Thus, by explicitly representing both levels of the hierarchy, compound nouns provide one way of helping children violate mutual exclusivity.

A series of studies by Au and Glusman (1990) addressed the kind of information that might enable young children to overcome their mutual exclusivity bias and treat a term as a second category label. The first study demonstrated that children and adults alike honor mutual exclusivity in a situation where they can readily avoid a second label for an object. Three-, 4-, and 5-year-old children and adults were taught a novel label for a novel object, for example, "This is a mido." Virtually all of the children and adults treated this new term as a category label – extending it to other objects like the one taught. Then while viewing an array of objects that included examplars of the just-learned object along with other objects, the children and adults were asked to find "all theris," where "theri" was a second novel label. In this situation, 94% of the children and 100% of the adults adhered to mutual exclusivity in interpreting the second label. That is, no midos were selected as possible instances of "theri." After observing the subjects' spontaneous interpretation of the second term, the experimenter then asked explicitly whether the mido could be a theri. Here, too, the majority of subjects honored mutual exclusivity, with 72% of the children and 62% of the adults saying no. Most of the subjects who said no justified their response by saying, for example, "It can't be a theri because it's a mido."

Thus, this first study established that adults as well as children prefer an interpretation of a second label that maintains mutual exclusivity. The remaining studies examined two circumstances under which mutual exclusivity might be readily violated. The first was one in which it was made clear that the category labels were to be hierarchically organized, and the second was one in which it was made clear that the terms came from two different languages.

Au and Glusman (1990) hypothesized that children will accept two category labels for the same object when it is made clear that the names come from different levels of a hierarchy but that they will avoid giving an object two labels within a single level of the hierarchy. To test this, 4- and 5-year-old children were shown an array of toy animals and nonanimals and asked to find all of the animals. One of the animals (e.g., one of two lemurs) was then pointed out while the experimenter said, "This is a mido." Later, another experimenter asked the child to find all of the theris while the child looked at the array of toys. As predicted, the children were able to learn the term *mido* and apply it correctly to both members of the category (to two lemurs). When later asked for all of the theris, virtually all of the children honored mutual exclusivity by finding an interpretation of *theri* that did not overlap with *mido*. Thus, when there was no information about how to organize these two labels with respect to one another and when both terms could well have had basic-level interpretations, the children preserved mutual exclusivity. However, also as predicted, when the terms could readily be interpreted at different levels of a hierarchy, the children did accept two category terms (*mido* and *animal*) for the same objects. Virtually all of the children correctly selected all of the animals when asked to find the animals, including the two lemurs. Thus, these children spontaneously allowed two category labels for the same object, and when explicitly asked, they agreed that a mido could be an animal. Au and Glusman argue that the reason the children violated mutual exclusivity here is that it was made clear to them that the two terms could refer to different levels of the hierarchy. Note that in this case the children were dealing with a hierarchy, *animal*, for which they already had many known violations of mutual exclusivity. Most of the conceptual work that goes into deciding whether to violate mutual exclusivity probably was already accomplished for *animal*. This does not argue against Au and Glusman's point, but rather suggests that it will not in general be so easy to clarify for children how category terms are hierarchically organized.

One situation in which mutual exclusivity might be readily violated is one in which an object is labeled in two different languages. If it is made clear to children that the second label comes from a different language, they should be willing to accept it. To test this hypothesis, bilingual adults and children were first taught a novel label for an object by an adult speaking English. For example, they were taught that a lemur was called a "mido." As in the earlier studies, the subjects had to select the midos. Later a Spanish-speaking adult asked for the "theris." Recall that in the earlier studies close to 100% of the subjects treated *theri* as mutually exclusive with *mido*. Now when the words came from different languages, the children and adults chose objects randomly. Thus, they did not show any bias to avoid giving a second label to an object when the label was in another language. This same pattern of results held for monolingual 4-year-olds as long as it was made clear to them that the second term was in a different language. Thus, by at least 4 years of age, children recognize that mutual exlcusivity is a bias that operates within but not between languages. Anecdotal reports and diary data suggest that bilingual children may recognize this much earlier – shortly after the start of language acquisition (see review by Clark, 1987).

Apparent evidence against mutual exclusivity

In this section I will try to reconcile the present hypothesis that children use the mutual exclusivity assumption as an initial guide to figuring out the meanings of novel terms with several recent arguments against mutual exclusivity.

In many cases, the studies that supposedly provide evidence against mutual exclusivity might well have been presented in the preceding section on how children override the mutual exclusivity assumption. That is, many of the data that have been taken as evidence against children using mutual exclusivity consist of cases in which mutual exclusivity has been violated (e.g., Gathercole, 1987; Merriman, 1987; Mervis, 1987); but as I argued earlier violations of mutual exclusivity in a child's lexicon may imply that the child was capable of overriding the assumption rather than that mutual exclusivity was not used at all.

Mervis (1987) argues, for example, that mutual exclusivity is a late-developing principle that depends on several other insights about language that children take time to discover. According to Mervis (1987) early language learners do not honor mutual exclusivity, and she supports her argument with cases in which children comprehended two category terms for the same object. Although there is no doubt that the examples Mervis provides are violations of mutual exclusivity, it could well be that the children were provided with enough information to enable them to overcome their mutual exclusivity bias. In fact, Mervis provides evidence for the same children's initial reluctance to violate mutual exclusivity, although she does not discuss it in this way. Mervis (1987) reports that early language learners often ignore a new name for an old object. Initial rejection of a second label is just what would be expected on the mutual exclusivity hypothesis. Moreover, Mervis (1989) reports:

> Very young children do not often correct adult labels. However, those corrections that are offered almost always occur in situations in which the adult has used the adult-basic label for the object; the child responds by providing the child-basic label. Often the child precedes his or her label with "No!" In other cases, the child's tone makes it clear that he or she intends to contradict the adult. (Mervis, 1989, p. 14)

In other words, one of the few situations that impels these early language learners to correct an adult is one in which the adult violates mutual exclusivity. Although these children may become convinced that a second label is appropriate, their initial rejection of second labels for objects is motivated by their mutual exclusivity bias.

An experimental study on the learning of second labels for objects was taken by Banigan and Mervis (1988) as evidence that 24-month-olds do not honor the mutual exclusivity assumption, but here again they failed to distinguish between initial attempts to honor mutual exclusivity and subsequent ability to learn second labels. In this study, 24-month-olds were taught labels for objects for which they already knew a label. For example, children who would have called a vest a *jacket* were taught *vest;* children who would have called goggles *glasses* were taught the word *goggles.* What Banigan and Mervis (1988) emphasize is that the children were capable of learning second labels for these objects, thus violating mutual exclusivity. What I would like to emphasize, however, is how difficult it was to teach these young children the second labels. There were four training conditions. In the first condition, the children were simply taught the label for the object, for example, "This is a vest." The children were not able to learn the second label under this *label-only* condition. Unfortunately, the study did not include a control group in which children were taught a first label for a novel object under the label-only condition. But given the age of the children, who were well past the average age of the vocabulary spurt, it is very likely that they would have been quite successful at acquiring object labels under this condition. Providing labels is a highly typical way of teaching object labels to young children. Nevertheless, these children were unable to learn second object labels in this way. In the next condition, children heard a label and a description, for example, "This is a vest. It doesn't have sleeves" (the experimenter pointed to the sleeve opening). Under this *label and description* condition, the children were still unable to learn the second label for the object. In a third condition, the distinctive property was demonstrated to the children while the label was provided, for example, "This is a vest. You see your shirt sleeves when you wear a vest." The experimenter held the vest up to her chest and ran her fingers through each arm. This resulted in some learning. Finally, the fourth condition, which included labeling, description, and demonstration, was the only condition in which there was an appreciable degree of learning.

Thus, given how hard it was to teach children a second label for an object compared with what we would expect for learning a first label, this study provides support for the mutual exclusivity bias. Moreover, it would constitute evidence for the use of mutual exclusivity in 24-month-olds that could not be explained by a propensity to fill lexical gaps. Compared with first label learning, where simply labeling an object is very likely sufficient to enable 2-year-olds to learn a new object label, second label learning requires extensive information about the referent.

Merriman and Bowman (1989) present a series of studies designed to test whether young children honor mutual exclusivity. This work is not subject to the objection just raised because the authors quite clearly distinguish between the initial versus subsequent acceptance of a second label. In a comprehensive and thoughtful review, they conceptualize mutual exclusivity as a default assumption that children may make, but one that can be violated under certain circumstances. They detail several different ways in which children could attempt to preserve mutual exclusivity. On the basis of several experiments they conclude that children do not honor the mutual exclusivity assumption until they are $2\frac{1}{2}$ years old. To accept this conclusion, however, requires that the experimental procedures they used were appropriate for very young children. Unfortunately, there are several problems with the studies that make it hard to interpret the results from the youngest children.

In the first two studies Merriman and Bowman (1989) tested whether very young children could use mutual exclusivity to reject a second label for a known object and treat it as a label for a novel object instead. Would 2-year-olds shown a doll and a garlic press, for example, and asked to "put your finger on the garlic press" be able to eliminate doll as the possible referent of *garlic press* and therefore choose the garlic press? If children did select the novel object in this situation, one would have to be sure that this was not due to a novelty preference. Markman and Wachtel (1988) dealt with this problem by having a control condition in which the children were simply asked to "pick one." In the control condition, the children showed no systematic preference for the novel object, choosing it at chance levels. Merriman and Bowman (1989) used a different way to control for novelty, one that unfortunately introduced a powerful confound. In an attempt to equalize objects for their familiarity, they allowed children to play for five minutes with all of the novel objects they would see in the experiment but with none of the familiar objects. So when it came time, for example, to ask a child to touch the garlic press, that child would have been playing with the garlic press for several minutes but would see the doll for the first time. The result was that 2-year-olds preferred the objects they had not yet had a chance to play with, which were always objects with known labels. Given young children's known tendency to tire of objects they have been exposed to (witness habituation studies), providing differential exposure to novel versus known objects is not an appropriate way to control for novelty. Rather than assuming that these very young children systematically preferred to violate mutual exclusivity, it is much more plausible to assume that they preferred to play with a fresh toy rather than one they had been playing with for a while. Note also that success in this task could be achieved by a motivation to fill a lexical gap (Merriman & Bowman, 1989) and would not require mutual exclusivity. Failure here would thus imply a lack of motivation to fill lexical gaps. Given that 2- to $2\frac{1}{2}$-year-olds often request labels for objects, this seems unlikely.

In two other studies, designed to test a different implication of the mutual exclusivity hypothesis, a precondition was that the subjects had to remember which objects had been labeled by the experimenter in a training phase. The 2-year-olds did not show evidence of honoring mutual exclusivity in these studies, but they also failed to remember which objects had been labeled. Thus, the information-processing demands of the experimental test were too taxing for the youngest children.

In sum, Merriman and Bowman's (1989) measures of mutual exclusivity were too taxing and thus overly conservative measures of very young children's use of mutual exclusivity. The $2\frac{1}{2}$-year olds were capable of maintaining mutual exclusivity despite these problems, but the 2-year-olds were not.

Whether or not mutual exclusivity is available to children about to enter the naming explosion is thus not yet known. Perhaps mutual exclusivity emerges later, as Mervis (1987) and Merriman and Bowman (1989) claim. The evidence and arguments they base this claim on are problematic, however, and it could well be that much younger children will show evidence of honoring mutual exclusivity when they are tested under more favorable circumstances. Mervis's (1987, 1989) report of younger children ignoring or refusing to accept a second label for a known object suggests that mutual exclusivity is used by children as young as 18 to 24 months of age.

Domain specificity of the constraints

In terms of the general theme of this volume, the relation between language and thought, one question that arises from this work is whether these constraints are specific to language or whether they arise out of more general cognitive biases. To date, we know so little about these issues that we can only begin to speculate. Also, there is no reason to believe that the constraints are equivalent in their domain specificity. Some may be unique to language or, more precisely, unique to lexical acquisition, while others may apply more widely. Some very general biases may operate to reduce the hypothesis space across a variety of domains, whereas others may operate only in the case of word learning. If the criterion for domain specificity were that the bias appear in no other domain, I doubt that any of the lexical constraints discussed so far would qualify. Keil (1990), however, suggests a weaker criterion, namely, that constraints are domain-specific if they are content-dependent, meaning that they apply only to types of knowledge that meet certain structural descriptions. This leaves open the possibility that a given constraint could be applicable in more than one domain, yet still not be domain-general. From this perspective, Keil (1990) wrestled with the question of whether the lexical constraints that have been postulated should be considered domain-specific. He found it hard to decide and concluded that they might be, but also pointed out reasons to be unsure. With these caveats in mind, I will comment briefly on the domain specificity of each of the three lexical constraints discussed in this chapter: the whole-object, taxonomic, and mutual exclusivity assumptions.

The whole-object assumption

Do children interpret novel labels as referring to whole objects because objects are in general very salient, or is their attention to objects heightened in the presence of a novel word? Clearly, objects are perceptually salient. Moreover, Spelke (1988, 1990) has demonstrated that infants have a richly interconnected set of beliefs about physical objects including the expectations that objects are cohesive, bounded, and spatiotemporally continuous. Thus, objects may have a privileged conceptual as well as perceptual status in babies. Yet imagine a child watching a colorful, pulsating neon object twirling around in an interesting way. It is very likely that the color and motion of the object would be attended to as well as the object per se. If so, what would happen if the object were labeled? Would the child interpret the label as referring to the brilliant color, the pulsating rhythm, the interesting motion, or the object itself? The whole-object assumption predicts that the child would interpret the novel label as a label for the object even when the nonlinguistic salience of properties was greater than that of the object. In other words, the constraint is presumed to operate in language learning even when it fails to coincide with what is salient nonlinguistically. Although the whole-object assumption has not yet been subjected to this stringent a test, Baldwin's (1989) and Backscheider and Markman's (1990) studies suggest that in those cases where color or a dynamic activity are made salient to children, the children will still interpret the label as a label for objects. Perhaps the whole-object assumption in word learning capitalizes on a cognitive bias to parse the world in terms of objects, and labeling objects may exaggerate this more general tendency, strengthening it enough to promote objects to the preferred interpretation of a novel label even in those cases where properties are otherwise more salient.

The taxonomic assumption

Markman and Hutchinson's (1984) original evidence for the taxo-nomic assumption suggests that this assumption may be specific to word learning. In fact, the impetus for studying this word-learning constraint was the observation that children treat words as referring to objects of like kind although they often organize objects accord-ing to their thematic relationships in classification and other tasks. At the same time, children notice and use taxonomic relations in domains other than language learning. One important domain where something like the taxonomic assumption very likely operates is in-ductive projection from one object to another. Children are almost certainly more likely to make inductive generalizations from one ob-ject to another of like kind than to one that is strongly associated with it. For example, after having learned that a poodle has incisors, a child should be more likely to conclude that a collie has incisors than that a bone does, even though dog and bone are strongly as-sociated. Such comparisons have not been made, but there is ample evidence that children draw inductive projections to objects of like kind (tempered by their knowledge of the domains, the hierarchical levels, and implicit theories [Carey, 1985; Gelman, 1988; Gelman & Markman, 1986; Keil, 1979]) and, to my knowledge, no evidence that children project properties to objects that are thematically re-lated. Thus, inductive inferences about object properties are also governed by a version of the taxonomic assumption that mitigates the strong version of domain specificity but is consistent with the weaker version – that the taxonomic assumption operates only in some select domains.

The mutual exclusivity assumption

The mutual exclusivity assumption resembles a number of other biases that have been postulated in other cognitive domains. Whether this similarity is superficial or whether it reflects a common source for these biases across domains is not yet clear. For now, however, mu-tual exclusivity appears to be the most likely to qualify as domain-general. In this section I present a partial list (from Markman & Wachtel, 1988; Markman, 1989) of some of the other domains in which biases comparable to mutual exclusivity appear.

Other linguistic constraints. One possibility is that mutual exclusivity is not limited to word learning but is used more broadly in language acquisition. Or to be more accurate, mutual exclusivity could result from a more general principle, either a one-to-one mapping principle (Slobin, 1973, 1977) or the uniqueness principle (Pinker, 1984; Wexler & Culicover, 1980) applied to word learning. Slobin's (1973, 1977) one-to-one operating principle of language acquisition is that children expect a one-to-one mapping between underlying semantic structures and surface forms. Although this principle was formulated for morphemes in a sentence, if it were extended to category terms it would result in the mutual exclusivity of the terms. That is, each category term would be referred to by only one category term.

The motivation for the uniqueness principle is to help account for the way children acquire grammatical rules in the absence of negative feedback (Pinker, 1984; Wexler & Culicover, 1980). If children are not informed that a given grammatical rule they have hypothesized is wrong, how can they reject erroneous hypotheses and settle on the correct grammar for their language? Pinker (1984), following Wexler and Culicover (1980), argues that in some cases, the need for negative evidence can be eliminated if children assume the uniqueness principle. That is, when children are faced with a set of alternative structures fulfilling the same function, they should assume that only one of the structures is correct unless there is direct evidence that more than one is necessary. Children require more evidence to accept a construction with a uniqueness violation than a construction that does not violate the assumption.

Mutual exclusivity is consistent with the uniqueness principle as applied to category terms. As in the domain of syntax, if children start out biased and assume that terms are mutually exclusive, they should require more evidence to accept a construction that violates mutual exclusivity. The problem of lack of negative evidence is not so acute for word learning as it is for the acquisition of grammar (see Markman & Wachtel, 1988, for a more detailed argument), but nevertheless children may still be able to make use of the mutual exclusivity assumption to reject certain hypotheses about a word's meaning because it would violate mutual exclusivity, even if no neg- ative evidence were provided.

Multiple representation. Mutual exclusivity may not be limited to lan- guage. It could derive from children's beliefs about objects and not just their beliefs about object labels. Children might believe that an object has only one identity, that is, that it can be only one kind of thing and that its identity is revealed by its label. Flavell (1988) ar- gues that young children assume that each thing in the world has only one identity, an assumption that adults may share. Unlike adults, however, children do not understand that each thing may never- theless be represented in more than one way. According to Flavell (1988), this limitation on multiple representation is revealed in a number of diverse tasks, including visual and conceptual perspec- tive taking and understanding the appearance–reality distinction, along with assuming mutual exclusivity of category terms.

A domain-general constraint on systematization. A final possibility is that mutual exclusivity or some more general principle that subsumes mutual exclusivity is a domain-general constraint – appearing widely in various manifestations across many diverse domains. Karmiloff- Smith (1979; Karmiloff-Smith & Inhelder, 1975) and Carey (1978) have argued that children may begin acquiring knowledge in a domain by learning basic concepts in relative isolation, but after a while are driven to try to organize and systematize their knowledge. Mutual exclusivity is a simple, primitive form of systematization. Basically it works to keep relations between elements distinct and to maxi- mize predictability from one element to another. Some implications of such a general one-to-one mapping bias are that it would lead children to expect perfect correlations between elements in a do- main; it would lead them to reject counterexamples and exceptions to general rules; and it would lead them to exaggerate regularities in their environment. The mutual exclusivity assumption in lan- guage, then, could be one instantiation of a widespread attempt to find simple, regular relations among elements in a domain.

Conclusions

The evidence on the whole-object, taxonomic, and mutual exclusiv- ity assumptions suggests that children use at least two of these assumptions by the average age of the naming explosion. By 18 months of age children assume that a novel label refers to the object as a whole – not to its substance, parts, color, size, shape or other property. They also extend a novel term to objects of the same kind as the one first labeled, rather than to objects that are related or associated with the named object in some other way. Young preschoolers can use mutual exclusivity to avoid making redundant hypotheses. They can use either mutual exclusivity or a bias to fill lexical gaps as an indirect means of figuring out the referent of a novel word. Finally, they can use mutual exclusivity to learn terms that refer to a part or the substance or other properties of objects, rather than just learning terms for the object itself. Mutual exclusivity thus enables children to override the whole-object assumption. It is not yet known how early in their lives children first use the mutual exclusivity assumption. Much of the evidence against the existence of this assumption is in fact evidence that quite young children have the capacity to override mutual exclusivity when given enough information. Just as mutual exclusivity helps children overcome the limitations of the whole-object assumption, other kinds of evidence help them overcome the limitations of mutual exclusivity. These constraints can be overridden when they conflict with other constraints or when enough evidence is provided in the input that contradicts the bias.

These assumptions guide children's initial hypotheses, eliminate numerous hypotheses from consideration, and thereby help solve the inductive problem posed by word learning. By drastically reducing the number of hypotheses children must consider, they make the inductive problem soluble. Very often these constraints lead children to make correct hypotheses about what a novel word might mean. But they are not infallible and in fact lead children to make errors. A commonly reported anecdote, for example, is that young children believe that *hot* is the term for stove. Parents warn children, "Don't touch that; it's hot," and the whole-object assumption leads children to interpret *hot* as the label for stove. The mutual exclusivity assumption makes it more difficult for children to learn subordinate and superordinate terms if they already know a basic-level label for an object. On the whole, the assumptions are advantageous, but problems arise. Children must then be capable of overriding the constraints. This system must be flexible enough to avoid the problems that would arise if the constraints were too rigid and completely insensitive to counterevidence but powerful enough to guide children in their initial hypotheses about what words mean.

References

Au, T. K. (1990). Children's use of information in word learning. *Journal of Child Language, 17,* 393–416.

Au, T. K., & Glusman, M. (1990). The principle of mutual exclusivity in word learning: To honor or not to honor? *Child Development, 61,* 1474–1490.

Au, T. K., & Laframboise, D. E. (in press). Linguistic contrast as corrective feedback in color name acquisition. *Child Development.*

Au, T. K., & Markman, E. M. (1987). Acquiring word meanings via linguistic contrast. *Cognitive Development, 2,* 217–236.

Backscheider, A., & Markman, E. M. (1990). *Young children's use of the taxonomic assumption to constrain word meanings.* Unpublished manuscript.

Baldwin, D. A. (1989). Priorities in children's expectations about object label reference: Form over color. *Child Development, 60,* 1291–1306.

Baldwin, D. A., & Markman, E. M. (1989). Mapping out word–object relations: A first step. *Child Development, 60,* 381–398.

Banigan, R. L., & Mervis, C. B. (1988). Role of adult input in young children's category evolution: II. An experimental study. *Journal of Child Language, 15,* 493–505.

Bauer, P. J., & Mandler, J. M. (1989). Taxonomies and triads: Conceptual organization in one-to-two-year olds. *Cognitive Psychology, 21,* 156–184.

Bloom, L. M. (1973). *One word at a time: The use of single word utterances before syntax.* The Hague: Mouton.

Bloom, L., Lifter, K., & Broughton, J. (1985). The convergence of early cognition and language in the second year of life: Problems in conceptualization and measurement. In M. Barrett (Ed.), *Children's single-word speech* (pp. 149–180). New York: Wiley.

Bolinger, D. (1977). *Meaning and form.* London: Longman Group.

Bowerman, M. (1987). Commentary: Mechanisms of language acquisition. In B. MacWhinney (Ed.), *Mechanisms of language acquisition* (pp. 443–466). Hillsdale, NJ: Erlbaum.

Bretherton, I., Bates, E., McNew, S., Shore, C., Williamson, C., & Beeghly-Smith, M. (1981). Comprehension and production of symbols in infancy: An experimental study. *Developmental Psychology, 17,* 728–736.

Bridges, A. (1986). Actions and things: What adults talk about to 1-year-olds. In S. A. Kuczaj (Ed.), *The development of word meaning* (pp. 225–255). New York: Springer.

Carey, S. (1978). The child as word learner. In M. Halle, J. Bresnan, & A. Miller (Eds.), *Linguistic theory and psychological reality* (pp. 264–293). Cambridge, MA: MIT Press.

Carey, S. (1985). *Conceptual change in childhood.* Cambridge, MA: MIT Press.

Carey, S., & Bartlett, E. (1978). Acquiring a single new word. *Papers and Reports on Child Language Development, 15,* 17–29.

Clark, E. V. (1973). What's in a word? On the child's acquisition of semantics in his first language. In T. E. Moore (Ed.), *Cognitive development and the acquisition of language* (pp. 65–110). New York: Academic Press.

104   E. M. Markman

Clark, E. V. (1983). Meanings and concepts. In J. H. Flavell, & E. M. Markman (Eds.), *Handbook of child psychology: Vol. 3: Cognitive development* (pp. 787–840). New York: Wiley.

Clark, E. V. (1987). The principle of contrast: A constraint on language acquisition. In B. MacWhinney (Ed.), *The 20th Annual Carnegie Symposium on Cognition* (pp. 1–33). Hillsdale, NJ: Erlbaum.

Corrigan, R. (1983). The development of representational skills. In K. W. Fischer (Ed.), *Levels and transitions in children's development* (pp. 51–64). San Francisco: Jossey-Bass.

Dockrell, J. (1981). *The child's acquisition of unfamiliar words: An experimental study.* Unpublished doctoral dissertation, University of Stirling, Stirling, Scotland.

Dromi, E. (1987). *Early lexical development.* Cambridge University Press.

Flavell, J. H. (1988). The development of children's knowledge about the mind: From cognitive connections to mental representations. In J. W. Astington, P. L. Harris, & D. R. Olson (Eds.), *Developing theories of mind* (pp. 244–267). Cambridge University Press.

Gathercole, V. C. (1987). The contrastive hypothesis for the acquisition of word meaning: A reconsideration of the theory. *Journal of Child Language, 14*, 493–531.

Gelman, S. A. (1988). The development of induction within natural kind and artifact categories. *Cognitive Psychology, 20*, 65–95.

Gelman, S. A., & Markman, E. M. (1986). Categories and induction in young children. *Cognition, 23*, 183–208.

Gelman, S. A., Wilcox, S. A., & Clark, E. V. (1989). Conceptual and lexical hierarchies in young children. *Cognitive Development, 4*, 309–326.

Golinkoff, R. M., Hirsh-Pasek, K., Baduini, C., & Lavallee, A. (1985, October). *What's in a word?: The young child's predisposition to use lexical contrast.* Paper presented at the Boston University Conference on Child Language, Boston.

Halliday, M. A. K. (1975). Learning how to mean. In E. H. Lenneberg & E. Lenneberg (Eds.), *Foundations of language development: A multidisciplinary approach* (Vol. 1, pp. 239–265). New York: Academic Press.

Heibeck, T., & Markman, E. M. (1987). Word learning in children: An examination of fast mapping. *Child Development, 58*, 1021–1034.

Hutchinson, J. E. (1984). *Constraints on children's implicit hypotheses about word meanings.* Unpublished doctoral dissertation, Stanford University, Stanford, CA.

Hutchinson, J. E. (1986, April). *Children's sensitivity to the contrastive use of object category terms.* Paper presented at the Stanford Child Language Research Forum. Stanford University, Stanford, CA.

Huttenlocher, J., & Smiley, P. (1987). Early word meanings: The case for objects names. *Cognitive Psychology, 19*, 63–89.

Karmiloff-Smith, A. (1979, June). *Language as a formal problem-space for children.* Paper presented at the MPG/NIAS Conference "Beyond Description in Child Language," Nijmegan, Holland.

Karmiloff-Smith, A., & Inhelder, B. (1975). If you want to get ahead, get a theory. *Cognition, 3*, 195–211.

Keil, F. C. (1979). *Semantic and conceptual development: An ontological perspective.* Cambridge, MA: Harvard University Press.

Keil, F. C. (1990). Constraints on constraints: Surveying the epigenetic landscape. *Cognitive Science, 14*, 135–168.

Landau, K. B., Smith, L. B., & Jones, S. S. (1988). The importance of shape in early lexical learning. *Cognitive Development, 3,* 299–321.

Lock, A. (1980). *The guided reinvention of language.* New York: Academic Press.

Markman, E. M. (1987). How children constrain the possible meanings of words. In U. Neisser (Ed.), *Concepts and conceptual development: Ecological and intellectual factors in categorization* (pp. 255–287). Cambridge University Press.

Markman, E. M. (1989). *Categorization and naming in children: Problems of induction.* Cambridge, MA: MIT Press.

Markman, E. M., & Callanan, M. A. (1983). An analysis of hierarchical classification. In R. Sternberg (Ed.), *Advances in the psychology of human intelligence* (Vol. 2, pp. 325–365). Hillsdale, NJ: Erlbaum.

Markman, E. M., & Hutchinson, J. E. (1984). Children's sensitivity to constraints on word meaning: Taxonomic versus thematic relations. *Cognitive Psychology, 16,* 1–27.

Markman, E. M., & Wachtel, G. F. (1988). Children's use of mutual exclusivity to constrain the meanings of words. *Cognitive Psychology, 20,* 121–157.

McShane, J. (1979). The development of naming. *Linguistics, 17,* 879–905.

Melkman, R., Tversky, B., & Baratz, D. (1981). Developmental trends in the use of perceptual and conceptual attributes in grouping, clustering and retrieval. *Journal of Experimental Child Psychology, 31,* 470–486.

Merriman, W. E. (1987, April). *Lexical contrast in toddlers: A reanalysis of the diary evidence.* Paper presented at the biennial convention of the Society for Research in Child Development, Baltimore.

Merriman, W. E., & Bowman, L. L. (1989). The mutual exclusivity bias in children's word learning. *Monographs of the Society for Research in Child Development, 54* (3–4, Serial No. 220).

Mervis, C. B. (1987). Child-basic object categories and early lexical development. In U. Neisser (Ed.), *Concepts and conceptual development: Ecological and intellectual factors in categorization* (pp. 201–233). Cambridge University Press.

Mervis, C. B. (1989). *Early lexical development: The role of operating principles.* Unpublished manuscript, Emory University, Atlanta, GA.

Nelson, K. (1973). Structure and strategy in learning to talk. *Monographs of the Society for Research in Child Development, 38* (1–2, Serial No. 149).

Nelson, K. (1974). Concept, word and sentence: Interrelations in acquisition and development. *Psychological Review, 81,* 267–285.

Nelson, K. (1988). Constraints on word learning? *Cognitive Development, 3,* 221–246.

Nelson, K., & Lucariello, J. (1985). The development of meaning in first words. In M. Barrett (Ed.), *Children's single-word speech* (pp. 59–86). New York: Wiley.

Pinker, S. (1984). *Language learnability and language development.* Cambridge, MA: Harvard Unviersity Press.

Quine, W. V. O. (1960). *Word and object.* Cambridge: MIT Press.

Rescorla, L. A. (1980). Overextension in early language development. *Journal of Child Language, 7,* 321–335.

Slobin, D. I. (1973). Cognitive prerequisites for the development of grammar. In C. A. Ferguson & D. I. Slobin (Eds.), *Studies of child language development* (pp. 45–54). New York: Springer.

Slobin, D. I. (1977). Language change in childhood and in history. In J. Macnamara (Ed.), *Language learning and thought* (pp. 185–214). New York: Academic Press.

Snyder, L. S., Bates, E., & Bretherton, I. (1981). Content and context in early lexical development. *Journal of Child Language, 8*, 565–582.

Soja, N., Carey, S., & Spelke, E. (1985, April). *Constraints on word learning.* Paper presented at the biennial convention of the Society for Research in Child Development, Toronto.

Spelke, E. S. (1988). Where perceiving ends and thinking begins: The apprehension of objects in infancy. In A. Yonas (Ed.), *Perceptual development in infancy: Minnesota Symposium on Child Psychology* (pp. 197–234). Hillsdale, NJ: Erlbaum.

Spelke, E. S. (1990). Principles of object perception. *Cognitive Science, 14*, 29–56.

Suchman, R. G., & Trabasso, T. (1966). Color and form preference in young children. *Journal of Experimental Child Psychology, 37*, 439–451.

Taylor, M., & Gelman, S. A. (1988). Adjectives and nouns: Children's strategies for learning new words. *Child Development, 59*, 411–419.

Taylor, M., & Gelman, S. A. (1989). Incorporating new words into the lexicon: Preliminary evidence for language hierarchies in two-year-old children. *Child Development, 60*, 625–636.

Waxman, S. R. (1990). Linguistic biases and the establishment of conceptual hierarchies: Evidence from preschool children. *Cognitive Development, 5*, 123–150.

Waxman, S. R., & Gelman, R. (1986). Preschooler's use of superordinate relations in classification. *Cognitive Development, 1*, 139–156.

Wexler, K., & Culicover, P. (1980). *Formal principles of language acquisition.* Cambridge, MA: MIT Press.

Woodward, A. L., & Markman, E. M. (in press). Constraints on learning as default assumptions: Comments on Merriman and Bowman's "The mutual exclusivity bias in children's word learning." *Developmental Review.*

4. Convergences between semantic and conceptual organization in the preschool years

SANDRA R. WAXMAN

> The gentleman who is discriminating about his wine . . . can consistently apply nouns to the different fluids of a class and he can apply adjectives to the differences between the fluids.
> Gibson and Gibson (1955, p. 35)

Our enduring fascination with issues concerning language and thought may derive from our sense that these are uniquely human capacities. Despite years of devoted tutoring, even our closest genealogical relatives have yet to acquire the complex and creative linguistic systems that human infants master within the first few years of life (Petitto & Seidenberg, 1979; Premack, 1971). And although members of other species surely manifest sophisticated conceptual and representational capacities, these appear to be accessible to them only under restricted conditions (Rozin, 1976). Findings like these lend substance to the intuition that humans are uniquely endowed with the capacity to build complex, flexible, and creative linguistic and conceptual systems.

Recent research has documented the remarkable rate at which very young children naturally acquire language and develop rich conceptual systems. Researchers estimate that by the time children reach 2 years of age, they learn an average of six new words each day (Templin, 1957). They also have at their command a rich variety of

The preparation of this chapter was supported, in part, by a fellowship from the Spencer Foundation and the National Academy of Education. Further support for much of the research came from grants from the Milton Fund (Harvard University) and the John D. and Catherine T. MacArthur Foundations. I am indebted to M. Callanan, D. G. Hall, and E. Shipley for their helpful discussions of this work and to the editors of this volume for their careful reading of the manuscript. I also thank the preschool children, teachers, and parents who contributed to this work. Requests for reprints should be sent to Sandra R. Waxman, Department of Psychology, Harvard University, Cambridge, MA, 02138.

conceptual relations (e.g., taxonomic, thematic, and associative relations) with which they organize and categorize the objects and events they encounter in their lives.

It is conceivable that these concurrent linguistic and conceptual advances are more than coincidental. After all, there is an essential conceptual component in even the simplest act of naming. Whenever we apply a single common label (e.g., *animal*) to a set of disparate instances (e.g., a dog, a horse, and a flamingo) we have, in fact, classified these together. And when we use different labels for each of these instances (e.g., *dog, horse*), we reveal our appreciation of their conceptual distinctions as well.

Moreover, the mastery of new words and new concepts appears to go hand in hand. Oftentimes, hearing an unfamiliar word launches a search for the concept to which it refers. For example, I recently read an article that made passing mention of Frances Wright's discovery of the *spherule*. The new word piqued my curiosity and led me to inquire into its meaning. Conversely, it is possible for an idea to germinate before its linguistic realization. This was undoubtedly the case for Professor Wright, who envisioned the concept of the spherule first and only later gave it a name to communicate the concept to others.

Observations like these fuel the intuition that human language and conceptual organization are essentially linked, but they leave open many questions concerning the nature of this relation (see R. Brown, 1986, for an excellent overview of research programs addressing language–thought questions). It is vital that we articulate our research questions precisely if we are to find satisfying answers regarding the complex relations between language and thought.

My approach has been to focus on questions concerning the relation between word learning and conceptual organization in one specific area of development. In my research program, I have been concerned primarily with the early establishment of object categories at various hierarchical levels (e.g., flamingo, bird, animal) and the labels we use to describe them. On the basis of evidence obtained from several different experimental paradigms and gleaned from several different cultures and language communities, I have taken the position that there are powerful, yet precise, relations that link language with conceptual development and promote the formation of conceptual hierarchies. More specifically, I have argued that in the process of word learning, children are guided by implicit biases that direct their attention to taxonomic relations among objects and classes of objects.

In this chapter, I bring together psychological, linguistic, and ethnobiological evidence to support this position. I begin by describing several characteristics of hierarchical systems of organization. I then amplify this psychological perspective by integrating it within the larger context of cross-cultural and cross-linguistic work. Here, I draw primarily on the work of ethnobiologists to argue that cross-cultural and cross-linguistic data can inform our current views on the relations between linguistic and conceptual organization. Turning next to developmental issues, I argue that early in development, linguistic and conceptual organization are wedded and that children use syntactic form class (e.g., noun, adjective) to help them determine the meaning of novel nouns. Nouns highlight higher-order taxonomic relations (e.g., animal, furniture) and adjectives highlight specific lower-order distinctions (e.g., Siamese cats vs. tabby cats). In this way, linguistic information guides the establishment of conceptual hierarchies. Finally, I articulate more precisely the claim that certain aspects of human development may unfold under the influence of constraints or biases.

Hierarchical systems of organization

A hallmark of human conceptual organization is its flexibility. We readily place objects in different kinds of classes, depending on the task at hand. For example, I may group a flamingo taxonomically with an oriole (because both are birds); I may also classify a flamingo taxonomically with a bear (because both are animals). Alternatively, I may group that same flamingo with a kumquat (because both thrive in warm climates) or even with the sunset (because both are pink). Amidst this conceptual flexibility, one type of organization – hierarchical systems of taxonomic classes – has been consistently singled out by scholars from diverse disciplines for its power and efficiency.

Hierarchical systems are composed of a series of taxonomic classes that vary in their scope (e.g., flamingo, bird, and animal) and together form a hierarchy in which lower-order classes are nested within higher-order classes. Hierarchical systems are governed by two organizing principles, the *hierarchical* and *contrastive* principles (Inhelder & Piaget, 1964; Miller & Johnson-Laird, 1976).

The hierarchical principle is concerned with logical inclusion relations among classes at various levels of abstraction and is based on the logical principles of *transitivity* and *asymmetry*. Transitivity captures the fact that if the members of Class C are a subset of Class B, and if the members of Class B are a subset of Class A, then the members of Class C are necessarily included in Class A. Asymmetry captures the fact that the inferences licensed by hierarchical systems are unidirectional. Inferences regarding class membership are licensed in ascending order within a hierarchy. Any member of a lower-order class (e.g., a flamingo) is, by definition, included in each of its higher-order classes (e.g., *birds, animals*). In this way, the principle of asymmetry ensures that higher-order classes are larger than any of their constituent subsets. The direction of the asymmetry is reversed when one considers class properties, as opposed to class membership. Properties are "inherited" in descending order within a hierarchy; any property that can be predicated of a higher-order class can also be predicated of its constituent subclasses. For instance, because we know that all fruits have seeds, we can infer that a papaya has seeds.

The hierarchical principle governs vertical relations among classes at different levels of abstraction; the contrastive principle maintains horizontal relations among classes at any given level of abstraction. Considered horizontally, the classes within a hierarchy are contrastive or mutually exclusive. This relation is sometimes known as "direct contrast," and the entire collection of classes immediately included within a single higher-order class constitutes a contrast set. For example, *tulip, rose,* and *daisy* comprise a portion of the contrast set immediately included in the higher-order class *flower*.

The hierarchical and contrastive principles provide the structural framework for hierarchical systems and make possible a rich set of inferences, both inductive and deductive. For example, if we encounter a novel item and learn that it is an animal, we can deduce that it eats. If we encounter a novel item and learn that it is, say, a dog, we can induce that it is an animal and shares other properties with members of that class (Blewitt, 1990). Further, when we discover a new property of a single item (e.g., that Fido has a heart rate that is much faster than that of a human), we tend to attribute that property to other class members as well (Gelman, 1988; Gelman & Coley, Chapter 5, this volume).

Therefore, by placing an object within a hierarchical system, we open up "a whole vista of possibilities for 'going beyond' the category by virtue of the . . . relationships linking one category to the others" (Bruner, Goodnow, & Austin, 1956, p. 13). As a consequence, hierarchical systems serve as the natural domain of induction (Gelman, 1988; Miller & Johnson-Laird, 1976; Shipley, 1989) and "give us the greatest command of our knowledge already acquired and lead most directly to the acquisition of more" (Mill, 1843, p. 432).

Conceptual modifications within hierarchical systems

Hierarchical systems are structured and powerful, but they are not carved in stone. On the contrary, they are supple enough to be revised as we incorporate new knowledge (Quine, 1969). As a result, our conceptual hierarchies are productive, flexible constructions that evolve throughout the course of development. Indeed, there is a fluid relationship between our systems of knowledge and our theories within a given domain (see Murphy & Medin, 1985, for a discussion of the relationship between theories and conceptual structure; see Carey, 1985, for an example of the development of theories and classification of the concept *animal*).

In this section, I describe three types of modifications that bear directly on the construction of hierarchical systems: new distinctions, new generalizations, and reorganizations. First, throughout development, we learn to make new distinctions within existing classes. For example, many adults who have little expertise with flowers distinguish one broad class of *roses*. With increasing experience, they may come to appreciate distinctions within this broad class and to capture these by creating categorical subclasses (e.g., tea roses vs. climbing roses). Similarly, at one time astronomers considered *stars* to be a homogeneous class, but with increasing experience, they discerned several distinct kinds, including single, double, and pulsing stars. Notice that neither flower novices nor early astronomers failed to establish hierarchical systems of organization. The point here is that earlier, more elementary hierarchies are often simply less elaborate than those established later on the basis of additional knowledge and experience.

Second, we often generalize to create new higher-order classes and, in so doing, establish increasingly elaborate hierarchies. Many examples of this phenomenon come from the field of biology. For example, biologists group shrimps, moths, and spiders together as members of the class *arthropod*; nonbiologists may not appreciate this higher-order relation. Other examples come from studies of folk biology (e.g., Berlin, Breedlove, & Raven, 1973). For example, in most cultures, two kingdoms (corresponding roughly to our plant and animal kingdoms) are recognized. As a result of extensive and detailed examinations, some Western biosystematicians now discern five biological kingdoms. Note that although the precise number of classes within a contrast set (here, the number of kingdoms) may differ, both biosystematicians and folk biologists have constructed hierarchical systems of organization.

Conceptual reorganizations represent a third type of modification within hierarchical systems. In conceptual reorganizations, no new classes (be they higher- or lower-order) are established. Instead, it is the relations among existing classes that are modified. One class (e.g., *whales*), previously classified in one way (e.g., as fish), may later (and perhaps more accurately) be classified in a different way (e.g., as mammals). Following the logical principles of class inclusion, the discovery that a particular whale is a mammal (because it shares properties characteristic of mammals) motivates a systematic reorganization in which all whales are reclassified as mammals.

These three kinds of conceptual modification illustrate the dynamic and creative nature of human classification. In some cases, modifications have only a local effect. In others, the modifications are more dramatic and may lead to a radical restructuring of the conceptual hierarchy for an entire domain (Carey, 1985; Kuhn, 1962). In general, this discussion of conceptual modification illustrates some possible routes by which young children's rudimentary classification systems may change or become more detailed over time (also see Chi, 1983; Waxman & Shipley, 1987; Waxman, Shipley, & Shepperson, 1990). By virtue of conceptual modifications, we incorporate new information, clarify relations among classes, and strive to fashion increasingly accurate bases for logical reasoning throughout development.

Some caveats concerning conceptual hierarchies

Although there is little doubt that hierarchical systems play a very important role in human cognition, two controversial points bear mention. The first is that precisely because human conceptual organization is so flexible, identifying any one type of conceptual organization (e.g., taxonomic hierarchies) is not tantamount to discovering the sole means of conceptual representation underlying the organization of the human mind. A rapidly accumulating body of research has revealed the importance of non-taxonomic systems of organization. These include script-based, or contextual, categories (Hunn, 1985; Mandler, Fivush, & Reznick, 1987; Nelson, 1987; Nelson & Gruendel, 1981), "taskonomies" (Dougherty & Keller, 1985), part–whole organizations (Tversky & Hemenway, 1984), kinship groupings (Casson, 1975), and ad hoc or utilitarian groupings (Barsalou, 1983; Dougherty & Keller, 1985; Hunn, 1985).

Evidence for these alternative systems of organization may be interpreted in one of two ways. If one takes the view that taxonomic hierarchies represent *the* structure of the mind, the considerable evidence for alternative forms of conceptual organization is damning. However, the existence of such alternative organizations is completely compatible with the position that hierarchies, although powerful and ubiquitous, are not the only system of organization in the repertoire of human conceptual representation.

The second controversial point concerns not the hierarchical relations among classes, but the internal structure of the constituent classes. The shortcomings of the classical theory of concepts, in which class membership is presumed to be determined by simple perceptual features, are now well known. Although criticisms have come from many quarters for many different reasons, no comprehensive description of the internal structure and representation of classes has yet taken its place (see Smith & Medin, 1981, for a thorough review of these issues, including discussions of feature-based, prototype-based, and exemplar-based representations). For the purposes of this chapter, I restrict my focus to the hierarchical relations among classes; issues concerning internal structure are not treated here.

These controversies notwithstanding, the psychological evidence attests to the prominent position of hierarchical systems in the repertoire of human cognition. This position is firmly grounded in converging results from many different experimental sources, including classification, reaction time, multidimensional scaling, labeling, habituation, and memory procedures (see Smith & Medin, 1981, for a representative sample of this work). Yet this body of work derives almost exclusively from research in Western cultures (for some notable exceptions see Luria, 1976; Saxe, 1982; Saxe, Gearhart, & Guberman, 1984; Wagner, 1974). If hierarchical systems are fundamental to human cognition, and not an artifact of Western culture, they should be evident universally.

I therefore turn now to a comprehensive body of anthropological research aimed at elucidating the classification schemes of Western and non-Western peoples alike. In this field, as in psychology, there is ample debate surrounding the subject of hierarchical systems, but the weight of the evidence supports the view that hierarchies are established universally (e.g., Frake, 1962; for arguments to the contrary, see Burling, 1964, Dupré, 1981, and Lancy, 1983). Moreover, the anthropological record reveals striking convergences between the hierarchical systems we create and the linguistic conventions we use to describe them.

Ethnobiological evidence

The field of ethnobiology, a formal discipline within cultural anthropology, is devoted to the study of the linguistic and conceptual systems created by people from diverse cultures to describe the organisms and classes of organisms that occupy the natural world. Scientific interest in "folk biology" was ignited by Berlin and his colleagues (Berlin, 1973; Berlin et al., 1973, 1974; Hunn, 1975). Ethnobiologists have since focused on specific segments of classification systems (e.g., Hage & Miller's, 1976, description of the Shoshoni's nomenclature for birds), as well as more exhaustive, large-scale studies of entire biological classification systems (e.g., Berlin et al., 1973). Consequently, there is now a body of research documenting the existence of hierarchical systems in such disparate cultures and surroundings as the American Southwest (Wyman & Bailey, 1964), Mexico (Berlin et al., 1974; Hunn, 1977), Thailand (Stanlaw & Yoddumnern, 1985), the Phillipines (Conklin, 1954), China (Anderson, 1967), and the New Guinea highlands (Bulmer & Tyler, 1968).

In ethnobiology, directed interviews with adult native informants have served as the primary research tool. The traditional approach has been to construct that part of the lexicon in a given language community that is devoted to describing the natural world and to use this lexicon as a window onto the underlying conceptual framework. Notice that in this field of research, language is accorded a special status, for it is assumed to provide the most direct observable access to underlying cognitive phenomena.[1]

On the basis of his seminal work with the Tzeltal Indians, Berlin abstracted two basic patterns concerning the nature of folk biological knowledge (Berlin et al., 1973). The first concerns the derivation of the basic principles of folk taxonomic classification from our perceptions of the morphological properties of objects in the natural world.[2] The second concerns the hierarchical organization of folk biological knowledge. Berlin's characterization of hierarchical systems embraces the hierarchical and contrastive principles described earlier (e.g., Miller & Johnson-Laird, 1976) and provides a point of contact between anthropology and psychology.

Ethnobiological rank

In an effort to interpret and compare the many different observed systems of folk knowledge, Berlin created a model, or idealized, folk taxonomy. This archetypical taxonomy, which is designed to include all of the categories of natural objects recognized in a given culture, incorporates a maximum of six, and a minimum of three, hierarchical levels or ranks. Beginning at the most inclusive level, these include the Unique Beginner, Life Form, Intermediate, Generic, Specific, and Varietal ranks.

This six-tiered schema does not match perfectly the three levels of abstraction (i.e., superordinate, basic, subordinate) that figure prominently in the psychological literature (Rosch, Mervis, Gray, Johnson, & Boyes-Braem, 1976). However, this mismatch is merely superficial, for there is a fundamental correspondence at one particular hierarchical level that unites the findings in psychology with those in anthropology.

Basic level. In both disciplines, one level has received special attention. This level, known as the basic or generic level (in psychology and anthropology, respectively), occupies a midlevel position within a hierarchical system and corresponds roughly to our notion of a biological species. The basic level appears to be privileged in several regards. First, according to Berlin (1966), classes at this level "cry out to be named." In all cultures examined to date, no matter how primitive or advanced, there are labels for basic-level classes. Oftentimes, higher- and lower-order classes remain unnamed. Moreover, children's earliest vocabularies contain predominantly object terms, and of these, most are at the basic level (Anglin, 1977; Mervis & Crisafi, 1982; Nelson, 1974).

Furthermore, the classes at the basic level tend to be stable over time and fairly consistent across cultures (but see Dougherty, 1978, for a critique of this view).[3] In contrast, researchers in anthropology and psychology share the view that the number and composition of higher- and lower-order classes are a function of the experience and familiarity of the people doing the classifying and may well vary across cultures (Dougherty, 1978; Randall, 1976; Rosch, 1975). Finally, even when a linguistic community (like our own) has established labels for higher- and lower-order classes, the basic-level label maintains its special status: Basic-level labels are the ones most readily supplied by adults in identification and labeling tasks (Callanan, 1985; Chapter 12, this volume; Shipley, Kuhn, & Madden, 1983; Smith & Medin, 1981). Thus, although many names may apply to a given object, the basic-level name seems truest.

R. Brown (1958) suggested that this privileged position may reflect the psychological utility of the basic level. Rosch and her colleagues (Rosch, 1975; Rosch et al., 1976) built on this line of reasoning to operationalize the notion of the basic level and to demonstrate its psychological utility.

One caution is in order here: The "basic-level advantage" is a robust empirical phenomenon. However, although many theoretical explanations have been advanced, none of these alone has proved sufficient (see Armstrong, Gleitman, & Gleitman, 1983; Mervis, 1987; Murphy & Medin, 1985; Smith & Medin, 1981).

Convergences between classification and nomenclature

From the vantage point of psychology, Berlin's signal contribution was his insight concerning the intricate and systematic relations between classes at various levels and their labels. In brief, Berlin asserted that each level within a taxonomy is associated with a particular linguistic form.

Central to Berlin's analysis is his discussion of the *lexeme*, or lexical item, of which he distinguishes two types: primary and secondary. Classes at the basic or generic level tend to be labeled with morphologically simple primary lexemes. Primary lexemes are "unique, single word expressions which . . . are semantically unitary and linguistically distinct" (Berlin et al., 1973). Examples from American English folk biology are nondecomposable nouns such as *orchid* and *whale*.

In many folk biological systems, the more abstract classes (e.g., those at the Unique Beginner and Intermediate levels) are not linguistically encoded. The psychological status of these unnamed classes, or *covert categories*, will be discussed later. If any linguistic pattern can be detected at these higher-order levels, it is that nouns tend to serve as labels. But in contrast to the nouns that typify the basic-level labels, the nouns for higher-order classes tend to have a more complex morphology. In part, this complexity is an inevitable consequence of linguistic constructions such as compounding (for a full discussion of morphological complexity and derivations see Lyons, 1977; Marchand, 1969).

Classes at the less inclusive levels (the Specific and Varietal ranks, or subordinate level) are labeled with secondary lexemes (Berlin et al., 1973; Brown, Kolar, Torrey, Truong-Quang, & Volkman, 1976), which typically include a modifier used in conjunction with a primary lexeme to denote a particular type of the category described by the primary lexeme. Modifier–noun phrases like *cymbidium orchid* and *humpback whale* are secondary lexemes in American English folk biology.

Further, these parallels between linguistic form and hierarchical level are in evidence in signed, as well as in spoken, languages. In American Sign Language (ASL), many superordinate-level terms are created by compounding basic-level terms in such a way as to create a new, morphologically complex noun. For example, the sign for *musical instrument* is a compound noun composed of the basic-level signs *guitar, piano, violin*. Like spoken languages, ASL employs different linguistic devices to mark subordinate-level classes. Here, the basic-level terms are typically modified by "size and shape specifiers" (SASSes) to denote a distinct subtype (Newport & Bellugi, 1978).

One difference between spoken and signed languages is relevant to our discussion here. In ASL, modifiers like the SASSes are signed simultaneously with the basic-level form. However, in spoken language, the modifier and noun are distinct lexical items. Over time, as a new subcategory gains utility in a given language community, the original modifier–noun phrase typically becomes nominalized. In essence, the phrase is replaced with a single lexical item. For this reason, it is interesting to chart the etymology of subordinate-level terms. For example, *terrier* is derived from the Latin *terra* because this dog was known specifically for its ability to search underground for small game.

Although these correlations between classification and nomenclature are not perfect, they certainly fuel the intuition that language and thought are interrelated in hierarchical systems of organization. The data from ASL are especially intriguing, because sign languages employ an entirely different perceptual modality (visuomotor) than do spoken languages (auditory–vocal). Thus, these convergences between linguistic form and category level appear to be inherent in the design of human language and are not due simply to the particular modality through which a given language is conveyed.

Does this interrelation contribute to the development of semantic and conceptual organization? Unfortunately, very little ethnobiological work has adopted a developmental perspective (for two exceptions see Dougherty, 1979; Stross, 1973). We therefore return to the psychological literature, this time focusing on early word learning and the development of hierarchical systems. More specifically, we ask whether *particular* linguistic forms expedite the acquisition of taxonomic classes at *particular* hierarchical levels.

Development of hierarchical systems

Young children acquire a wealth of information in their first few years, and conceptual hierarchies are especially tailored for this enterprise. It therefore stands to reason that children might begin to build hierarchical systems early in development and use them in the service of learning. However, this is emphatically not the position embraced by traditional developmental theorists, who based their work on the assumption that preschool children lack the requisite cognitive capacity to construct hierarchical systems (Bruner et al., 1956; Inhelder & Piaget, 1964; Vygotsky, 1962). Yet in recent years, it has become increasingly clear that children do establish hierarchies early in development and that language plays a decisive role in this development. What is the evidence for this view? There is no doubt that children appreciate at least some taxonomic classes, notably those at the *basic* level (Anglin, 1977; Mervis & Crisafi, 1982; Rosch et al., 1976). Children make their first forays into labeling and classifying objects at just the taxonomic level that adults, across cultures, find most salient. Across languages, children acquire basic-level terms with remarkable speed and proficiency, well before they master higher- and lower-order category terms (Anglin, 1977). And one of the most robust findings in the literature on cognitive development is that children succeed in classifying objects at the basic level long before they do so at nonbasic levels. Thus, for adults as well as for children, the basic level appears to occupy a psychologically privileged position.

However, children's early successes at the basic level stand in sharp contrast to their difficulty in imposing taxonomic relations at nonbasic levels under most circumstances (Anglin, 1977; Mervis & Crisafi, 1982). Therefore, the most intriguing developmental questions are those concerning development beyond the basic level.

In my research program, I accept as a given the "primacy" of the basic level and go on to ask how children advance beyond it to form the higher- and lower-order classes that comprise hierarchical systems. And it is precisely here, at nonbasic levels, that subtle yet powerful biases linking word learning and conceptual development have become evident.

Theoretical motivations

Before describing the empirical work related to these biases, it is worthwhile outlining briefly the theoretical motivation for proposing that such biases exist. Recall that within the first few years of their lives, young children demonstrate an appreciation of a variety of conceptual relations, including taxonomic, thematic, event-related, and ad hoc groupings. Concurrent with these conceptual advances, they make equally impressive gains in language acquisition. These simultaneous achievements have presented something of a puzzle to developmental psychologists, for although conceptual flexibility affords remarkable creativity, it could, in principle, complicate the task of word learning.

Given their appreciation of myriad possible relations among objects, how do children single out the taxonomic relations central to the construction of conceptual hierarchies? This question is particularly engaging when it is posed in light of the developmental research suggesting that young children actually prefer thematic and associative relations over taxonomic relations (Inhelder & Piaget, 1964; Smiley & Brown, 1979; Vygotsky, 1962). How, then, do children learn that a given word (e.g., *flamingo*) may apply to a particular object and may be extended to other members of that class (e.g., other flamingos), but not to thematic relations (e.g., a flamingo and sand), salient properties of the object (e.g., its long neck or unusual color), or an action in which it is engaged (e.g., feeding its young)?

Children's seemingly effortless solution to the logically difficult problem of mapping words to their appropriate meanings has led to the hypothesis that when learning the meaning of a novel word, children do not sample randomly from among all the possible interpretations. Instead, the data suggest that children restrict their focus to a circumscribed set of possible meanings. In particular, children's expectations about a new word's meaning appear to be guided by the syntactic status of the word itself.

Several different research laboratories have provided evidence that young children appreciate formal distinctions among syntactic categories (e.g., noun, adjective, determiner) and use these distinctions to help them discern the *semantic* content of novel words (R. Brown, 1957; Clark, Gelman, & Lane, 1985; Gelman & Markman, 1985; Gelman & Taylor, 1984; Hall & Waxman, 1990; Katz, Baker, & Macnamara, 1974; Naigles, Gleitman, & Gleitman, in press; Taylor & Gelman, 1988; Waxman, 1990). That is, children's expectations about a novel word's meaning are guided by the syntactic environment in which that word is introduced.

To understand how children's expectations about word meaning support the establishment of taxonomic relations and conceptual hierarchies, we will first consider the evidence pertaining to the superordinate level (e.g., animals, clothing, food).

Establishing superordinate relations: the role of nouns

Under most circumstances, preschool children have difficulty sorting objects at the superordinate level (Gelman & Baillargeon, 1983; Inhelder & Piaget, 1964). In fact, they seem to view superordinate classification tasks as an invitation to create stories and scenes rather than to impose a taxonomic classification. However, when children are introduced to novel words for superordinate-level classes, their performance changes dramatically.

To illustrate this phenomenon, R. Gelman and I compared preschoolers' superordinate-level classification with, and without, novel labels (Waxman & Gelman, 1986). First, we introduced children to three handpuppets who were "very picky and only liked a certain kind of thing" and enlisted the children's assistance in finding items for each puppet. To get the children started, we displayed three typical members (e.g., a dog, a horse, and a cat) of each superordinate-level class under investigation (e.g., *animal*) to give them an idea of the "kinds of things" each puppet favored.

In one condition, the *instance* condition, children were left to sort the remaining pictures (these were various members of the classes *animals, clothing,* and *food*) with no further instructions. As one might expect on the basis of traditional developmental literature, 3-year-old children had difficulty forming superordinate-level classes when they were presented with the instances alone. In fact, children in the instance condition performed only slightly better than we would have expected if they had distributed the items to the puppets randomly.

In the *novel-label* condition, the children encountered the same typical instances, but in addition the experimenter introduced the Japanese label for each superordinate class (e.g., "These are 'dobutsus,' these are 'gohans,' and these are 'kimonos' "). Although these Japanese terms were completely unfamiliar to our children, they had a dramatic effect: Children in the novel-label condition formed superordinate classes readily.

As a control, we asked another group of children to classify the same sets of objects, but we gave these children the familiar English superordinate labels (e.g., "These are animals, these are clothes, and these are food"). Performance in the *English label* and novel-label conditions was indistinguishable. Therefore, we can conclude that introducing preschool children to novel nouns motivates them to classify as successfully as children who have been prompted with the English labels for these superordinate-level classes.

Clearly, the introduction of a novel label effectively alerted preschool children to the taxonomic relations among items and licensed the induction of superordinate-level categories. This phenomenon, which has been referred to alternatively as the *noun-category bias* (Waxman, 1989; Waxman & Kosowski, 1990) or the *taxonomic assumption* (Clark, Chapter 2, this volume; Markman, 1989; Chapter 3, this volume), has now been demonstrated using both triad tasks (Markman & Hutchinson, 1984) and classification procedures (Waxman & Gelman, 1986). Taken together, these findings support the claim that when interpreting the meaning of novel nouns, children focus on categorical relations.

This intriguing result has generated several further questions. The first concerns the age at which children evidence this affinity between nouns and superordinate-level relations. The second concerns the specificity of the taxonomic bias. Are taxonomic relations highlighted in the context of word learning in general, or is the taxonomic focus reserved for novel nouns in particular?

To begin to answer these questions, T. Kosowski and I designed an experimental procedure specifically for research with 2-year-old children (Waxman & Kosowski, in press). This was essential because 2-year-old children often become sidetracked and falter in most classification tasks (Sugarman, 1982; Waxman, 1987). And although triad tasks, like those designed by Markman and Hutchinson, are simple enough to be applied to 2-year-olds, these toddlers, unlike older children, are virtually unable to articulate *why* they have chosen one particular item as opposed to another. Without such justifications, the data from these tasks are difficult to interpret unambiguously. (Because Markman & Hutchinson's experiments included older preschool children, this did not present an obstacle in their work.)

To circumvent these procedural difficulties, we developed a five-item match-to-sample task in which we supplemented children's first choices with second choices rather than with justifications. We created a picture book in which each page constituted a trial (Waxman & Kosowski, in press). On each page, there were five pictures, a target (e.g., a cow) and four alternatives. Two of these alternatives were members of the same superordinate-level class as the target (e.g., a fox and a zebra); the remaining two alternatives were thematically related to the target (e.g., a barn and milk).

The experimenter sat with each child individually to read the book. In the *no-word* condition, she pointed to the target and said, "See this? Can you find another one?" In the *novel-noun* and *novel-adjective* conditions, in addition to pointing to the target, she labeled it with a novel word. These conditions differed from one another only in the syntactic context in which the novel words were presented. In the novel-noun condition, she said, for example, "See this 'fopin'? Can you find another 'fopin'?" In the novel-adjective condition, she said, for example, "See this 'fopish one'? Can you find another one that is 'fopish'?"

After they had gone through the book once, the experimenter encouraged the children to read it a second time. On each page, she reminded the children of their first choice and asked them to select another of the remaining alternatives. In this way, despite the fact that 2-year-olds are unable to justify their selections, we were able to supplement their first choices with second choices.

If children select both of the superordinate category members and none of the thematic alternatives, it is likely that they have established a taxonomic criterion and have applied it consistently. If novel nouns highlight superordinate category relations in 2-year-old children, we would expect children in the novel-noun condition to prefer the taxonomically related alternatives. If this bias is specific to novel nouns, children in the novel-adjective condition, like those in the no-word condition, should demonstrate no such preference.

The results of this experiment were straightforward. Performance in the novel-adjective and no-word conditions were indistinguishable from one another and from the pattern expected if children had selected items randomly. Only in the novel-noun condition did children consistently favor category relations. Thus, it is not word learning, per se, that highlights superordinate relations. Instead, superordinate relations gain priority only in the context of learning novel nouns.

For the purpose of charting the development of the noun–category bias across the preschool years, we conducted companion studies with 3-year-old children and found a pattern of results that was virtually identical to that obtained with the 2-year-olds. Therefore, whatever the origin of the noun–category bias, it is clearly in place by the time children are 2 years of age.

We interpreted the consistent difference between performance in the novel-noun and other conditions as evidence for an abstract bias that leads children to focus their attention on category relations when learning the meaning of novel nouns. To make this argument compelling, we had to rule out a competing hypothesis: that children "translated" the novel nouns into known category terms (e.g., *dog*) and the novel adjectives into known attributes or descriptive phrases (e.g., *furry thing* or *brownish one*) and then used these translations to guide their item selections.

To rule out the possibility that the powerful effect of the nouns was the result of children's "translations," we showed another group of 2- and 3-year-old children our picture book and explicitly asked them to translate our novel terms into English. We explained that although our puppet had "his own special language," he wanted to learn to speak English. In the novel-noun condition, the experimenter pointed to the target item on each page and said, for example, "See this? Zupe [the puppet] calls this a 'dobin.' What do you think 'dobin' means?" In the novel-adjective condition, she asked, for example, "See this? Zupe calls this a 'dobish' one. What do you think 'dobish' means?" As a control, we asked another group to label the targets, but did not provide them with novel words. For example, the experimenter asked, "See this? Tell Zupe what we call this."

Children in all three experimental conditions translated the novel terms (whether nouns or adjectives) into familiar basic-level nouns. Clearly, when they are explicitly asked to translate, preschool children treat novel nouns and adjectives similarly. Note that if the children had relied on these translations in the preceding experiments, their performance in all three conditions would have been indistinguishable. But this was not the case. The children made systematic and reliable distinctions between these syntactic categories. We therefore conclude that the children's item selections were not mediated by direct translation of the novel terms into English.

The experiments described thus far reveal that children as young as 2 years are sensitive to the syntactic environment in which novel words are introduced. They expect novel nouns, but not novel adjectives, to highlight superordinate-level relations, even in the presence of thematic alternatives. Moreover, the effect of the novel noun is powerful enough to guide both a first and a second set of choices.

Notice, however, that these findings are based solely on English-speaking children. This is a serious limitation, for if these phenomena reflect a fundamental relation between language and conceptual development, they should be evident in all children, independent of the language they are learning. Therefore, to ascertain whether the systematic patterns we have observed in our English-speaking preschoolers are evident in other languages as well, we have recently embarked on a series of cross-linguistic developmental experiments (Waxman, Senghas, Ross, & Benveniste, 1990).

Cross-linguistic developmental studies

Our aim in this series is to detect developmental universals in the relation between word learning and conceptual development and, at the same time, to document any differences due to the particulars of the language being acquired. To date, our sample includes preschool children from two different language communities. Our unilingual French speakers are from Montreal, Canada, and our unilingual Spanish speakers are from Buenos Aires, Argentina. We are limited, at this early stage in our research program, to languages that are closely related to one another. However, despite their commonalities, there are also variations in the grammars of English, French, and Spanish that may bear on the questions at hand.

There is, for example, a linguistic difference between English, on the one hand, and French and Spanish, on the other. In the latter languages, because categories have associated with them a particular gender, the words (nouns, adjectives, determiners, etc.) that refer to these categories carry gender markings as well. It is possible that the gender markings associated with the various object terms influence young children's interpretations of novel words.

Moreover, in Spanish and French, nouns are typically dropped if the subject is recoverable from the context. Under such circumstances, adjectives essentially stand in for the noun and convey nominal information. Consider, for example, a scenario in which there are six coffee mugs, each of a different size. In English, we would distinguish these linguistically by pairing the noun *mug* with an adjective. That is, to request the largest mug, we might ask for *the big mug* or *the big one*. In Spanish, such constructions are ungrammatical. Instead, the noun is dropped, leaving the determiner and adjective to refer to the intended mug. For example, we might request *la grande*, where *grande* is the adjective. Likewise, in French, we might indicate the smallest mug by asking for *la petite*.

We wondered if as a result of this aspect of French and Spanish grammar, novel adjectives might produce a different effect in these languages that they had in our English-speaking sample. In particular, we wondered whether in French and Spanish, nouns and adjectives might produce very similar results.

To address these possibilities, we adapted the five-item match to the sample procedure developed by Waxman and Kosowski (1990) to accommodate the particular requirements of our different populations and their structurally different languages. To examine the possible influence of gender markings in these languages, we took two distinctly different routes. On half of the pages (trials), we included only items that shared a common gender designation. For example, a representative page in French included the following items (all masculine): a squirrel (target), a cat, a fox, an acorn, and a tree. On these pages, because we eliminated the possibility that children could select items on the basis of gender, the French and Spanish speakers' task was wholly comparable to the task confronting their English-speaking age-mates.

On the remaining trials, however, we varied the gender composition of the items in the following manner: We selected one thematic and one taxonomic alternative that matched the target in gender, and one taxonomic and one thematic alternative that conflicted with the target's gender. For example, a representative Spanish trial included a banana (target, feminine), an apple (feminine), a lemon (masculine), a girl (feminine), and monkey (masculine). On these trials, it was possible for children to select items on the basis of gender agreement. In the current example, one gender-matched choice is related taxonomically to the target (the apple); the other gender-matched choice is related thematically to the target (the girl). If, however, children were to select on the basis of taxonomic relations, they would have to overlook gender agreement to do so. In the current example, one taxonomically related choice (the apple) matches the target in gender; the other taxonomically related choice (the lemon) does not match. Thus, these mixed-gender trials allowed us to examine whether children in a novel-noun condition would override gender agreement to select both taxonomically related items.

The French-speaking preschoolers. With the French-speaking preschoolers, our results were identical to those obtained with our English-speaking sample. Children in the novel-adjective and no-word conditions demonstrated no particular preference for taxonomically, thematically, or gender-related items. However, as we predicted, French-speaking children in the novel-noun condition chose predominantly taxonomically related items. This effect seemed to be stronger for the 2- and 3-year-olds than for the 4-year-olds. Furthermore, there was no evidence that children relied on gender matching in making their selections.

The Spanish-speaking preschoolers. Our preliminary results with the Spanish-speaking children have been very interesting. Like their English- and French-speaking age-mates, Spanish-speaking preschoolers in the novel-noun condition demonstrated a strong noun–category bias. They exhibited a strong preference for the taxonomically related items on both their first and their second trials. The Spanish-speaking children in the no-word condition showed no particular preference for thematic, taxonomic, or gender-matched stimuli. The essentially random performance in this condition replicates the results obtained with our other two language samples. However, unlike our French- and English-speaking children, the Spanish-speaking children in the novel-adjective conditions did display a systematic inclination toward the taxonomically related items.

Before concluding that this inclination reflects a linguistic difference in the status of adjectives in Spanish, we address two alternative hypotheses. First, we must determine whether this effect could have been due to the particular items used in the study with the Argentine children. To examine this hypothesis, we conducted a companion experiment, using the stimuli designed for the Spanish speakers with a new group of English-speaking children. Our results are very much like those obtained earlier with our English-speaking sample. Namely, children in the novel-adjective condition did not show a strong inclination toward taxonomic relations. Like children in the no-word condition, English-speaking children hearing novel adjectives appeared to show no preference for taxonomic or thematic relations.

The second hypothesis concerns the wording of the instructions to the Argentine children. Perhaps there was some ambiguity regarding the introduction of the adjectives that could account for these very preliminary cross-linguistic differences. We are currently testing this hypothesis. Therefore, any firm conclusions regarding this issue must await additional data.

Although our cross-linguistic developmental program of research is only in its infancy, it has already begun to reveal some very strong similarities as well as some compelling differences in development. The noun–category bias is evident as early as 2 years of age in all three languages we have studied. And on the basis of Gentner's (1982) extensive review of the noun and predicate systems across languages, I suspect that this may be a universal phenomenon that guides development from the very onset of language acquisition.

Across languages, children's earliest words are predominantly nouns (see Gentner, 1982, for a review). Further, nouns function in a similar fashion across these languages, picking out primarily objects and classes of objects. Finally, there is linguistic evidence that nouns are organized differently in the lexicon than are other syntactic classes (Huttenlocher & Lui, 1979).

The members of the predicate system (e.g., adjectives, verbs, adverbs) seem to have a more fluid status, and there is considerable cross-linguistic variation as to what information is conveyed as part of one predicate and what is conveyed as part of another (Gentner, 1982; Talmy, 1975, 1985). Unlike those of nouns, the syntactic status and semantic role of these predicates are much less distinct. I suspect that the noun–category bias is evident very early in development, but that the role of adjectives (and other predicates) may emerge later in development and may vary according to the language being acquired.

The preceding experiments with English-, French-, and Spanish-speaking children provide strong empirical support for the claim that by the age of 2, there is a close affiliation between nouns and superordinate category relations. Does this linkage extend to other hierarchical levels, or is it specific to the superordinate level? The psychological as well as ethnographic literature gives us reason to suspect that nouns exert different influences at different hierarchical levels. This is because the "cognitive processes" involved in forming superordinate-level generalizations among basic-level classes are genuinely different from those involved in generating subordinate-level distinctions within a basic-level class.

Establishing subordinate relations: The role of adjectives

Psychologists have appealed to different explanations for the relative difficulties encountered in forming superordinate- as opposed to subordinate-level classes (e.g., Rosch, 1973). At the superordinate level, where class members vary widely in appearance and function, classes have little internal coherence, or *within-category similarity*. Nouns may augment the internal coherence of abstract superordinate-level classes by drawing together the disparate members. The ethnographic record is compatible with this line of reasoning. Recall that the linguistic labels for basic and higher-order classes tend to be primary lexemes. Single nouns may amplify the commonalities and internal coherence among the distinct members and, in this way, facilitate the establishment of superordinate-level classes.

However, highlighting commonalities is not likely to promote the establishment of subordinate distinctions. At subordinate levels, where members of different classes closely resemble one another, class membership is easily confused. For example, Clydesdale and Palamino horses have a great deal in common, both in appearance and in function. Thus, to foster the formation of distinct subordinate-level classes, one must highlight not the commonalities within a particular class, but the categorical distinctions between classes.

The fact that different cognitive mechanisms may be required to establish superordinate- as opposed to subordinate-level classes may have a direct bearing on the types of linguistic labels that will highlight each. It is possible that although nouns facilitate the establishment of superordinate-level classes, they may fail to do so at subordinate levels. At the subordinate level, where categorical distinctions, not commonalities, must be amplified, adjectives may play a crucial role.

Once again, this prediction accords well with the ethnographic data. Here we find a strong tendency for subordinate-level classes (or Varietal and Specific ranks) to be marked by secondary lexemes, which are composed of a head noun referring to the basic (or Generic) level and a modifier to distinguish a salient characteristic of the subtype.

To examine the possibility that particular linguistic constructions (e.g., nouns vs. adjectives) expedite the establishment of taxonomic classes at particular levels within a hierarchy (superordinate vs. subordinate), we conducted a series of experiments to compare in a systematic way the effect of introducing either novel nouns or novel adjectives at multiple hierarchical levels (Waxman, 1990). We asked each child to classify pictures of objects at all three hierarchical levels (subordinate, basic, and superordinate) within the two different natural object hierarchies (animals and food) depicted in Figure 4.1.[4] Notice that these classes conform to the hierarchical and contrastive principles. Considered vertically, the lower-order classes are nested within subsequently higher-order classes; considered horizontally, the classes are mutually exclusive.

The experimental procedure was similar to the one utilized in the superordinate-level classification task described earlier in this chapter (Waxman & Gelman, 1986). Once again, to ensure that the children understood that they were to sort the items into classes, the experimenter first set out three small dolls and explained that they were "very picky and only liked a certain kind of thing." She then

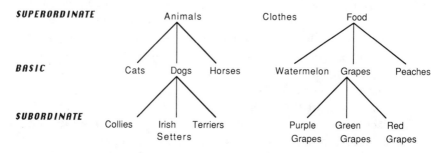

Figure 4.1. A hierarchical system of natural object categories.

revealed three typical members of each contrastive class to indicate the "kinds of things each puppet would like," leaving these clue photographs in full view during the experiment proper.

We assigned 3- and 4-year-old subjects to one of three experimental conditions (no word, novel noun, novel adjective). In the no-word condition, the experimenter simply drew attention to these clue photographs as she set them out, saying, "This doll likes this, and this, and this, and other things like that," as she placed the appropriate clue photographs beneath each doll. The instructions in the novel-noun and novel-adjective conditions were identical to those in the no-word condition, with only one exception: Here the experimenter provided a novel label in conjunction with the clue photographs. For example, in the novel-noun condition, she said, "This doll likes this, and this, and this, and other things like that. She calls these 'akas.' But this doll [indicating a second doll] likes this, and this, and this, and other things like that. She calls these 'dobus.'" In the novel-adjective condition, the novel words were presented in an adjectival context. For example, the experimenter labeled the classes as "These are the 'akish ones,' these are the 'dobish ones,' and these are the ones that are 'kimish.'"

The most interesting results to emerge from this series concerned the specific effects of the novel labels. As we had expected, we found very different effects at the different hierarchical levels. Let us first consider the influence of the novel nouns. At the superordinate level, the novel nouns facilitated taxonomic classification. This, of course, was expected on the basis of the work described earlier in this chapter (Markman & Hutchinson, 1984; Waxman & Gelman, 1986; Waxman & Kosowski, 1990). At the subordinate level, where we expected the nouns to have very little influence, they actually made taxonomic classification more difficult. Children in the novel-noun condition classified less well at the subordinate level than did their peers in the no-word condition.

Of course, this is not to say that labels have no effect on the establishment of subordinate classes. Recall that the findings from ethnobiology as well as those from American Sign Language revealed a tendency across languages for subordinate classes to be marked with modifier–noun phrases or secondary lexemes. On the basis of these findings, we suspected that novel adjectives would facilitate the establishment of subordinate-level classes.

Our predictions concerning the role of novel adjectives at the subordinate level were borne out by the data. Unlike novel nouns, novel adjectives supported subordinate, but not superordinate, classification. Children in the novel-adjective condition classified very successfully at the subordinate level. Yet novel adjectives exerted no demonstrable effect at either the basic or superordinate level. Thus, novel adjectives produced a systematic pattern of results, but one that was quite distinct from the pattern engendered by the novel nouns.

In this series, we found that the 3-year-old children were swayed to a greater extent by the novel words than were the 4-year-olds. This is consistent with the view that children may be most sensitive to the influence of novel words early in development, before they have established elaborate hierarchical systems. It would certainly be worthwhile pursuing this intuition by examining these phenomena in children younger than 3 years of age.

Fostering subordinate-level classification: The joint contributions of word-learning biases and existing knowledge

One unexpected result of the preceding experiment was particularly puzzling. We had expected the novel nouns to have very little influence at the subordinate level, but they actually interfered with subordinate classification. That is, children in the novel-noun condition had more difficulty forming subordinate-level classes than did their age-mates in the no-word condition. This enigmatic finding, which has since been replicated (Waxman & Shipley, 1987), underscores the complexity of relations linking language and conceptual organization; for although novel nouns promote the establishment of some classes (notably, those at the superordinate level), they hinder the formation of others (those at the subordinate level). But why should novel nouns promote some taxonomic relations and obscure others?

E. Shipley and I designed a series of experiments to address this question (Waxman, Shipley, & Shepperson, 1990).[5] We suspected that the detrimental effect of introducing novel nouns at the subordinate level was related to children's lack of knowledge concerning subordinate-level distinctions (Chi, 1983). Our reasoning was as follows: If children have not yet established categorical subclasses, novel nouns should highlight taxonomic relations at the basic level and, as a consequence, interfere with the establishment of new subclasses. But if children *have* begun to establish subclasses, novel nouns might be taken to refer to the emerging subclasses. In this case, novel nouns should no longer interfere with subordinate-level classification.

To test this hypothesis, we supplied 3-year-old subjects with factual information concerning the subordinate-level distinctions. For example, pointing to an angelfish, the experimenter explained that "this kind of fish changes color to hide from enemies, and has fused teeth." She offered different facts about salmon and trunkfish. All of the facts were true, but could not be detected perceptually by studying the stimuli themselves. We then observed the effect of introducing novel nouns, by comparing children in a novel-noun condition with others in a no-word condition. In the novel-noun condition, the experimenter labeled each target with a novel noun. In the no-word condition, she supplied the facts, but no labels, for the subclasses.

As we had predicted, when we provided children with specific information to distinguish the relevant subclasses, novel nouns no longer presented an obstacle in subordinate classification. In this experiment, we detected no difference between performance in the no-word and the novel-noun conditions. Because the specific information emphasized the categorical distinctions among the subclasses, it reduced children's tendency to interpret the novel nouns at the basic level. As a result, the children no longer encountered difficulty when novel nouns were introduced at the subordinate level.

However, parents and teachers do not always accompany novel subordinate-level terms with such substantial distinguishing information. How, then, do children learn to make subordinate-level distinctions and to label them appropriately? To answer this question, we drew on the literature on parental labeling strategies. Parents employ a systematic strategy known as *anchoring at the basic level* when they introduce young children to subordinate-level distinctions (Adams & Bullock, 1986; Callanan, 1985, 1989; Chapter 12, this volume). They use the novel nouns (e.g., *salmon*) in conjunction with the familiar basic-level term (e.g., "This is a salmon. It's a fish").

In the next experiment, we followed the parents' lead. We explicitly mentioned the basic-level labels. In addition, we provided children with information about general properties shared by members of the basic-level classes. We then observed the effect of introducing novel nouns for the subordinate-level classes. In the no-word condition, the experimenter pointed to three targets (one from each contrastive class), saying, "We've got three fish here. This one, this one, and this one. Fish breathe by taking water into their mouths [etc.]." In the novel-noun condition, she introduced the same basic-level labels and information, but in addition labeled each target with a novel noun. For example, she said, "We've got three fish here. This is a 'tosa,' this is an 'aka,' and this a 'kita' [pointing to each target]. Fish breathe by taking water into their mouths [etc.]."

Once the novel nouns were introduced together with the known basic-level terms and basic-level information, they no longer interfered with subordinate-level classification. In fact, in this experiment, children in the novel-noun condition sorted more items correctly than did their age-mates in the no-word condition. We suspect that by anchoring the novel terms at the basic level, we effectively ruled out the possibility that the children would try to interpret the novel nouns at the basic level.

These experiments illustrate an important point: Children's bias to interpret novel nouns as referring to taxonomic relations does not operate in a vacuum. Rather, their interpretation of novel nouns depends crucially on the status of their existing knowledge regarding the classes under consideration, their existing vocabularies, and the conditions under which the words are introduced (see also Callanan, Chapter 12, this volume). Either by providing new information about distinct kinds or by ruling out basic-level interpretations of the novel nouns, we can focus children's attention on subordinate-level distinctions within a known basic-level class. And once they are so focused, children are able to take novel nouns as referring to these emergent subordinate-level classes.

Parallels in ethnobiology and developmental psychology

Taken together, the findings from developmental psychology and ethnobiology provide support for the claim that there is a precise link between linguistic and conceptual systems of organization. This link appears to be evident throughout development and across a wide range of object categories. Across diverse cultures and languages, there is a strong tendency to use nouns to refer to higher-order classes and adjectival phrases, with the head noun referring to the familiar basic-level class, to refer to subordinate-level classes.

In addition to their common interests and findings, researchers in ethnobiology and developmental psychology also encounter common obstacles when it comes to interpreting data. In large part, this is because neither conceptual organization nor linguistic structure is amenable to direct observation. As a consequence, researchers in both fields must depend on overt behaviors (such as intrinsic common responses, labeling, or classification) to draw inferences concerning the covert organization of the mind. Although we now have sophisticated and precise tools of measurement, inferences of this sort are as much a challenge to modern cognitive scientists as they were to our predecessors. Therefore, we must take care not to mistake the map (here, the measurements) for the territory itself (the mind).

Problems of measurement and inference

In both ethnobiology and psychology, our assessment of the presence or absence of a particular category is based on subjects' behavior when they are faced with a variety of discriminable stimuli. For example, when subjects group objects together in a classification task, or when they produce or accept a common label for a group of different objects, we infer that their common response reflects an underlying conceptual category. This inferential logic is also evident in the behavioral techniques and physiological measures that have gained wide acceptance in infancy research (see Reznick, 1989, for a current review of methods employed in infancy research). For example, Mervis (1985) systematically charted one particular observable behavior (bringing an object to the mouth and blowing) to describe one infant's category, *horn*.

To be sure, these measures have yielded important insights into categories and their development. However, they also raise some critical problems of interpretation. First, a subject's failure to provide a common response toward a given set of objects does not necessarily warrant the conclusion that the subject fails to appreciate the category in question. For example, although I appreciate the category *animal*, I may not provide a common behavioral response to all members of the class. I may run from a tiger, but not from a lamb. Or, to take a more physiological measure, I may produce an elevated galvanic skin response when faced with a tiger, but not with a lamb.

Conversely, the fact that a subject does produce a common response (be it a verbal label, a physical grouping of objects, or an observable behavior such as blowing) does not necessarily warrant the conclusion that the subject appreciates the category in question. For example, I may produce a common response (rapid running) to a tiger and to a bus that is about to depart without me.

The question of when, and on what basis, to credit subjects with an appreciation of a category, particularly an unnamed category, has generated extensive debate, particularly in ethnobiological circles. On one side of the debate are those who insist that only if a category is named by native informants can it be said to have the status of a conceptual category within a culture (C. H. Brown, 1977; Burling, 1964; Hunn, 1977). Others (Berlin, 1978; Kay, 1971; Taylor, 1984) maintain that this interpretation is too restrictive and that "although a name may be an unambiguous indicator of a category, the absence of a label does not necessarily imply the absence of a category" (Berlin, 1978, p. 12).

To support the position that a category, though unnamed, is not unrecognized requires other sources of evidence. Berlin provided such evidence in his study of Tzeltal. Although there are no overt labels for the Unique Beginner rank *plant* or *animal* in Tzeltal, other linguistic indices suggest that these conceptual categories are indeed recognized by members of this Mayan Indian language community. For example, Tzeltal speakers consistently describe the plant domain phrasally as "those things that don't move, don't walk, possess roots, and are planted in the earth." Further, all plants take the Tzeltal classifier *tehk*; all animals take the classifier *koht* (Berlin et al., 1973; see Allan, 1977, for a thorough discussion of classifiers).

Although this argument is persuasive, it is not unimpeachable. There is no compelling reason to accept the premise that a group of objects whose labels occur with a particular classifier term constitute the same sort of class as do a group of objects that take a common label. For example, in Dyirbal (an aboriginal Australian language), a common classifier, *balan,* accompanies the labels referring to women, fire, scorpions, and other dangerous things (Lakoff, 1988). Yet the mechanisms or principles linking this diverse set of items together appear to be quite different from those linking taxonomic classes such as *plant* and *animal.* Therefore, the argument that groups of objects denoted by common classifiers have the same status as those picked out by common labels stands on tenuous ground.

The issue of covert categories has been discussed primarily in the ethnobiological literature, but it has implications in developmental psychology as well. For example, it is a well-documented finding that children acquire basic-level labels before they acquire superordinate- and subordinate-level labels (Anglin, 1977; Mervis & Crisafi, 1982; Waxman, 1990). Thus, early in development, the nonbasic levels often remain unnamed. Most developmental psychologists appear to accept tacitly the premise that a failure to label does not necessarily constitute a failure to appreciate a conceptual grouping.

In fact, there is an interesting parallel between ethnobiologists' treatment of classifier terms and developmental psychologists' treatment of children's overextensions. Early in semantic development, children typically fail to label superordinate-level classes such as *animal, clothing,* and *vehicle.* Yet they tend to extend a basic-level term (e.g., *car*) to other objects within the same superordinate-level class (e.g., *vehicle*) (Rescorla, 1980). These apparently rule-governed overextensions have sometimes been taken as hints that children are cognizant of such superordinate categories, despite their failure to label them. Additional support for this position has come from preschoolers' performance on other behavioral measures (including oddity tasks, semantic clustering techniques, and habituation procedures). However, it remains an open question whether these early groupings share the same status as labeled classes.

Biases in development

The focal point of this chapter has been the hypothesis that there are powerful convergences between hierarchical systems of organization and the linguistic devices we use to describe them. Languages encode the categories, relations, and ideas we deem salient and help us to transmit these to others. In brief, I have asserted that hierarchical systems are a universal and fundamental aspect of human cognition and that implicit biases in word learning foster their development.

The notion that certain aspects of human psychological development unfold under the influence of constraints or biases has generated considerable debate. For this debate to be constructive, it is crucial that the theoretical position itself and its attendant claims be made clear. The essential position is that children approach the task of learning and development equipped with certain biases or predispositions. Children find themselves immersed in an enormously rich and varied world. Each day they encounter a continual stream of new objects and witness new events. Biases serve as guideposts; they help children to organize these encounters into coherent systems.

Notice that the argument for biases or constraints is not meant to provide a complete account of human psychological development. This theoretical approach does not, in any sense, preclude the examination of other important sources and mechanisms of development. Researchers working from this theoretical perspective do not envision human development as an inflexible procession toward a single, predetermined goal. Nor are they committed to the view that discovering a particular bias in development (e.g., the noun–category bias) is tantamount to discovering that a mature system is "there" from the start. On the contrary, central to this approach is the conviction that children are active learners who seek out information from the world around them. Biases provide direction for development, but leave ample opportunity for the elaboration and variation that comes with children's important interactions with the people, objects, and events that constitute their world.

These other sources of development are essential, for the categories we construct are not rigidly fixed by innate predispositions, by linguistic structures, or by objective reality. They vary with experience and evolve over time. For example, although the noun–category bias highlights taxonomic relations and facilitates the early development of hierarchical systems, it does not dictate precisely which categories a given child will establish. This will be a function of that child's perceptual endowments, her existing knowledge and theories, and the particular constellation of objects she encounters.

Further, there are fundamental questions concerning the nature and origins of these biases in development. It is important that we determine whether the biases we have discussed are learned during the process of language development, or whether they are part of a child's innate endowment. Infants do not appear to use syntactic context to affix meaning to a new word at the very onset of language acquisition. Before the "naming explosion" (at approximately 17 to 24 months), they appear to interpret most words, independent of their syntactic status, as referring to objects and categories of objects.

An anecdote may illustrate this point: A 15-month-old repeatedly tried to get a hold of a broom (an item for which she had no label) while her mother was sweeping the floor. Frustrated in her domestic efforts, the mother offered the toddler her "own broom" (actually, a hand-sized fireplace sweeper), placing emphasis on the word *own*. The toddler repeated the stressed syllable *own* and, for six weeks thereafter, consistently labeled her small broom and all others *own*.

Later, as children begin to appreciate the formal distinctions among various syntactic form classes (Gordon, 1987; Valian, 1986), they begin to rely on syntactic information to determine the meaning of novel words. At this point, they begin to interpret nouns, but not adjectives and other predicates, as referring to category relations. On the basis of my research with children as young as 2 years of age learning English, French, and Spanish, I have speculated that the noun–category bias may be innate, but that children's interpretation of adjectives may arise at a later point in development, may vary across languages, and may be dependent on the particulars of the language being acquired.

Finally, this rapidly accumulating body of research has set the stage for a whole new line of inquiry concerning the interrelations among the various proposed biases (e.g., among the noun–category bias [Waxman, 1989; Waxman & Kosowski, 1990], the principle of mutual exclusivity [Markman, Chapter 3, this volume; Merriman & Bowman, 1989], and the principle of contrast [Clark, Chapter 2, this volume]). For example, there is evidence that children are constrained to interpret the first word for a novel object as referring to the basic-level kind (Markman, Mervis), but that the second word applied to an object is not so constrained. Once they have acquired a basic-level kind term, children are free to interpret words acquired later in a host of ways. These may include higher- and lower-order terms (Taylor & Gelman, 1988, 1989; Waxman, 1990), property terms (Au, 1990), and various restricted terms (e.g., life-phase and context-restricted terms) (Hall & Waxman, 1990; Macnamara, 1986). How are the various proposed biases coordinated such that children rapidly derive the meanings of new words and, at the same time, work out the relations among new words? Further research on this important question is certainly warranted (see Waxman, 1990).

Conclusions

Language exerts a strong influence in the early establishment of hierarchical systems. Basic-level classes emerge early in development, are remarkably consistent across cultures, and tend not to be affected by the introduction of novel terms, whether they be nouns or adjectives. However, at nonbasic levels, where categories vary considerably across cultures and throughout development, language exerts a definite and constructive influence. For very young children, nouns highlight higher-order category relations (e.g., animals, furniture) and adjectival phrases mark specific, lower-order distinctions (e.g., Ribier grapes, Thompson grapes). These implicit word-learning biases streamline the acquisition of word meaning and, at the same time, promote the establishment of hierarchical systems of organization.

Notes

1. Within cultural anthropology, examinations of language still occupy a privileged position as overt indices of implicit cognitive activity. In recent years, there has been a growing trend toward developing other measures of cognitive activity (see Dougherty, 1985).
2. This entails three assumptions: (a) that there is structure in the natural world (a fact that biologists have long embraced), (b) that human perceptual abilities are sensitive to this structure (a position which psychologists since Rosch and Gibson have embraced but which is problematic; see Carey, 1983), and (c) that our underlying conceptual representations echo this perceptible, real-world structure (this third assumption is a most controversial one).
3. Determining which level is the *basic* level is, at least in part, a function of the salience, or cultural significance, attached to a particular domain by the members of the society. For example, taxa of the Generic rank may be most salient to people who interact frequently with their biological environment and whose subsistence depends on it. But for those

of us living in an urban, industrialized world, categories at the Life Form or Intermediate rank may be judged to be at the basic level. See Dougherty (1978) and Rosch (1978) for this position.
4. In one experiment, the children classified pictures of objects at four (rather than three) hierarchical levels. See Waxman (1990) for a complete account of this series of experiments.
5. To begin this series of experiments, we conducted an initial study, the purpose of which was to select stimuli that preschool children could recognize as individual members of their respective basic-level classes but that were not yet organized into distinct kinds or subclasses. In other words, we wanted to be sure that preschool children's existing knowledge regarding the subclasses we selected was indeed limited. On the basis of this preliminary study, we selected three subordinate-level contrast sets, including types of dogs (collies, terriers, and Irish setters), types of grapes (Ribier, Thompson, and Foch), and types of fish (angelfish, salmon, and trunkfish).

References

Adams, A. K., & Bullock, D. (1986). Apprenticeship in word use: Social convergence processes in learning categorically related nouns. In S. A. Kuczaj II & M. D. Barrett (Eds.), *The development of word meaning: Progress in cognitive development research* (pp. 155–197). New York: Springer.
Allan, K. (1977). Classifiers. *Language, 53*(2), 285–311.
Anderson, E. N. (1967). *The ethnoicthyology of the Hong Kong boat people.* Unpublished doctoral dissertation, University of California, Berkeley.
Anglin, J. M. (1977). *Word, object, and conceptual development.* New York: Norton.
Armstrong, S., Gleitman, L. R., & Gleitman, H. (1983). What some concepts might not be. *Cognition, 13,* 263–308.
Au, T. K. (1990). Children's use of information in word learning. *Journal of Child Language, 17,* 393–416.
Barsalou, L. W. (1983). Ad hoc categories. *Memory and Cognition, 11,* 211–227.
Berlin, B. (1966). Folk taxonomies and biological classification. *Science, 154,* 273–275.
Berlin, B. (1973). The relation of folk systematics to biological classification and nomenclature. *Annual Review of Systematics and Ecology, 4,* 259–271.
Berlin, B. (1978). Ethnobiological classification. In E. Rosch & B. B. Lloyd (Eds.), *Cognition and categorization* (pp. 9–26). Hillsdale, NJ: Erlbaum.
Berlin, B., Breedlove, D., & Raven, P. (1973). General principles of classification and nomenclature in folk biology. *American Anthropologist, 75,* 214–242.
Berlin, B., Breedlove, D. E., & Raven, P. H. (1974). *Principles of Tzeltal plant classification.* New York: Academic Press.
Blewitt, P. (1990). *Understanding categorical relations: The earliest level of skill.* Unpublished manuscript.
Brown, C. H. (1977). Folk botanical life-forms: Their universality and growth. *American Anthropologist, 79,* 317–342.
Brown, C. H., Kolar, J., Torrey, B. J., Truong-Quang, T., & Volkman, P. (1976). Some general principles of biological and non-biological folk classification. *American Ethnologist, 3,* 73–85.

Brown, R. (1957). Linguistic determinism and the part of speech. *Journal of Abnormal and Social Psychology, 55,* 1–5.

Brown, R. (1958). *Words and things.* Glencoe, IL: Free Press.

Brown, R. (1986). *Social psychology: The second edition.* New York: Free Press.

Bruner, J. S., Goodnow, J. J., & Austin, G. A. (1956). *A study of thinking.* New York: Wiley.

Bulmer, R., & Tyler, M. (1968). Karam classification of frogs. *Journal of Polynesian Society, 77,* 333–385.

Burling, R. (1964). Cognition and componential analysis: God's truth or hocus-pocus? *American Anthropologist, 66,* 20–28.

Callanan, M. A. (1985). How parents label objects for young children: The role of input in the acquisition of category hierarchies. *Child Development, 56,* 508–523.

Callanan, M. A. (1989). Development of object categories and inclusion relations: Preschoolers' hypotheses about word meanings. *Developmental Psychology, 25,* 207–216.

Carey, S. (1983). Constraints on the meanings of natural kind terms. In T. Seiler & J. Wannenmacher (Eds.), *Concept development and the development of word meaning* (pp. 126–146). New York: Springer.

Carey, S. (1985). *Conceptual change in childhood.* Cambridge, MA: MIT Press.

Casson, R. W. (1975). The semantics of kin term usage: Transferred and indirect metaphorical meanings. *American Ethnologist, 2,* 229–238.

Chi, M. T. H. (1983). Knowledge-derived categorization in young children. In D. R. Rogers & J. A. Sloboda (Eds.), *The acquisition of symbolic skill* (pp. 327–332). New York: Plenum Press.

Clark, E. V., Gelman, S. A., & Lane, N. M. (1985). Compound nouns and category structure in young children. *Child Development, 56,* 84–94.

Conklin, H. C. (1954). *The relation of Hanunoo culture to the plant world.* Unpublished doctoral dissertation, Yale University, New Haven, CT.

Dougherty, J. W. D. (1978). Salience and relativity in classification. *American Ethnologist, 5,* 66–80.

Dougherty, J. W. D. (1979). Learning names for plants and plants for names. *Anthropological Linguistics, 21(6),* 298–315.

Dougherty, J. W. D. (1985). *Directions in cognitive anthropology.* Urbana: University of Illinois Press.

Dougherty, J. W. D., & Keller, C. M. (1985). Taskonomy: A practical approach to knowledge structures. In J. W. D. Dougherty (Ed.), *Directions in cognitive anthropology* (pp. 161–174). Urbana: University of Illinois Press.

Dupré, J. (1981). Natural kinds and biological taxa. *Philosophical Review, 90,* 66–90.

Frake, C. O. (1962). The ethnographic study of cognitive systems. In T. Gladwin & W. C. Sturtevant (Eds.), *Ahtropology and human behavior* (pp. 72–85). Washington, DC: Anthropological Society of Washington.

Gelman, R., & Baillargeon, R. (1983). A review of some Piagetian concepts. In J. H. Flavell & E. M. Markman (Eds.), *Cognitive development* (Vol. 3, pp. 167–230, of P. H. Mussen [Gen. Ed.], *Handbook of child psychology*). New York: Wiley.

Gelman, S. A. (1988). The development of induction within natural kind and artifact categories. *Cognitive Psychology, 20,* 65–95.

Gelman, S. A., & Markman, E. M. (1985). Implicit contrast in adjectives vs. nouns: Implications for word-learning in preschoolers. *Journal of Child Language, 12,* 125–143.

Gelman, S. A., & Taylor, M. (1984). How 2-year-old children interpret proper and common names for unfamiliar objects. *Child Development, 55,* 1535–1540.

Gentner, D. (1982). Why nouns are learned before verbs: Linguistic relativity versus natural partitioning. In S. Kuczaj (Ed.), *Language development: Language, thought, and culture* (pp. 301–334). Hillsdale, NJ: Erlbaum.

Gibson, J. J., & Gibson, E. J. (1955). Perceptual learning: Differentiation or enrichment? *Psychological Review, 62,* 32–41.

Gordon, P. (1987, April). *Determiner and adjective categories in children's grammars.* Paper presented at the biennial meeting of the Society for Research in Child Development, Baltimore.

Hage, P., & Miller, W. R. (1976). 'Eagle' = 'bird': A note on the structure and evolution of Shoshoni ethnoornithological nomenclature. *American Ethnologist, 3*(3), 481–488.

Hall, D. G., & Waxman, S. R. (1990). *On the acquisition of restricted and unrestricted nouns.* Unpublished manuscript.

Hunn, E. S. (1975). A measure of degree of correspondence of folk to scientific biological classification. *American Ethnologist, 2,* 309–327.

Hunn, E. S. (1977). *Tzeltal folk zoology: The classification of discontinuities in nature.* New York: Academic Press.

Hunn, E. (1985). The utilitarian factor in folk biological classification. In J. W. D. Dougherty (Ed.), *Directions in cognitive anthropology* (pp. 117–140). Urbana: University of Illinois Press.

Huttenlocher, J., & Lui, F. (1979). The semantic organization of some simple nouns and verbs. *Journal of Verbal Learning and Verbal Behavior, 18,* 141–162.

Inhelder, B., & Piaget, J. (1964). *The early growth of logic in the child.* New York: Newton.

Katz, N., Baker, E., & Macnamara, J. (1974). What's in a name? A study of how children learn common and proper names. *Child Development, 45,* 469–473.

Kay, P. (1971). On taxonomy and semantic contrast. *Language, 47,* 866–887.

Kuhn, T. (1962). *The structure of scientific revolutions.* Chicago: University of Chicago Press.

Lakoff, G. (1988). *Women, fire, and dangerous things: What categories reveal about the mind.* Chicago: University of Chicago Press.

Lancy, D. F. (1983). *Cross-cultural studies in cognition and mathematics.* New York: Academic Press.

Luria, A. R. (1976). *Cognitive development: Its cultural and social foundations.* Cambridge, MA: Harvard University Press.

Lyons, J. (1977). *Semantics.* Cambridge University Press.

Macnamara, J. (1986). *A border dispute: The place of logic in psychology.* Cambridge, MA: MIT Press.

Mandler, J. M., Fivush, R., & Reznick, J. S. (1987). The development of contextual categories. *Cognitive Development, 2,* 339–354.

Marchand, H. (1969). *The categories and types of present-day English word-formation* (2nd ed.). Munich: Beck.

Markman, E. M. (1989). *Categorization and naming in children.* Cambridge, MA: MIT Press.

Markman, E. M., & Hutchinson, J. E. (1984). Children's sensitivity to con-

Semantic and conceptual organization in preschoolers 143

straints on word meaning: Taxonomic vs. thematic relations. *Cognitive Psychology, 16,* 1–27.

Merriman, W. E., & Bowman, L. L. (1989). The mutual exclusivity bias in children's word learning. *Monographs of the Society for Research in Child Development, 54* (3–4), Serial No. 220, 1–123.

Mervis, C. B. (1985). On the existence of prelinguistic categories: A case study. *Infant Behavior and Development, 8,* 293–300.

Mervis, C. B. (1987). Child-basic categories and early lexical development. In U. Neisser (Ed.), *Concepts and conceptual development: Ecological and intellectual factors in categorization* (pp. 201–233). Cambridge University Press.

Mervis, C. B., & Crisafi, M. A. (1982). Order of acquisition of subordinate-, basic-, and superordinate-level categories. *Child Development, 53,* 258–266.

Mill, J. S. (1843). *A system of logic, ratiocinative and inductive.* London: Longman Group.

Miller, G. A., & Johnson-Laird, P. N. (1976). *Language and perception.* Cambridge, MA: Belknap.

Murphy, G. L., & Medin, D. L. (1985). The role of theories in conceptual coherence. *Psychological Review, 92,* 289–316.

Naigles, L., Gleitman, H., & Gleitman, L. R. (in press). Children acquire word meaning components from syntactic evidence. In E. Dromi (Ed.), *Linguistic and conceptual development.* Norwood, NJ: Ablex.

Nelson, K. (1974). Variations in children's concepts by age and category. *Child Development, 45,* 577–584.

Nelson, K. (1987, April). *Where do taxonomic categories come from?* Paper presented at the biennial meeting of the Society for Research in Child Development, Baltimore.

Nelson, K., & Gruendel, J. M. (1981). Generalized event representation: Basic building blocks of cognitive development. In M. E. Lamb & A. L. Brown (Eds.), *Advances in developmental psychology* (pp. 131–158). Hillsdale, NJ: Erlbaum.

Newport, E. L., & Bellugi, U. (1978). Linguistic expression of category levels in a visual–gestural language: A flower is a flower is a flower. In E. Rosch & B. B. Lloyd (Eds.), *Cognition and categorization* (pp. 49–71). Hillsdale, NJ: Erlbaum.

Petitto, L. A., & Seidenberg, M. S. (1979). On the evidence for linguistic abilities in signing apes. *Brain and Language, 8,* 72–88.

Premack, D. (1971). Language in chimpanzee? *Science, 172,* 808–822.

Quine, W. V. (1969). Natural kinds. *Ontological relativity and other essays* (pp. 114–138). New York: Columbia University Press.

Randall, R. A. (1976). How tall is a taxonomic tree? Some evidence for dwarfism. *American Ethnologist, 3,* 543–553.

Rescorla, L. (1980). Overextension in early language development. *Journal of Child Language, 7,* 321–335.

Reznick, J. S. (1989). Research on infant categorization. *Seminars in Perinatology, 13*(6), 458–466.

Rosch, E. H. (1973). On the internal structure of perceptual and semantic categories. In T. E. Moore (Ed.), *Cognitive development and the acquisition of language* (pp. 111–144). New York: Academic Press.

Rosch, E. (1975). Universals and cultural specifics in human categorization.

In R. Brislin, S. Bochner, & W. Honner (Eds.), *Cross-cultural perspectives on learning* (pp. 177–206). New York: Halsted Press.

Rosch, E. (1978). Principles of categorization. In E. Rosch & B. B. Lloyd (Eds.), *Cognition and categorization* (pp. 27–48). Hillsdale, NJ: Erlbaum.

Rosch, E., Mervis, C. B., Gray, W. D., Johnson, D. M., & Boyes-Braem, P. (1976). Basic objects in natural categories. *Cognitive Psychology, 8,* 382–439.

Rozin, P. (1976). The evolution of intelligence and access to the cognitive unconscious. In J. M. Sprague & A. A. Epstein (Eds.), *Progress in psychobiology and physiological psychology* (pp. 245–280). New York: Academic Press.

Saxe, G. B. (1982). Culture and the development of numerical cognition: Studies among the Oksapmin of Papua New Guinea. In C. J. Brainerd (Ed.), *Children's logical and mathematical cognition* (pp. 157–176). New York: Springer.

Saxe, G. B., Gearhart, M., & Guberman, S. R. (1984). Education and cognitive development: The evidence from experimental research. *Monographs of the Society for Research in Child Development, 44*(Serial No. 178).

Shipley, E. F. (1989). Two kinds of hierarchies: Class inclusion hierarchies and kind hierarchies. *Genetic Epistemologist, 17,* 31–39.

Shipley, E. F., Kuhn, I. F., & Madden, E. C. (1983). Mothers' use of superordinate category terms. *Journal of Child Language, 10,* 571–588.

Smiley, S. S., & Brown, A. L. (1979). Conceptual preference for thematic or taxonomic relations: A nonmonotonic trend from preschool to old age. *Journal of Experimental Child Psychology, 28,* 249–257.

Smith, E. E., & Medin, D. L. (1981). *Categories and concepts.* Cambridge, MA: Harvard University Press.

Stanlaw, J., & Yoddumnern, B. (1985). Thai spirits: A problem in the study of folk classification. In J. W. D. Dougherty (Ed.), *Directions in cognitive anthropology* (pp. 141–159). Urbana: University of Illinois Press.

Stross, B. (1973). Acquisition of botanical terminology by Tzeltal children. In M. S. Edmonson (Ed.), *Meaning in Mayan languages* (pp. 107–142). The Hague: Mouton.

Sugarman, S. (1982). Developmental changes in early representational intelligence: Evidence from spatial classification strategies and related verbal expressions. *Cognitive Psychology, 51,* 309–348.

Talmy, L. (1975). Semantics and syntax of motion. In J. Kimball (Ed.), *Syntax and semantics* (Vol. 4, pp. 181–238). New York: Academic Press.

Talmy, L. (1985). Lexicalization patterns: Semantic structure in lexical forms. In T. Shopen (Ed.), *Language typology and syntactic description* (Vol. 3, pp. 57–149). Cambridge University Press.

Taylor, M., & Gelman, S. A. (1988). Adjectives and nouns: Children's strategies for learning new words. *Child Development, 59,* 411–419.

Taylor, M., & Gelman, S. A. (1989). Incorporating new words into the lexicon: Preliminary evidence for language hierarchies in 2-year-old children. *Child Development, 60,* 625–636.

Taylor, P. M. (1984). "Covert categories" reconsidered: Identifying unlabeled classes in Tobelo folk biological classification. *Journal of Ethnobiology, 4*(2), 105–122.

Templin, M. C. (1957). *Certain language skills in children: Their development and interrelationships.* Minneapolis, MN: University of Minneapolis Press.

Tversky, B., & Hemenway, K. (1984). Objects, parts, and categories. *Journal of Experimental Psychology: General, 113,* 169–193.

Valian, V. V. (1986). Syntactic categories in the speech of young children. *Developmental Psychology, 22,* 562–579.

Vygotsky, L. (1962). *Thought and language.* Cambridge, MA: MIT Press.

Wagner, D. A. (1974). The development of short-term and incidental memory: A cross-cultural study. *Child Development, 48,* 389–396.

Waxman, S. R. (1987, April). *Linguistic and conceptual organization in 30-month-old children.* Paper presented at the biennial meeting of the Society for Research in Child Development, Baltimore.

Waxman, S. R. (1989). Linking language and conceptual development: Linguistic cues and the construction of conceptual hierarchies. *Genetic Epistemologist, 17*(2), 13–20.

Waxman, S. R. (1990). Linguistic biases and the establishment of conceptual hierarchies: Evidence from preschool children. *Cognitive Development, 5,* 123–150.

Waxman, S., & Gelman, R. (1986). Preschoolers' use of superordinate relations in classification and language. *Cognitive Development, 1,* 139–156.

Waxman, S. R., & Kosowski, T. D. (1990). Nouns mark category relations: Toddlers' and preschoolers' word-learning biases. *Child Development, 61,* 1461–1473.

Waxman, S. R., Senghas, A., Ross, D., & Benveniste, L. (1990). *Word-learning biases in French- and Spanish-speaking children.* Unpublished manuscript, Harvard University, Cambridge, MA.

Waxman, S. R., & Shipley, E. F. (1987, April). *Interactions between existing knowledge and language in subordinate classification.* Paper presented at the biennial meeting of the Society for Research in Child Development, Baltimore.

Waxman, S. R., Shipley, E. F., & Shepperson, B. (1990). *Establishing new subcategories: The role of category labels and existing knowledge.* Unpublished manuscript.

Wyman, L. C., & Bailey, F. L. (1964). *Navaho Indian ethnoentomology* (Publications in Anthropology no. 12). Albuquerque: University of New Mexico.

5. Language and categorization: The acquisition of natural kind terms

SUSAN A. GELMAN AND JOHN D. COLEY

What is striking about human categories is their diversity. They range from the simplest classification of a face or color to the most carefully constructed taxonomic grouping. Considering this diversity, many are struck by the apparent gap between the simple, intuitive categories formed by children and the complex, theory-laden categories of educated adults (e.g., Inhelder & Piaget, 1964; Quine, 1969; Vygotsky, 1962).

In this chapter we first argue that despite a number of salient differences between children's categories and those of adults, there are important parallels between the two: Both are informed by an ability to overlook salient appearances, an attention to nonobvious properties, and the potential to draw many new inferences about the unknown. Both the initial groupings of the prescientific child and the most thoughtful, theory-laden classifications of the adult extend knowledge in important ways. To use Quine's terminology, both children and adults form "theoretical kinds." Second, we address the role of language in the formation of theoretical kinds. Although the structure of everyday object categories (e.g., *dog*, *hammer*, *oak tree*, and *computer*) is traditionally thought to result from the structure of the world and/or the nature of human perception and cognition, we will present evidence that language is also critical and that how objects are named helps determine the structure of the categories they fall into.

The chapter has three sections. In the first, we set forth our as-

This work was supported in part by NICHD Grant HD-23378 and a Spencer Fellowship to the first author and an award from the W. K. Kellogg Foundation through the Presidential Initiatives Fund of the University of Michigan. We thank Andrea Backscheider, Lawrence Barsalou, Douglas Behrend, James Byrnes, Grant Gutheil, Chuck Kalish, Frances Kuo, and Karl Rosengren for their thoughtful comments on a previous draft.

sumptions about the nature of categories for adults. We review recent analyses suggesting that categories are enriched and informed by intuitive theories, summarizing arguments from psychology, philosophy, and linguistics to converge on the point that human categories extend far beyond observable similarities. In the second section, we demonstrate that this analysis of adults can be extended fruitfully to children. Contrary to most standard views of children, and despite children's relatively modest scientific knowledge, many of their categories have theory-laden properties. In the final section, we examine the role of language in the formation and structure of children's theory-laden categories.

Natural kinds as theory-laden categories

One critical feature of human categorization is that in forming categories we strive to incorporate our theories about, and explanations of, the world (Quine, 1969). Quine distinguishes between *intuitive kinds* (e.g., groupings based on color), which even rats form with ease, and *theoretical kinds* (e.g., the classification of bats as mammals rather than as birds), which require a restructuring of our innate sense of similarity. Theoretical kinds result from our attempts to understand the environment, not simply to organize and catalog it. Such categories hang together to the extent that they can explain and predict phenomena, instead of simply describing them. Mill (1843) aptly explained this function as follows: "Classification . . . is a contrivance for the best possible ordering of the ideas of objects in our minds; . . . in such a way as shall give us the greatest command over our knowledge already acquired, and lead most directly to the acquisition of more" (p. 432). In the rest of this section, we provide recent arguments and evidence that theoretical kinds are indeed central to much of adult thought.

Theory-laden categories

Arguments for the importance of theories in adult categories begin with the observation that similarity alone cannot explain why things belong to a given category. In order to calculate similarity, it is necessary to have a theory of which features are important and how they should be weighted. Murphy and Medin (1985) present two arguments for the inadequacy of similarity for categorization (see also Goodman, 1972). First, the similarity of any two objects depends on which properties of the objects are under consideration. As they point out, "Any two entities can be arbitrarily similar or dissimilar by changing the criterion of what counts as a relevant attribute" (p. 292). Two seemingly disparate objects, such as a blender and a sparrow, could be considered highly similar if certain attributes are highlighted. For example, both are less than 10,000 years old, both weigh less than 2,000 kilograms, both can be found in North America, both are visible without magnification, and so on. Second, even if the set of possible attributes is somehow constrained, similarity judgments depend on the relative importance of those attributes. There is no theory-neutral weighting of properties. For example, both habitat and method of breathing may be important attributes for classifying species. If habitat is given more weight, humpback whales might be classified with fish. But if breathing method is considered more important, humpback whales would be considered mammals. Similarity alone is insufficient to hold categories together because it does not by itself provide adequate constraints on category membership.

Rips (1989) provides empirical evidence for the distinction between similarity judgments and categorization, showing that judgments of similarity and category membership vary independently, and therefore similarity cannot completely account for categorization. In one experiment, adult subjects said that an unknown object three inches in diameter[1] was more *similar to* a quarter than a pizza, but more *likely to be* a pizza than a quarter. Presumably, theoretical beliefs concerning the range of possible sizes for pizzas and quarters determined the subjects' category judgments. In another experiment, subjects read stories about animals undergoing accidental transformations (e.g., following exposure to toxic chemicals). For example, the birdlike "sorp" (eats seeds and berries, lives in a nest, has two wings, two legs, feathers, etc.) was rated by a control group as much more similar to a bird than to an insect and much more likely to be a bird. After exposure to the chemicals, the sorp was transformed into an insectlike creature (it began to eat only the nectar of flowers, took shelter by sticking to the underside of leaves, sprouted new wings made of transparent membranes, developed two more pairs of legs and a brittle shell, etc.), but it was still able to mate and produce normal sorp offspring. After reading this tale, the subjects rated the transformed sorp as more similar to an insect than a bird, but still more likely to be a bird, despite the changes. On the basis of these and other experiments, Rips argues that the independence of the categorization and similarity responses shows that one cannot be reduced to the other.

The claim, then, is that category membership is dictated not by perceptual similarity but by deep or predictive properties. Categories are psychologically coherent not because of surface similarity among members, but because of explanatory theories that underlie them. "Concepts are viewed as embedded in theories and are coherent to the extent that they fit people's background knowledge or naive theories about the world" (Medin & Wattenmaker, 1987, p. 58). So, to return to our previous examples, whales are mammals because they share properties with other mammals that modern biology deems important, such as type of metabolism and method of reproduction. Conversely, sparrows and blenders do not form a coherent category because we are hard pressed to come up with an explanatory theory linking the two. Note that *theory* here refers to "any of a host of 'mental explanations' [including scripts, rules, and causal explanations], rather than a complete, organized, scientific account" (Murphy & Medin, 1985, p. 290).[2]

The theory view is perhaps best understood when contrasted with other possible positions. Some have argued a *nominalist* position, that human categories represent an essentially arbitrary framework imposed on the world. This implies that the psychological act of categorization is one of invention, as described by Bruner, Goodnow, and Austin (1956):

> Science and common-sense inquiry alike do not discover the ways in which events are grouped in the world; they invent ways of grouping. . . . Do such categories as tomatoes, lions, snobs, atoms, and mammalia exist? In so far as they have been invented and found applicable to instances of nature, they do. They exist as inventions, not as discoveries. (p. 7)

Nominalists argue that every object has many more discriminable attributes than we could take into account in any categorization and that therefore we must select which attributes to consider. Because attention to different attributes could lead to different categories, categorization is essentially an inventive act.

Others have argued a *realist* position, that categories are direct reflections of a structured world. This perspective is typified by the work of Rosch and Mervis (1975), who contend that "division of the world into categories is not arbitrary. The basic category cuts in the world are those which separate the information-rich bundles of attributes which form natural discontinuities" (p. 602). Realists hold that objects naturally fall into groups, and in such groups members are similar to one another and dissimilar to members of other groups. On this account, the attributes important for categorization exist in the environment as correlated bundles (for reviews see Mervis & Rosch, 1981; Rosch, 1978).

The nominalist position stresses the arbitrary nature of categories; the realist position places heavy emphasis on perceptual features devoid of context or explanation. The theory-laden position supplants this controversy, making use of both the notion of inventiveness in categorization and the notion of constraints inherent in the environment. For example, the theory-based grouping of bats as mammals is partly an inventive decision (because they could be classified differently), yet follows from our attempts to capture regularities in the environment (e.g., deeper qualities, such as means of bearing young). Our categories must be consistent with patterns in the environment, yet are not limited to perceptually salient features. Perceptual cues often signal the presence of these deeper qualities, but are not themselves the basis of category structure.

Properties of natural kind categories

Taking a broad view, theories are important for nearly all human categories (Murphy & Medin, 1985). For example, even an ad hoc category such as *things to take out of a burning house* (including children, jewelry, paintings, and book manuscripts; see Barsalou, 1983) gains coherence by means of a theory or goal that tells us what people value. Without considering the underlying goal that holds these items together, they have no similarities to speak of. But when the goal that relates category members is explicitly stated, the category becomes coherent. Subjects can even judge the typicality of category instances (as in more traditional categories, such as *birds*).

Nonetheless, on an intuitive level it would seem that categories vary in their theory-ladenness. Although many categories have psychological coherence, only some categories attempt to carve nature at its joints. Although many categories depend on theories, only a subset promotes an inexhaustible set of nonobvious inferences and warrants scientific investigation. It is useful here to invoke a distinction between natural kinds (e.g., *tiger, lemon, gold, electron*) and other categories (e.g., *chair, box, things to take out of a burning house*) (Locke, 1706/1965). What are the properties that distinguish natural kinds from other, less theory-laden categories? Below we present six properties that characterize natural kinds: rich inductive potential, nonobvious basis, essence, existence of anomalies, division of linguistic labor, and corrigibility. These interrelated properties convey the psychological nature of natural kinds. They are derived from discussions of natural kinds in philosophy and linguistics by Kripke (1971, 1972), Mill (1843), Putnam (1970, 1973), Quine (1969), Schwartz (1977, 1979), and others. Our aim is to detail with some precision what natural kind concepts are like in ordinary language.

Rich inductive potential. People construct categories with the implicit (perhaps unconscious) goal of learning as much as possible about the objects being classified (Jevons, 1877; Mill, 1843; Ruse, 1969). For example, if we learn that X is a "cat," we infer that it has many important properties in common with other cats, including diet, body temperature, genetic structure, and internal organs. We can even induce previously unknown properties. For example, if we discover that one cat has a substance called "cytosine" inside, we may then decide that other cats also contain this substance. Theory-laden categories encourage us to discover more similarities among the objects being classified than we would ever discover otherwise.

Indirect evidence for the importance of inductive potential can be found by examining which kinds of groupings we prefer over others. For example, we classify animals by shape and covering because these properties reliably predict other, more central properties such as habitat, diet, and means of locomotion. We would probably not even think to classify animals solely by color (e.g., considering brown cats, brown bears, and brown birds to be members of the same species, but white cats, white bears, and white birds to be members of another species), because color is not predictive of many other properties for animals.

Nonobvious basis. Natural kind categories promote inductive inferences in part because they capture deep similarities that are not always immediately obvious (see Wellman & Gelman, 1988). As we have seen, theories dictate which similarities count as important. One striking example is that of marsupial mice – small, ratlike animals that are classified as kangaroos because they have pouches and lack placentas (Quine, 1969). Marsupial mice are classified on the basis of underlying properties; they are not classified according to their most obvious surface features.

The importance of nonobvious features holds not only for unusual instances (such as marsupial mice), but also for more everyday entities. For example, we expect all tigers to have a particular genetic structure, chemical makeup, and bone structure in common, not just stripes; we expect all water to have a certain chemical structure in common, not just potability and transparency. Nonobvious features are also critical for understanding two other ubiquitous phenomena: developmental change (note the difference between a caterpillar and a butterfly, an ugly duckling and a beautiful swan, or an infant and adult human) and sexual dimorphism (males and females of many species differ radically in size, outer coloring, and/or morphology). Common nonobvious features lead us to classify caterpillars and butterflies together, or peacocks and peahens together, despite contrasting outward appearances.

Essence. Medin (1989; Medin & Ortony, 1989) has suggested that adults believe that certain categories have an essence, or a unique underlying property that is *responsible* for other similarities that category members share (Goosens, 1977). He calls this belief "psychological essentialism." In contrast to essentialism, which is a metaphysical claim about the structure of the world, psychological essentialism is a claim about human cognition. For example, although tigers share many properties (a certain DNA structure, bone structure, chemical makeup, appearance, and behavior), people may believe that DNA is the essence of a tiger because it causes the other properties. We do not even need to know what the essence is to believe it exists (see the subsection on the division of linguistic labor), although we presume that science will discover the essence eventually.

Although the notion of an essence is objectionable from an evolutionary perspective (because having an essence implies that the essence – and so the category – is immutable; Mayr, 1988), it has appeared repeatedly throughout recorded history (Kelly, 1989). Nonscientific cultures also appear to treat categories as embodying an essence. Using folk taxonomies as evidence, Atran (1987a, p. 197) suggests that there is "a (universal) presumption to the effect that visible organic types have underlying natures and that these essences provide a principle of natural causality for manifest organic regularity. . . . Cross-culturally, people presume that living kinds have (possibly unknown) natures with propensities responsible for the readily perceived regularities of those kinds."

Existence of anomalies. Because nonobvious features are critical to category membership, natural kind categories include anomalies, or members that differ greatly from the category prototype and may outwardly seem not to belong (Putnam, 1970; Quine, 1969). For example, we readily accept that birds include ostriches and penguins, or that fish include eels and flounder. Some of the properties that are usually used to identify category members can be missing, but we will still agree that the object is a member of the category if there is reason to believe that the more essential, more explanatory properties still hold. Albino dwarf tigers might lack many of the properties we usually associate with tigers: They would not have stripes, they would not be ferocious, they would probably look and act more like domestic cats than tigers. Because hidden properties are more important for natural kinds, surface similarity is only a fallible guide to category membership.

Division of linguistic labor. The average speaker recognizes that theory-laden knowledge is critical for the appropriate use of natural kind terms, even when that same speaker does not possess the underlying theoretical knowledge. Thus, one does not have to be an expert to treat categories as natural kinds. This point is critical, because it suggests that theories are considered integral to natural kinds and are not simply an accidental by-product of schooling or expertise. Putnam (1973) explains this as follows:

> The features that are generally thought to be present in connection with a general name – necessary and sufficient conditions for membership in the extension, ways of recognizing whether something is in the extension, etc. – are all present in the linguistic community *considered as a collective body*; but that collective body divides the "labor" of knowing and employing these various parts of the "meaning" of [e.g.,] "gold." (p. 125)

Thus, the basis of a category label can go far beyond what is known by most users of the word. For example, many of us do not know the difference between elms and beeches, but a botanist does. Even though we may not know what makes these trees different, we assume there is an underlying distinction that an expert would know. Putnam makes the analogy with tools requiring cooperative activity for their use (e.g., steamships) as contrasted with tools that can be used by an individual (e.g., hammers). He suggests that many words function like cooperative tools.

Corrigibility. Natural kind categories are always open to revision (Putnam, 1970, 1973; Quine, 1969). As long as theories are open to change, categories too will be open to change. For example, whales used to be considered fish, but as people learned more about them, they reclassified them as mammals. The category changed because people sought a grouping that would reflect deeper properties such as body temperature and breathing patterns. In one sense all categories are corrigible in that they undergo historical change. To give a recent example, in the NCAA basketball tournament, shots from beyond 18 feet, 8 inches were classified as "two-point shots" before the 1987 tournament and as "three-point-shots" thereafter. However, in a stricter sense corrigibility implies that classifications were previously either in error or incomplete. In this sense, the categories of basketball shots are not corrigible: It is not true that shots beyond 18 feet, 8 inches were actually three-point shots before 1987 and that the NCAA classification was wrong. In contrast, whales are and always have been mammals (at least according to current theories), and previous classifications of whales as fish were incorrect.

Which categories are natural kinds?

The epitome of natural kinds are scientific concepts, which by definition have a persistent commitment to go beyond similarity (see also Kelly, 1989). For example, in the modern conception of species, the mechanisms underlying the observable similarities and differences across species are primary (Ghiselin, 1969). As a consequence, surface similarities at times become irrelevant, taking a back seat to the underlying mechanisms, such as genealogy, reproductive isolation, or chromosomal structure. Ghiselin characterizes modern conceptions of species as follows: "Instead of finding patterns in nature and deciding that because of their conspicuousness they seem important, we discover the underlying mechanisms that impose order on natural phenomena, . . . then derive the structure of our classification systems from this understanding" (1969, p. 83). As this example illustrates, the modern species concept in biology is notable for its search for inductive potential, appeal to nonobvious properties, incorporation of anomalies, and so forth. These are qualities that are not evident in ad hoc categories such as *things to take out of a burning house.*

We propose that there are striking parallels between scientific natural kind categories (such as biological species concepts) and a subset of ordinary categories. In suggesting this analogy, we distinguish category content from category function. Clearly, content differences exist between scientific and ordinary classifications (Dupré, 1981; Morris, 1979). Ordinary people lack extensive scientific knowledge, so many words in ordinary language fail to map precisely onto scientific categories. For example, pterodactyls are not technically dinosaurs, but they are included in a box of "Dinosaur Honey Graham Cookies" sold commercially and in a collection of "dinosaur magnets" at an Ann Arbor store selling kitchen accessories. Similarly, the lay distinction between fruit and vegetables has no biological correlate. It should not be surprising that the content of ordinary language categories at times fails to mesh with the classifications of science, especially given that scientific categories are continually changing with the addition of new information.

However, the properties that make a category a natural kind concern how the category functions and do not determine which particular properties are critical for category membership. Despite differences in content, many categories function in similar ways for both scientists and nonscientists. Ghiselin (1969, pp. 87–88) notes that "the purpose of a [scientific] classification is not the accurate pigeonholing or identification of enzymes or dried specimens, but the assertion of meaningful propositions about laws of nature and particular events." Or in Stephen Jay Gould's words, "Classifications are theories about the basis of natural order, not dull catalogues compiled only to avoid chaos" (1989, p. 98). Similarly, in everyday life much – perhaps most – of what we learn is by inference (Holland, Holyoak, Nisbett, & Thagard, 1986), and categories provide an invaluable framework for such inferences. So although the content of the *dinosaur* category probably varies between expert and novice, the function remains the same, and most likely both novice and expert would expect deep, nonobvious similarities among dinosaurs.

Thus, natural kind categories are common in ordinary language. Many categories of naturally occurring objects or substances (e.g., *fish, roses, gold*) have all six properties, for ordinary adults. Even more abstract categories can have many natural kind properties. For many people *intelligence* is one such example: It has rich inductive potential (an intelligent person will probably perform well in school, have a successful career, etc.), a nonobvious basis (intelligence cannot be judged by appearances), perhaps an essence (such as a "*g*" factor), a division of linguistic labor (those who administer IQ tests are considered best equipped to determine whether someone is truly a genius), corrigibility (as evidenced by long-standing debates as to whether intelligence is just one factor or many factors), even anomalies (e.g., "idiot savants," who are geniuses of a sort yet seem not to be; learning-disabled children who may actually be very intelligent). Categories that have a full set of theory-laden properties can be considered natural kinds in that they aim to capture, as best as possible, the true structure of the world (see Jevons, 1877; Mill, 1843).

Many categories are assumed to be richly structured in the same way, even before all the evidence is in. For example, conceptions of certain disorders such as autism and dyslexia contain the hope that there is an underlying essence that, when discovered, will yield a rich array of inductive inferences concerning etiology, course of progression, and (ultimately) remedies. In other words, debates about how to define "autism" are not simply semantic, but rather concern which grouping will be most fruitful in discovering more about the problem.

Nonetheless, not all categories are theory-laden to the same degree. Categories that fall at the nontheory end of the continuum are sometimes referred to as artificial classifications, in that they are based on an arbitrary set of properties. They include categories defined by a single property, such as *white things* or *objects bigger than a breadbox* (see Mill, 1843). Ruse (1969) expresses this as follows: "An empty, arbitrary, or unreal concept yields nothing that was not already built into the definition" (p. 108). Because categories such as *white things* are structured around a single property with little predictive power, they fail to promote inductive inferences (e.g., if you learn something new about a white mouse, it is unlikely to generalize to a white fence), their basis is entirely obvious (resting solely on color), they have few if any anomalies (except for unusual viewing conditions, there are no white things that do not appear to be white), no division of linguistic labor (any intelligent, sighted person is qualified to determine what belongs in the category), no essence (there is no deeper property in common to all white things), and no corrigibility (we will never discover that light blue objects actually belong in the category of *white things*).

We propose that categories expressed in ordinary language vary along a continuum in the extent to which they can be considered natural kinds. Some categories (e.g., *computers*) have a nonobvious basis (it is its inner workings rather than outer appearance that makes something a computer), rich inductive potential (witness the emergence of the field of computer science), division of linguistic labor (a computer technician is better equipped to determine whether a new machine is a computer or some other device), even anomalies (such as cars with built-in computers), but probably do not have an underlying essence (since what makes something a computer changes over time). Other categories (e.g., *descendants of George Washington*) have a nonobvious basis (one cannot tell who belongs to the category by just looking), division of linguistic labor (a genealogist or other family members would be most accurate at identifying members of the category), and an essence (namely, a certain line of descent and genetic material), but little rich inductive potential or corrigibility. Still others (*objects weighing 256 grams*) may have a nonobvious basis, but few if any of the other theory-laden properties. And many common artifact categories (e.g., *cup, chair*) include anomalies (e.g., bowl-like cups, beanbag chairs) but none of the other theory-laden properties. In sum, there are a wide range of categories that have one or more theory-laden properties, including categories that are not traditionally thought of as embedded in theories. For example, the concept *run batted in* in baseball has many theory-laden properties, although in standard parlance it would be rare to say one has a "theory" of baseball (Siegler, 1989).

Knowing whether a category is a natural kind, an artificial classification, or something in-between has important consequences. The extent to which one considers a category to be theory-laden has direct ramifications for whether it is used to generate hypotheses and make inductive inferences. Cases of prejudice may arise when a rather limited distinction is assumed to be a natural kind distinction with an underlying essence. (For example, gender and race differences are heightened and exaggerated beyond their true basis, perhaps in conformity with the view that these are natural kind distinctions.)

Or in the case of medical disorders, if a disease is assumed to be an artificial classification rather than a natural kind (e.g., a rash), physicians will not bother to look for underlying commonalities.

The relation between theory and similarity

So far we have characterized "theory-based" natural kind categories in contrast to "similarity-based" categories. We have argued that human categories are not limited to perceptual similarity; they strive to capture how the world works. The world is complex, so the groupings we first notice do not always yield the deepest, most sophisticated level of understanding, but rather undergo change with increased knowledge and experience.

Nonetheless, perceptual similarity is often an important indicator of theoretically relevant variables. In other words, similarity and theory typically converge (see also Mayr, 1957; Medin, 1989). If our immediate perceptions were not extremely good cues for locating food, dangerous animals, or other members of our species, we would not survive. Presumably we evolved such that the perceptual similarities we find most salient are the ones most important for our survival. As Quine put it, "Our innate standards of perceptual similarity show a gratifying tendency to run with the grain of nature. This concurrence is accountable, surely, to natural selection" (1974, p. 19). Surface similarities may also lead us to look for deeper similarities.

Moreover, when similarity and theory do not converge, each is useful in its own way. The two are complementary sources of information. Similarity is most useful as a rough guide to identifying what something is, whereas theory provides the underlying basis of the classification. For example, birds are often identified by their feather color, yet feather color is not the causal force behind the classification. In the absence of more detailed knowledge, similarity is a powerful default, even for adults (see Chi, Feltovich, & Glaser, 1981). This distinction between the underlying basis of a category and reliable cues for identification emerges repeatedly in discussions of classification (see Atran, 1987b, conceptual identity vs. conceptual access; Miller & Johnson-Laird, 1976, and Smith & Medin, 1981, conceptual core vs. identification procedure; Sokal, 1977, establishing a category vs. allocating objects to the category).

In short, it is important to realize that there are two separate issues here. The first is: What information does one use to decide what something is? In the absence of an explicit label, the answer to that will nearly always be appearances – it may be uninformed overall similarity, it might involve attention to a theoretically important subset of features (e.g., those indicating animacy; see Massey & Gelman, 1988), or it may even be similarity that requires extensive training, as in reading medical x-rays and classifying them as x-rays of healthy versus x-rays of diseased tissue. The second issue is: What are the structure and consequences of a category? This is where an analysis of perceptual similarity is insufficient. Categories have implications that extend far beyond the features used to identify members.

Summary

The distinction between theory-laden and non-theory-laden categories has its roots in a distinction between *natural* and *artificial* systems of classification (Knight, 1981; Markman, 1989). Mill (1843) distinguishes between classifications that reflect patterns in nature (natural kinds such as *horse* or *animal*) and those we construct for our own convenience (artificial classes such as *white things*). Natural kinds pick up rich clusters of information that extend far beyond our original characterization; in contrast, artificial classes capture simply the property on which they are based (e.g., for *white things*, the property of being white). Artificial classifications name for the sake of expressing a certain quality. They do not change with the addition of new information, as do natural kinds. We discover natural classification systems; we construct artificial ones (Ghiselin, 1969).

A similar distinction has been proposed by Jevons (1877), who remarks that "deep correlations, or in other terms deep uniformities or laws of nature, will be disclosed by any well chosen and profound system of classification" (p. 676). Whereas natural classification systems aim to uncover a deeper reality, artificial classification systems are useful because of the ease and convenience with which they are put into practice. Although we strive for natural systems, we retain the artificial ones for our first attempts at classifying and when we need something convenient that will work most (though not all) of the time.

In this section we have proposed that natural kinds are theory-laden categories exhibiting the following six properties: rich inductive potential, nonobvious basis, underlying essence, anomalies, division of linguistic labor, and corrigibility. Categories vary along a continuum in the degree to which they embody these properties. The net implication is that a vast set of ordinary concepts requires attention to the nonobvious.

Children's understanding of natural kind categories

The view that many of adults' categories are theory-laden natural kinds raises a critical developmental question: How do children learn categories that have a nonperceptual basis, anomalous members, hidden essences, and/or the potential for unforeseen inductions? The standard developmental picture of young children might predict that they could not appreciate theory-laden, nonobvious concepts such as these. A vast array of research in cognitive development demonstrates that children attend to superficial appearances even when they are misleading (e.g., Bruner, Olver, & Greenfield, 1967; Flavell, 1963, 1977; Inhelder & Piaget, 1964; Livesly & Bromley, 1973; Peevers & Secord, 1973; Piaget, 1970; Smiley & Brown, 1979). For example, in Piaget's conservation task, children see a volume of liquid being poured from a short container to a tall container. Nothing is added or taken away, but preschoolers insist that there is more liquid in the taller container because it appears to have more. Given children's attention to appearances, many have argued that an appreciation for theory-laden categories may emerge later in development. As Neisser (1987) puts it, "It is intriguing to discover that the two major alternatives considered by category theorists – featural similarities and theory-based definitions – correspond to points on a developmental continuum" (p. 6).

Another potential difficulty with early natural kind categories is that children have a relatively sparse understanding of science. In a detailed study of children's biological knowledge, Carey (1982, 1985) suggests that an appreciation for natural kinds might not develop until about age 10. She explains as follows:

> First, the child may need a minimal understanding of the workings of science, in general, before he has the concept of a natural kind term. Second, the child (or adult) may need a minimal knowledge of a particular science before a natural kind term in the theory of that science is recognized as such. For instance, Putnam (1962) suggests that *atom* changed from a

classical term meaning "smallest indivisible particle of matter" to its present natural kind status only when enough physics was known for *atom* actually to refer to atoms. Young children are markedly deficient in both reflections of scientific knowledge – the understanding of science in general and of particular theories as well. (1982, pp. 383–384)

Carey argues that knowledge about science in general and scientific domains in particular is necessary for a theoretically based conceptual structure to emerge and that without this requisite knowledge, children's categories cannot be characterized as natural kinds.

Nonetheless, the problems with similarity-based categories proposed for adults (Murphy & Medin, 1985) apply equally (if not more so) to children. Children must have some basis for constraining or weighting the features in the environment if they are to construct categories that make any sense. Moreover, it would be particularly useful for children to realize the rich inductive potential of categories from an early age, when they are first learning and organizing large amounts of knowledge.

We propose that children do appreciate natural kind categories well before the onset of formal schooling or the acquisition of extensive domain-specific knowledge. In particular, children use language to help set up categories that function like adult natural kind categories – as if they were theory-based – even though children have not yet filled in the particulars of the theory.

Past studies are limited in what they tell us about children's understanding of natural kind categories. First, past work assumed that categories do not substantially differ from one another. On this view the study of one sort of category is generalized to all the child's classification schemes and abilities. Categories that were studied previously often included wholly perceptual and/or arbitrary groupings, rather than natural kinds. For example, children might be asked to reason about blue circles and red squares (see Inhelder & Piaget, 1964). The class of blue circles is merely a grouping based on perceptual attributes; it does not capture nonobvious similarities, nor does it draw on richer sorts of knowledge children have about the world. However, as discussed earlier, categories differ in the richness of their structure and resemblance to natural kinds. To avoid this limitation, the categories to be studied should include nonobvious similarities and should tie into world knowledge (e.g., natural kinds).

Second, past work typically assumed that category knowledge can best be tapped by asking children to sort or classify objects. Tasks used previously most often required children to construct a classification (e.g., "Put together the things that go together") – thus emphasizing similarity – rather than to reason about or draw inferences from a category – thereby emphasizing the nonobvious. When we ask children simply which objects belong together, we are neglecting the deeper questions of whether the grouped objects form a motivated category and what the consequences are of having such a category.[3] It seems clear that concepts comprise more than knowledge of which instances belong in a category (see, e.g., Salmon, 1981). Indeed, as argued earlier, inductions about completely new instances and properties reveal important aspects of category functioning.

In the remainder of this section we review developmental studies that avoided both of these difficulties. When the categories studied include natural kinds, and when children's deeper understanding is probed, these studies show that young children (ages $2\frac{1}{2}$ to 5 years) have an appreciation for categories that promote rich inductive inferences, share nonobvious properties that do not always correspond to outward appearances, have essential natures, and permit anomalous members. Although many of these features overlap, we separate them here for the sake of clarity. We will also consider whether for children, natural kind categories are subject to division of linguistic labor, and are subject to revision (exhibit corrigibility).

Rich inductive potential

Content versus function. Earlier we distinguished between content and function when comparing scientific and ordinary classification systems. Although scientific categories often differ from everyday categories in content, their functions are similar; both types of category serve to guide inferences beyond what is already known. Here we propose a similar relation between adults' and children's categories: Although children may rely on different bases for classification than adults (e.g., Inhelder & Piaget, 1964; Keil & Batterman, 1984; Smiley & Brown, 1979; Smith & Kemler, 1977; Vygotsky, 1962), their categories fulfill similar functions. Later we describe research demonstrating that for children as young as $2\frac{1}{2}$, categories promote extraordinarily rich inductive inferences and that this is true even in the absence of any perceptual support.

Categories and induction. As mentioned earlier, a major function of categories is to promote inferences beyond the obvious. There are two ways this happens. First, categories promote inferences about nonobvious properties, such as "produces insulin" or "has a spleen inside." Such properties are not readily apparent from the outward appearance of an object. Second, even category members that do not look much alike share important properties (e.g., both a robin and an ostrich lay eggs, have warm blood, etc.).

To examine children's understanding that categories promote inferences, Gelman and Markman (1986) devised a task designed to tap children's inductive inferences. *Induction* entails making an inference beyond what one knows with certainty and contrasts with *deduction*, in which conclusions follow with certainty from the premises (Skyrms, 1975).

Gelman and Markman (1986) presented preschool children and adults with pictures depicting a wide range of natural kind categories, including snakes, dinosaurs, birds, squirrels, sand, gold, and diamonds, among others. Twenty sets of three pictures each were used. Each set was constructed so that the third picture closely resembled one of the first two pictures but was from the same category as the other. Thus, each item pitted perceptual similarity and category membership against one another. Of interest was whether children would draw inferences from one picture to another on the basis of outward appearance or natural kind category membership.

Two pictures from different natural kind categories (e.g., a colorful tropical fish and a gray dolphin) served as targets. These target pictures were named (in this case, *fish* and *dolphin*), and the subjects learned an unfamiliar nonobvious property about each. A broad range of important, nonobvious properties, concerning such things as behavior ("eats grass"), physical properties ("melts in an oven"), function ("has cold blood"), and origin ("comes from a mountain"), was used.[4] In this example, the children were told, "This fish [i.e., tropical fish] stays underwater to breathe" and "This dolphin pops above the water to breathe." (Pretesting confirmed that 4-year-olds did not previously know which property applied to each animal.) Children were then shown a test picture, in this case a gray shark. In all cases, the test picture belonged to the same category as one of the targets (the shark and the tropical fish are both fish) but looked much more like the target picture from the other category (the gray shark and the gray dolphin look much more alike than the shark and the tropical fish). Adult ratings were collected to confirm perceptual similarity relations. After being shown the picture of the shark and told that it was a fish, the subjects were asked whether it stayed underwater to breathe like the fish or popped above the water to breathe like the dolphin.

When adults performed this task (with more difficult properties, such as "This bird's heart has a right aortic arch only" for a flamingo), they based their inferences on category membership 86% of the time (i.e., they inferred that pictures from the same natural kind category shared novel nonobvious properties). As expected, this performance significantly exceeds what one would expect by chance. Furthermore, the subjects were highly confident of their answers, giving a mean confidence rating of 5.8 on a scale of 1 (*very unsure*) to 7 (*very sure*).

Given the excellent performance of adults, the performance of the preschool group was of particular interest. The results were strikingly similar to those of adults. Four-year-olds based 68% of their inferences on category membership despite the lack of perceptual support for such inferences. This figure was significantly above chance and significantly higher than the results of a control condition in which subjects were shown the labeled test pictures only (e.g., shark) and were asked the test questions (e.g., whether it breathed underwater or above the water). Moreover, 37% of the children consistently based their inferences on category membership across items, whereas none of the subjects consistently based their answers on appearances.

These results were replicated with younger children in a follow-up study. Gelman and Markman (1987) examined patterns of inferences in 3- and 4-year-olds using a slightly different procedure. For each of 10 picture sets, the task involved teaching subjects about a novel property of a single target picture (e.g., "See this cat? It can see in the dark") and then pairing the target with four test pictures in turn. The children were then asked whether the property was true of each test picture. There were four types of test pictures: (a) same category, similar appearance (e.g., a cat with markings similar to those of the target cat), (b) same category, dissimilar appearance (e.g., a cat with different markings, in a different position), (c) different category, similar appearance (e.g., a skunk with markings strikingly similar to those of the target cat), and (d) different category, dissimilar appearance (e.g., a dinosaur).

The experiment had three conditions designed to tease apart the effects of language and appearance. In the word and picture condition, all pictures were shown and named. In the word-only condition, all pictures were named but the target picture was not shown to the child. Instead, the experimenter simply said, for example, "I see a picture of a cat. This cat can see in the dark . . ." In the picture-only condition, all pictures were shown, but none were named.

The results support the view that children rely on natural kind category membership to guide their inferences (Figure 5.1). In the word and picture condition, the children drew more inferences to members of the same category with dissimilar appearances (64% overall) than to members of a different category with similar appearances (29% overall). For example, when told that a small brown snake lays eggs, they were more likely to infer that a large gray cobra lays eggs than to infer that a small brown worm lays eggs. Appearances were important within the target category: The children drew more inferences to similar members of the target category (e.g., another small brown snake) than to dissimilar members (e.g., a large gray cobra). However, no such trend was apparent outside the target category (the children drew as many inferences to a cow as they did to a small, brown worm).

As expected, in the word-only condition, the children also based their inferences on category membership and not appearances. It was only in the picture-only condition that they were more apt to draw inferences based on appearances. They drew more inferences to pictures similar in appearance to the target but from a different category (e.g., from a tan shell to tan stone of the same shape) than in the word and picture condition. And for pictures that differed in category membership from the target, they drew more inferences to those pictures similar in appearance (e.g., from a black and white striped cat to a skunk) than to those dissimilar in appearance (e.g., from a black and white striped cat to a dinosaur). Few significant differences were found between 3- and 4-year-olds, and none were found in the word and picture condition. By age 3, children use information about category membership to guide inferences.

In fact, children as young as age 2 are sensitive to the rich infer-

166   S. A. Gelman and J. D. Coley

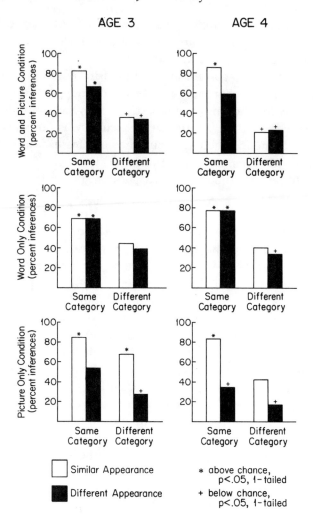

Figure 5.1. Results, by condition, from Gelman and Markman (1987).

ential power of natural kind categories (Gelman & Coley, 1990). Children ranging in age from 2,1 to 3,1 (mean age 2,8) were tested on a simplified version of the inference task already described. Specifically, for each of nine items, children were shown a target picture from a familiar category (e.g., a bluebird) and reminded of a familiar property that described it (e.g., "This bird lives in a nest"). This target picture was then set aside and not referred to again, but was left in view. Each subject was then shown four test pictures, one at

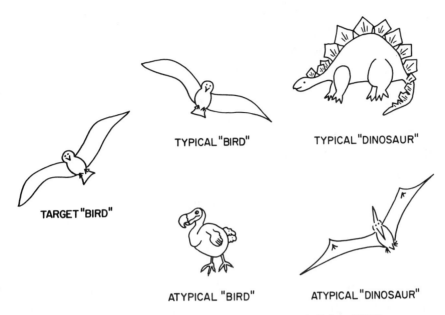

TYPICAL "BIRD"

TYPICAL "DINOSAUR"

TARGET "BIRD"

ATYPICAL "BIRD"

ATYPICAL "DINOSAUR"

Figure 5.2. Sample item set from Gelman and Coley (1990).

a time. These included (a) a typical instance of the target category (another bluebird), (b) an atypical instance of the target category (a dodo), (c) a typical instance of a contrasting category (a stegosaurus), and (d) an atypical instance of the same contrasting category (a pterodactyl) (see Figure 5.2 for a sample set). Furthermore, the atypical instance of the contrasting category was perceptually quite similar to the target picture, whereas the atypical instance of the target category was not (e.g., the pterodactyl looked like the target bluebird, but the dodo did not). Perceptual similarity was confirmed by adult ratings. Finally, for half the subjects, category membership was conveyed via verbal labels (e.g., "This is a bird"); the other half heard no labels.

As expected, subjects performed well on the typical items in both conditions (overall, 75% correct). For example, the subjects reported that the bluebird lived in a nest and the stegosaurus did not, whether or not these pictures were labeled. For the atypical items, however, the subjects who heard the labels drew correct inferences at a level significantly above chance (69% correct), whereas those who did not hear a label performed significantly below chance (42% correct). For example, the children inferred that a dodo, labeled *bird*, lived in a nest like the target bird, but that a pterodactyl, labeled *dinosaur*, did not. When pictures were not labeled, 2-year-olds were more likely to infer that the pterodactyl lived in a nest and that the dodo did not. These results also held up when the performance of individuals was examined. In the label condition, 6 of 11 children consistently based their inferences on category membership (i.e., they answered on the basis of category membership for 26 or more of the 36 trials); none based their inferences consistently on appearances. In the no-label condition, one child responded on the basis of category membership, whereas 6 of 11 consistently answered on the basis of appearances.

Thus, for children as young as age 2, category membership promotes important inferences.[5] This is a remarkable achievement, given the age of the subjects, their lack of formal scientific training, and their otherwise persistent attention to salient perceptual features.

Control studies. Because category membership in these studies was conveyed by language, children's performance could conceivably have been due to a simple "same word–same property" strategy. That is, the children may have had a response bias to say that category members were alike just because the experimenter had labeled them with identical words. This seemed unlikely, because the task required the children to say the property explicitly (not just to point), and because the children gave many sensible justifications (Table 5.1). Nonetheless, several control studies, described later, show that the children were not answering solely on the basis of hearing the same word for two pictures.

In some cases, children drew appropriate categorical inferences without identical labels. Four-year-olds performed well when category information was conveyed by synonymous rather than identical labels (e.g., the target was referred to as a "puppy" and the test picture was referred to as a "baby dog"; Gelman & Markman, 1986). Children in this condition based their inferences on category membership 63% of the time, which is significantly above chance.

Children sometimes drew category-based inferences even in the absence of labels. In the no-label condition of Gelman and Markman (1987), in which none of the pictures was named, children occasionally figured out category membership on the basis of subtle perceptual clues and then proceeded to draw correct inferences (3-year-olds on 3 out of 10 items and 4-year-olds on 5 out of 10 items). For

Table 5.1. *Sample justifications of category-based choices*

A squirrel eats bugs, "because it's a squirrel."
A fish stays underwater to breath, "because he's a fish.'
The gold nugget melts like the gold bar, "because they're both the same thing."
A chunk of salt helps make snow melt, "because it's the same kind as this [fine-grained salt]."
A bug breathes air in, "because some bugs work like that."
A flower has tubes for water inside, because "every flower has tubes inside, so it does have tubes inside!"
The coral has to catch food, "because all corals do that."
A bug breathes air in, "because every bug breathes in and every leaf breathes out."
The dinosaur has cold blood, "'cause every dinosaur has cold blood, even when it's frozen."

example, the children did not draw inferences from a leaf insect to a leaf – despite a striking similarity between the two – because they attended to subtle features (e.g., the leaf insect had eyes and antennae, which the leaf lacked). When a separate group of children was later asked to name all the pictures used in the study, correct naming correlated highly ($r = .77$) with the children's ability to draw category-based inferences. Those pictures that the children named correctly (e.g., the leaf insect, which was typically called "a bug") were the ones for which the children also drew appropriate inferences.

In other cases, identical labels did not yield unwarranted inferences. In one control condition (Gelman & Markman, 1986), children were presented with a meaningless task for which category membership was irrelevant. In this task, the experimenter labeled and placed a different-colored chip on each of the two target pictures in each set. (The picture sets and labels were identical to those used in the induction task described earlier.) The children were then asked which color should go on the test picture. For example, if the tropical fish received a red chip and the dolphin received a blue chip, should the shark (labeled *fish*) receive a red or a blue chip? If children have a response bias to match pictures on the basis of the labels, the results should be identical to performance in the induction task. However, if performance in the induction task reflected the belief that natural kind categories share deep similarities, children would have no basis for deciding which color chip to select and performance on the control task should be at chance, with subjects choosing each color about half the time. Indeed, children's performance in this condition was not significantly different from chance.

Similarly, in another control condition, when 4-year-olds learned properties that should be more generalizable on the basis of appearance than category membership (e.g., "weighs 10 pounds"), they did not base inferences on categories over appearances (Gelman & Markman, 1986). Likewise, 2-year-olds who heard pictures labeled with adjectives describing temporary states (e.g., *sleepy*) instead of category names (e.g., *dinosaur*) performed just like those who had heard no labels at all (Gelman & Coley, 1990). See S. A. Gelman (1988) for further evidence that children are more likely to generalize enduring biological properties concerning, for example, internal structure, diet, or function (e.g., "has parts made out of calcium," "likes to eat alfalfa," "needs branchias to breathe") than transient properties dealing with temporary states or historical accident (e.g., "smells yucky," "fell on the floor this morning," "is a year old").

Thus, children do not blindly base their inferences on the similarity of words that are associated with each picture. Not all words promote categorical inferences, and not all categorical inferences require labels. Rather, children use category labels to guide inferences about important underlying properties.

Role of theories. Carey (1985) argues that a naïve theory of biology best explains children's patterns of inferences across basic-level animal categories. Rather than look at patterns of induction within basic-level natural kind categories, Carey has investigated how children project properties taught about one basic-level animal category to other categories differing in similarity to the target category. Subjects were taught that people, dogs, or bees had a spleen ("a green round thing") inside of them. When taught that people had spleens, young children inferred that other animals had spleens on the basis of their similarity to people. Mammals were most likely to have spleens, down through worms, which were the least likely. However, when children were taught that dogs or bees had spleens, the property was not generalized on the basis of similarity to dogs or bees. For instance, children generalized from people to aardvarks 76% of the time, but from dogs to aardvarks only 29% of the time. Similarly, children generalized from people to stinkbugs 52% of the time, but from bees to stinkbugs only 12% of the time. These results run counter to what one would expect if children were basing their inferences on similarity alone, since, for example, bees and stink-bugs are more similar to one another than are people and stinkbugs. Nonetheless, the findings can be explained if 4-year-olds hold the belief that people are the prototypical animals and thus the proto-typical possessors of animal properties. If 4-year-olds hold this the-ory, then animal properties taught about people should be readily generalizable, whereas those taught about more peripheral animals (dogs and bugs) should be less so. Further support for this inter-pretation is that children generalized from dogs to people only 18% of the time, whereas they generalized from people to dogs 71% of the time. Carey argues that "the prototypicality of people plays a much larger role in determining 4-year-olds' projection of having a spleen than does similarity among animals" (p. 128).

In a related experiment, Carey (1985) found that subjects as young as age 7 rated a mechanical toy monkey more similar to a person than to any of a number of pictured animals. However, these sub-jects rarely (12% of the time) attributed animal properties such as eating, sleeping, and having babies to the toy monkey. In fact, they attributed animal properties significantly less often to the mechan-ical monkey than they did to a worm, which was understandably rated as very dissimilar to a person. By age 7, children are aware that people and worms are alike in important ways that people and mechanical monkeys are not, despite similar appearances. Overall, Carey's work demonstrates that children do not base inductions across categories on perceptual similarity alone. Rather, such inductions are informed by children's emerging biological theories.

Taken together, these results demonstrate that children are in-deed sensitive to the importance of natural kind categories for pro-moting inferences beyond what can be perceived. By 2 years of age, language signals category membership, and categories promote rich inductions beyond what is observable. This is true even in the strongest case, in which category membership receives little per-ceptual support.

Knowledge of nonobvious properties

Nonobvious properties are especially important for natural kind cat-egories. Evidence from several domains points to the conclusion that children are knowledgeable about nonobvious properties and realize their importance for the way objects function.

Understanding of insides. Children's knowledge of unobservables is demonstrated by their relatively accurate descriptions of the insides of objects. Gelman and O'Reilly (1988) asked preschool and second-grade children whether a range of categories (*animals, plants, vehicles, clothing,* etc.) had the same insides. For example, children were asked whether each of the following had "the same kinds of stuff inside": (a) all dogs, (b) dogs and horses, (c) dogs and snakes, and (d) dogs and tractors. They were also asked to describe what each had inside. In explaining their answers, the children appropriately mentioned internal parts 65% of the time and external parts or functions only 12% of the time. Furthermore, on natural kind items children discussed natural kind parts (liquids, organs, bones) 35% of the time, whereas they mentioned artifact parts (stuffing, metal, fabric) only 1% of the time. This pattern was reversed for artifact items: The children appropriately mentioned artifact parts 59% of the time and mentioned natural kind parts only 4% of the time. Although not always accurate in detail ("[Carrots] have milk [inside]. Milk and wheat"; "Teddy bears have feathers inside"), the subjects knew what kinds of insides were appropriate for different kinds of items.

Similarly, R. Gelman (1987) asked preschool children what was on the inside and on the outside of various animate and inanimate objects, including humans, elephants, cats, dolls, and puppets. As in Gelman and O'Reilly (1988), children distinguished animals from inanimate objects on the basis of internal properties. They tended to say that animals had blood, bones, or other internal organs on the inside, whereas inanimate objects had material, mechanical devices, or nothing inside. Moreover, children seemed to believe a more general rule, that the inside of an animal causes its self-generated movement ("causal innards principle"). As evidence for this principle, R. Gelman found that children expected the insides of different animals to be very similar to each other and to differ from their outsides. In contrast, for inanimate objects children often reported that the insides were the same as the outsides (a "surface generalization rule"). For example, children might say that a doll has material on both the outside and the inside, whereas an elephant has skin outside and blood inside. Again, preschool children differentiate between animals and inanimate objects on the basis of nonobvious properties.

Children can also attend to internal composition when it conflicts with surface appearances. Gelman and Wellman (in press; cited in Gelman & Coley, 1989) showed children triplets of items in which the target item and one test item looked alike but were from different categories (e.g., a pig and a piggy bank), and the target item and the other test item did not look alike but were from the same category (e.g., the pig and a cow). For each pair of test items, children were asked two questions: In this example, "Which of these looks most like the pig?" and "Which of these has the same kinds of insides as the pig?" These questions required the subjects to switch their answers; the first required attention to surface similarity, and the second to the less obvious property of internal makeup. Four-year-olds performed better than 3-year-olds (78 vs. 58% correct), but both performed better than chance. Gelman and Wellman also conducted an analysis of error patterns that took into account how the children answered both questions for a given triplet (i.e., both the "looks like" and "has insides" questions). It is interesting that on this analysis children erred as often by saying that things that had the same insides not only had the same insides but also looked alike (e.g., the pig and the cow looked alike) as by saying that things that looked alike not only looked alike but also had the same insides (e.g., the pig and the piggy bank had the same insides). These results show that the children were able to consider both appearances and nonobvious properties in the same task and that not all errors were due to emphasizing outward similarity over category membership.

Children are also able to sort objects with identical outward appearances on the basis of internal, hidden (but remembered) characteristics. Deloache and Todd (1988) found that 5-year-olds could sort identical closed containers into two groups of six, depending on whether they had seen M&M candy or pegs put into each container before it was closed. Overall, the children succeeded with this sorting task on 78% of the trials. In a follow-up experiment, 5-year-olds were asked to form similar categories, but in this case two different-looking types of containers were used. Half of each type of container contained candy and half contained pegs. To succeed in this task, the subjects not only had to attend to nonobvious properties (i.e., remember which containers held which objects) but also had to ignore the salient appearances of the containers. Although this task was more difficult than the previous one (44% successful sorting overall), by the fourth trial the subjects were able to sort successfully on the basis of contents 62% of the time.

Even preverbal infants can attend to nonobvious properties. In another categorization task, Kolstad and Baillargeon (1989) examined infants' ability to categorize on the basis of both perceptual and functional properties. To do this, they habituated $10\frac{1}{2}$-month-old infants to series of events in which three brightly colored cylindrical containers were manipulated in a viewing box. In the experimental condition, subjects watched salt being poured into and out of the containers; in the control condition the movements were the same, but no salt was used. After habituation, the infants' looking times were recorded for two test events, either with a container that resembled the training containers but apparently had no bottom (a "tube" that actually had a transparent bottom) or with a floral-pattern box that did not resemble the training containers but did have an obvious bottom. Each test container was manipulated either with salt (experimental condition) or without salt (control condition). In the experimental condition, both containers actually held the salt. Infants in the experimental (salt) condition looked longer at the event involving the "bottomless" tube that held salt than at the event involving the box that held salt. Infants in the control (no salt) condition looked longer at the box event. The authors argue that in the experimental condition, the subjects focused on containment and therefore categorized the box with the other containers. The infants were surprised that the apparently bottomless tube actually held the salt and so gazed longer at that event. The control children had no reason to be surprised and therefore focused on perceptual similarity, classifying the tube with the other brightly colored cylinders and seeing the box as novel. Children as young as $10\frac{1}{2}$ months are not limited to categorization on the basis of perceptual similarity alone.

Understanding the animate–inanimate distinction. Massey and Gelman (1988) demonstrated that 3- and 4-year-old children can make a conceptual distinction between animals and inanimate objects on the basis of subtle perceptual cues. Children were shown photographs of unfamiliar objects from five categories – *mammals, nonmammalian animals, lifelike statues of mammals, wheeled vehicles,* and *complex rigid objects* – and were asked whether each object "could go down (up) a hill all by itself." The statues and the mammals looked more alike than did the mammals and the nonmammalian animals (e.g., praying mantis, tarantula). Overall, 4-year-olds were correct on 90% of the trials, and 3-year-olds on 78%. Twelve of 20 subjects reliably said that animals, but not inanimate objects, could go up and down a hill by themselves. The correct use of this "animacy" rule required attention to subtle cues rather than overall similarity. Five more subjects used a variant of the animacy rule, but sometimes denied that an animal could go up and down a hill by itself for practical reasons (e.g., the hill was too big). The authors concluded:

> Performance on this task cannot be attributed to simple perceptual prototypes or rules that are based on single perceptual features. Clearly, the children were using perceptual information, because pictures were their only direct source of information about these unfamiliar objects. However, the patterns in their answers are not predicted by the obvious perceptual similarities and dissimilarities among the items. (p. 316)

This finding is consistent with other work showing that children are knowledgeable about the distinction between animate and inanimate objects from an early age (e.g., Dolgin & Behrend, 1984; Gelman, Spelke, & Meck, 1983; Richards & Siegler, 1984, 1986).

Understanding of mind. Children's understanding of the mind is another realm in which an appreciation for unobservables is apparent. Wellman and Gelman (1988) note at least two ways that children's theory of mind demonstrates an appreciation for the nonobvious. First children, like adults, distinguish beween internal thought and external behavior. Wellman and Estes (1986) showed that children as young as age 3 correctly report that physical objects – and not thoughts or dreams of such objects – can be touched and manipulated, or seen by someone else. Second, children are aware that internal psychological states offer the best explanation of others' external behavior. For example, Wimmer and Perner (1983) show that 4-year-olds can correctly predict that a boy in a story will look for a cookie in a drawer because he *believes* the cookie is there, despite the fact that the subjects know the cookie has been moved to a cupboard. Through their differentiation between thoughts and objects and their use of beliefs to predict behavior, preschoolers show an understanding of the nonobvious.

In this section, we have shown that children's understanding in a variety of domains, including knowledge of objects' insides, animacy, and the mind reveals that children are aware of, and are able to attend to and use, nonobvious properties.

Psychological essentialism

Beyond appreciating unobservable but important properties that category members have in common, children also believe that members of a category share some unique underlying property that is *responsible* for the other similarities associated with category membership.

One way that this psychological essentialism can manifest itself is through a belief in innate potential. Recognition that an animal has the potential to develop into an outwardly different mature form (e.g., recognition that a tadpole has the potential of becoming a frog) is consistent with belief in a category essence. Recent work suggests that $4\frac{1}{2}$ to 5-year-olds believe that individuals have an innate potential, even before that potential visibly manifests itself (Gelman & Wellman, in press; cited in Gelman & Coley, 1989). In this study, children were shown an immature member of an animal or plant category (either a baby animal or a seed) and then were told that the baby or seed grew up in an environment better suited to another species (e.g., a cow that grew up on a pig farm and never saw another cow, or a seed that came from an apple but was planted in a flower pot). Next, the subjects were asked questions about what the baby animal or seed would be like when it grew up. Overall, 80% of the time children answered that the baby would have the characteristics expected given its category membership, despite the conflicting environment. For example, children answered that the baby cow would moo and have a straight tail when it grew up and that the apple seed would grow into an apple tree. These data provide preliminary evidence that children are essentialists. They assume that members of a category share an early-emerging (or innate) potential that can overcome a strong environmental influence.

Another way to examine psychological essentialism in children is to ask them to explain why objects have certain properties. If children explain such phenomena by appealing to intrinsic factors rather than external, imposed factors, they are showing indirect evidence of essentialism. Kremer and Gelman (1989) asked children questions such as "Why do rabbits have long ears?" and "Why do birds fly?" They found that 72% of 4-year-olds and 73% of first-graders spontaneously mentioned inborn dispositions, intrinsic nature, or growth at least once. For example, preschoolers answered that a rabbit has long ears because "the egg made the [rabbit's] ears so that it had them when it hatched," or birds fly "because that's the way birds are made." Moreover, children mentioned these factors significantly more often when explaining properties of natural kinds (e.g., rabbits, flowers, salt) than when explaining properties of human artifacts (e.g., cars, crayons, phones). Apparently, children appeal to essential properties such as inborn factors, instrinsic nature, and growth to explain why natural kind category members share certain attributes.

Essentialism also entails the belief that deeper properties are more important for category membership than are superficial ones. Nelson (1974) provides arguments and evidence that in the earliest stages of word learning children look for defining qualities of objects that extend beyond obvious similarity features. More recently, Keil (1986) examined these issues in older children. He presented children in kindergarten, second grade, and fourth grade with stories about animals that had appearances and habits characteristic of one natural kind (e.g., raccoons), but upon closer scrutiny (e.g., inspection through microscopes) were found to have a cluster of features of another natural kind (the raccoonlike animals actually had the internal organs of skunks, their parents and babies were skunks, etc.). Five-year-olds tended to maintain that the creatures were raccoons. Second- and fourth-graders and adults were willing to let discoveries override appearances; they tended to say that the creatures were skunks.

The relatively poor performance of 5-year-olds on this task seems to run counter to the claim that preschool children are psychological essentialists. However, Keil's task involved inferring categories from properties (e.g., "This animal has properties x, y, and z. Is it a skunk?"). Young children have been shown to find this sort of inference task much more difficult than the converse task of inferring properties from categories (e.g., "This animal is a skunk. Does it have properties x, y, and z?"), at least with gender categories (Gelman, Collman, & Maccoby, 1986). The performance of the younger subjects could reflect this difficulty rather than a lack of essentialism.

Another way to examine childhood essentialism is to ask children about transformations of objects. If an object has an essence that determines its category membership, then superficial changes in that object that do not affect its essence should not affect its category membership. Keil (1986, 1987) reports that by age 5, children correctly report the identity of an object when superficial transformations cross ontological boundaries. For example, when asked about a porcupine that became cactuslike in appearance (dyed yellowish green and injected with a substance that caused it to hibernate for years), 5-year-olds answered that the animal in question was still a porcupine. Results were different for transformations occurring within ontological boundaries. Five-year-olds tended to say, for example, that a raccoon that was shaved, painted black and white, and implanted with an odor sac was now a skunk. Reliance on appearances decreased with age; children became more essentialistic as they grew older. By second grade, children preserved category membership within ontological boundaries on a majority of their judgments. Again, the errors of younger children could be attributed to their difficulty in inferring the category of an object given properties of that object rather than a lack of essentialism.

Recent work hints at the kinds of properties children consider essential. Springer and Keil (1989) found that children predicted that unrelated members of an animal category would share abnormalities that were inborn, but not abnormalities that were acquired. For example, children reasoned that a bull was more likely to be born with a pink heart inside if other bulls that lived nearby had been born with pink hearts inside than if other bulls had a one-time accident that made their hearts pink. Children are aware that inborn features are more likely to be intrinsic to species, and therefore essential.

Although more work must be done, these studies offer some evidence that children approach concept learning with at least the roots of psychological essentialism.

Acceptance of anomalies

By 2 years of age, children have a rudimentary ability to accept anomalies that are explicitly labeled. In the studies reported earlier, nearly all the children accepted the anomalies presented (e.g., a long-eared squirrel or a birdlike flying fish). They occasionally commented on the anomaly (e.g., "That's a funny looking squirrel"), but generally they accepted it (Gelman & Coley, 1990; Gelman & Markman, 1987).

Nonetheless, children may have difficulty accepting category anomalies that are not explicitly pointed out or explained to them. We predict that anomalies would be difficult for children because they conflict with the belief that category members have much (including appearances) in common. In one study, 4-year-olds accepted anomalies that adults considered possible, such as "a rabbit that doesn't like carrots," only 26% of the time (Biderman, 1989). By age 6, children accepted such anomalies 53% of the time. (Adults accepted these "possible anomalies" 91% of the time.) Even when trick photographs depicting these anomalies were shown to the children, preschoolers still accepted fewer anomalies than 6-year-olds (55 and 90%, respectively). At both ages, children consistently distinguished between possible anomalies (such as the rabbit just mentioned) and impossible anomalies (such as "a whale that lives out of water"). Nonetheless, they were rather conservative in their judgments of whether anomalous category members were possible.

Overall, it appears that children have some ability to accept anomalous category members when presented with them, but otherwise tend to discount the possibility of their existence. Children learn to accept anomalous category members later than they learn that categories promote inferences, share nonobvious properties, and have essences.

Division of linguistic labor

There is informal evidence that children may recognize a division of linguistic labor in the meaning and use of category terms. In our previous work (e.g., Gelman & Markman, 1986, 1987; Gelman & Coley, 1990) children accepted the labels provided by the adult experimenter even when they were inconsistent with what they initially thought the names to be. One 2-year-old subject even articulated this principle to his mother after participating in one of our experiments. When discussing a sticklike snake shown in one picture, he said, "I thought it was a stick, but the man [i.e., the experimenter] said it was a snake." This initial understanding that linguistic knowledge may be greater among a subset of the community could arise out of children's early grasp of the asymmetry between children and adults, in both knowledge and authority. Unfortunately, to date we still lack any rigorous investigation of the development of this understanding.

Corrigibility

Theory-laden categories are subject to revision on the basis of new information. If children appreciate the corrigibility of categories, they should be willing to revise initial categorizations on the basis of new discoveries. This ability would include the capacity to accept category anomalies that were originally misclassified. We know of little direct evidence, but we expect this capacity to be late-developing. Corrigibility requires appreciating the limits of one's categories and contrasts with properties such as essentialism that stress the importance of categories for revealing hidden realities about the world. To the extent that one believes a category to be richly structured, nonarbitrary, and reflecting the natural order, it should be difficult to abandon, question, or restructure that category. Moreover, corrigibility implies flexibility, and there is some evidence that early cognitive structures may be relatively inflexible (Inhelder & Piaget, 1964; Keil, 1986, 1987). To examine the issue further, we need studies that provide children with new information that is inconsistent with their present category knowledge and to examine how readily children's categories change to incorporate the new information.

Summary

In this section we have presented evidence that children's natural kind concepts exhibit many of the properties we outlined for adults' natural kind concepts. Specifically, they promote rich inductive inferences, embody knowledge of the importance of unobservable properties, reveal the roots of psychological essentialism, and make some allowance for anomalous members. In the next section, we will outline our proposal for how children's categories come to possess these qualities.

The role of language in children's construction of natural kinds

We have shown that children's natural kind categories exhibit many of the same properties as the natural kinds of adults, although children have little in the way of explicit scientific training. The implication is that children do not require expertise, scientific training, or even an explicit theory to assume that categories are richly structured beyond surface similarity. How is this accomplished?

For adults, there are at least two ways that concepts may go beyond appearances without explicit theory. First, extensive experience can direct one's attention to nonobvious yet informative perceptual cues or feature correlations. For example, expert chick sexers learn to distinguish between male and female day-old chicks on the basis of years of experience with classifying and getting feedback from experts (Biederman & Shiffrar, 1987). They do not have an explicit biological theory to guide their classification. Rather, they learn the exceedingly subtle perceptual cues by extensive exposure and feedback. Given children's lack of extensive experience, perceptual learning does not offer a promising account of children's early appreciation of natural kinds, although it probably plays an increasing role in later development.

Second, conceptual change can be induced in adults without theory via language, without extensive knowledge or perceptual learning. For example, suppose that you initially believe that bamboo plants are members of the category *tree*. On learning that bamboo is actually a grass, you may modify your conceptual structure to classify bamboo as having deeper properties in common with other grasses than with trees (e.g., stem structure and rate of growth). This change would not necessarily be accompanied by any theoretical understanding of why bamboo is a grass.[6] Nor would it necessarily result from learning subtle perceptual distinctions – via either theory or pure experience – that betray bamboo's true identity. Rather, the label *grass* conveys the category identity. The assumption is that certain named categories capture deep similarities despite outward appearances and despite the nature of one's particular theory.

To what extent do children use language to help construct natural kind categories? There are two extreme models that may characterize the role of language in children's understanding of natural kinds. According to a *conceptual* position, language has no role in the way children organize their knowledge and experience; at most it reflects a conceptual understanding, but it does not shape it. In contrast, a *linguistic* position holds that language is the primary source of information about the structure of the world. On this view, children assume that things called by the same name are natural kinds, sharing deep similarities and a category essence. Words are primary; concepts are molded to fit the language.

Neither extreme position can account for the available data. We have already seen that providing a label can alter the way children reason about an object, thus arguing against the conceptual position. For example, calling a pterodactyl a "dinosaur" leads children to infer that it does not live in a nest, whereas without the name children assume that it does (Gelman & Coley, 1990). At the same time, words sometimes fail to promote inferences for children (see, e.g., the adjectives used in Gelman & Coley, 1990), thus arguing against a strong linguistic position. Indeed, there are many words in the adult language that children must at some point learn to distinguish from natural kind terms, including homonyms (*bat*), superordinates (*furniture*), simple adjectives (*striped*), and metaphors (*mouse*).

We hypothesize that children have several expectations that jointly determine when a word maps onto such a richly structured category. Without evidence to the contrary, children will assume that an object word maps onto a natural kind category. They will make this assumption as long as the set of objects named by the word is reasonably coherent (excluding, e.g., *red things*). Once children determine that a word names a natural kind, this conclusion is fairly robust and will persist even when they encounter anomalies that would seem to contradict the grouping. The coherence of the category plus the belief in hidden underlying similarities allows children to accept anomalies that are explicitly presented. For example, once a child decides that *bird* maps onto a natural kind category, when learning that a dodo is a bird the child will assume that it is the same kind of thing as other birds (an otherwise coherent category consisting of robins, sparrows, etc.). Thus, language is critical for reorganizing or restructuring categories away from groupings based on similarity alone. Objects that might otherwise not be considered members of a category will be classified (or reclassified) once the name is learned. In contrast, if a category lacks coherence when it is initially learned, then a child will not assume that the new word maps onto a natural kind. For example, a child will not consider *mammal* a natural kind term if it labels a diverse group including aardvarks, wallabies, bison, and ferrets.

Thus, children's expectations can be viewed as an interplay of three distinct assumptions. On this account, children's understanding of natural kinds is both linguistically and conceptually based. We are not saying that language determines the categories children have. Rather, children have certain expectations about categories and how they are named. These expectations together influence the nature of the categories a child constructs.

Hypothesis 1: Natural kind assumption

First, we propose that children assume that every object is a member of some natural kind category (i.e., with an underlying essence, potential to promote inferences, nonobvious properties, etc.). This can be thought of as a *theory placeholder* view (analogous to the *essence placeholder* notion of Medin & Ortony, 1989). The claim is that children have a broad expectation that objects will fall into kinds and that these kinds will share theoretically important properties whether or not those properties are currently known. The expectation that categories will have a deeper theoretical basis may precede the actually filling out of the substance of the theory. Hearing a name for the first time should be enough evidence for a child to infer that it is a natural kind term. However, this assumption is also possible without language and may operate prelinguistically (see Baldwin, Markman, & Melartin, 1989, for evidence that infants make inductions from unnamed categories).

Evidence. As detailed in the preceding section, preschool children treat a wide range of categories as having an essence, rich inductive potential, and nonobvious features. Even wholly novel categories can serve as the basis for induction (Davidson & Gelman, 1990). Evidence that children hold a general assumption that objects fall into natural kinds comes from the finding that children overgeneralize the inductive potential of categories. Recall that some categories – particularly simple artifact categories (e.g., *chairs, hammers*) – have few if any theory-laden properties. We would expect artifact categories to promote many fewer inferences than natural kind categories (see S. A. Gelman, 1988, for a discussion). Indeed, elementary school children and adults draw many fewer inferences within artifact categories (e.g., *televisions* or *cups*) than within natural kinds (e.g., *rabbits* or *flowers*). However, preschool children tend not to distinguish them, at times overgeneralizing their inductions from artifacts (S. A. Gelman, 1988; Gelman & O'Reilly, 1988). For example, preschool children are as likely to infer that different chairs have the same internal substance as they are to infer that different dogs have the same internal substance. It seems that young children have a general assumption that all objects belong to natural kind categories, an assumption that gets refined with age.

Hypothesis 2: Linguistic transparency

We hypothesize that children assume that every natural kind has a name and that names convey category membership and all the properties that go along with category membership. Coupled with the natural kind assumption, this implies that certain words may function like Kuhnian paradigms: "object[s] for further articulation and specification under new or more stringent conditions" (Kuhn, 1970, p. 23). That is, a word can serve to stake out a new category, which then must be explored in more depth, a "lure for cognition" (Brown, 1956).

Although there is no direct evidence that children assume that all natural kinds are encoded in language, clearly they do assume that at least some natural kinds are expressed in words. This is evident in the way words modify children's conceptions of the objects being labeled. As shown earlier, children draw inferences on the basis of familiar category labels. Without a label, they may decide that a dodo does not live in a nest; if they are told that it is a bird, they declare that it does. In a very real sense, then, our natural kinds are passed down to children through the language we speak. The naming practices of the culture are fundamental to the content of our natural kinds.

Hypothesis 3: Coherence

Children appear to assume that membership in a natural kind category is typically reflected in outward signs (i.e., those properties that are immediately apparent, including appearances and salient behaviors or traits). Objects that are more alike in a Roschian sense (Rosch, 1978) are more likely to share an essence. So, for example, objects with similar shapes, parts, functions, and textures would, on the child's first guess, probably belong to the same natural kind category.[7] The implication is that basic-level categories are likely to be natural kinds. At the same time, however, similarity is at best only a fallible guide to natural kind identity. Thus, similarity serves as a heuristic rather than a defining basis.

It is important to note that coherence operates on a category taken as a whole, not on individual instances. Thus, if trying to determine whether to draw an inference from Object A to Object B, a child would not simply calculate the similarity between the two objects. Rather, the child would determine whether A and B belong to members of the same natural kind category, using as a guide the coherence of the category that encompasses both A and B. If A and B receive the same name, the child could start by calculating the coherence of the category that receives that name, to determine whether it is a natural kind. Thus, even a very anomalous object could be a member of a highly coherent category (e.g., *dogs* may be considered highly coherent, even if a child also comes across a chihuahua). Or if two objects are highly similar but are known to belong to different natural kinds (e.g., a bird and a pterodactyl), children will not try to calculate the coherence of the grouping that includes both birds and pterodactyls and so will not assume that they have underlying properties in common.

Evidence. Children are aware that more coherent categories provide a better basis for induction than less coherent categories. Within a hierarchy, basic-level categories (e.g., *chairs*) are more coherent than superordinate-level categories (e.g., *furniture*) (see Waxman, Chapter 4, this volume). In one study (Gelman & O'Reilly, 1988), preschoolers, second-graders, and adults drew many inferences at the basic level and significantly fewer inferences at the superordinate level. When taught a new property of a familiar object (e.g., "This dog has leukocytes all through it"), they readily drew inductions to members of the same basic-level category (e.g., inferring that other dogs also have leukocytes inside). However, they drew few inferences to members of the same superordinate-level category (e.g., inferring that other animals – horses and snakes – have leukocytes inside) even when they were all explicitly labeled *animals*. (All items were pretested to make certain that even the youngest subjects knew both the basic- and superordinate-level names of these pictures.) For example, children tended to deny that a horse or a snake would have leukocytes inside like the dog, even when all three were repeatedly called *animals*.

There were also developmental differences, with preschoolers showing the most dramatic difference between basic and superordinate level. Thus, preschoolers showed the strongest tendency to distinguish coherent from less coherent categories. These results are consistent with the results of Carey (1985) and Inagaki and Sugiyama (1988), who also found few superordinate-level inferences (from the categories *animals* and *living things*) but did not provide labels for these categories. It may be that superordinate categories are more coherent for older children and adults than for younger children (Murphy & Medin, 1985).

More evidence for the importance of coherence comes from a series of studies by Davidson and Gelman (1990) examining children's inductive inferences within novel categories such as gnulike animals with trunks. The major finding was that category labels affected whether children drew inferences, but only when the words mapped onto coherent categories. There were two ways this could happen. First, a category could inherit coherence by means of language, when a set of novel pictures was named by a familiar natural kind term. For example, children drew many more inferences from one object to another when both were called "cows" than when both were called "zavs." Presumably, the category *cow* is already coherent, whereas the category *zav* is not. Second, a category gained coherence when there was some correspondence between the way sets of objects were named and their appearances. When naming and perceptual similarity were completely orthogonal to one another (e.g., when "zavs" were as dissimilar from each other as they were from "feps"), children ignored the labels and based their inferences strictly on appearances. However, when there was even a slight correlation between naming and appearance ("zavs" were more similar overall than were "zavs" and "feps"), children used both the labels and appearances as the basis of their inferences. It was not the similarity of pictures taken individually that determined whether children used a word as the basis of induction, but rather the coherence of the set of pictures given the same name. Thus, conceptual grasp of the category being named, and not just the label itself, influences children's expectations about a label.

In short, we propose that children start with an assumption about *categories*, that they are natural kinds and that natural kind categories are typically signaled by appearances. Children then look for words that express these categories. Once a word is found that expresses a natural kind, it can help organize new information, promote inferences, and so on. Note that children do not have a completely general assumption about language per se, but rather about how language and categorization interact.

When is a category coherent?

There is a critical interplay between coherence and linguistic transparency. Consider category anomalies, such as penguins. We might not at first include penguins within the *bird* category, but given the appropriate linguistic information we are willing to stretch the category to include them. So language can identify members of a category when appearances would not. Yet if the amount of stretching required is too great (e.g., stretching the *bat* category to include both flying bats and baseball bats), then linguistic transparency is overcome by lack of coherence.[8] A crucial question that remains concerns how the difficult cases get decided – how powerful is language, how powerful is conceptual coherence? At the least, we know that language can stretch (and compress) a category beyond what its boundaries would be on a purely nonlinguistic basis.

At this point we are just beginning to understand what category coherence consists of. However, it seems clear that three factors in particular could be especially useful in helping children determine whether a category is coherent: language form, parental input, and prototypes.

Language form. Language form ("part of speech") can give children a clue as to whether the category named is theory-laden. In particular, common nouns are much more likely to refer to theory-laden categories than are adjectives (see Markman, 1989, for a more detailed discussion of this possibility). If children are sensitive to linguistic form, then simply by knowing that *white* is an adjective and not a noun, a child could rule out the possibility that the class of *white things* is a theory-laden category. Certainly with familiar words, common nouns have a privileged position and promote many more inferences than adjectives (Gelman & Coley, 1990; Gelman et al., 1986).

Although we have no evidence concerning whether children would attend to language form per se to determine whether a completely novel word maps onto a natural kind (e.g., to determine that a "fep" could refer to a member of a natural kind, but a "fep one" could not), we do know that children from $1\frac{1}{2}$ years of age onward are sufficiently sensitive to linguistic form to distinguish a variety of parts of speech (Brown, 1957; Gelman & Markman, 1985; Gelman & Taylor, 1984; Gelman, Wilcox, & Clark, 1989; Gordon, 1985; Katz, Baker, & Macnamara, 1974; Taylor & Gelman, 1988, 1989; Waxman, 1990; Chapter 4, this volume).

Input. Parental naming strategies (the context in which a word is used; the range of exemplars selected when the name is used) could provide indirect cues as to which names are natural kind terms. For example, the way superordinates are introduced suggests that they are less central to the identity of an object than are basic-level terms. In particular, parents "anchor" superordinates at the basic level (e.g., when teaching *animal,* parents are more apt to say, "This is a cat; it is an animal" than simply "This is an animal") and generally fail to use superordinates to name just a single object (Blewitt, 1983; Callanan, 1989). Moreover, children's assumptions about the input may combine with the variations in input (Callanan, 1989). In this way, different ways of speaking to children may do more than teach new vocabulary; they may be a means of marking which words map onto richly structured natural kinds.

Prototypes. Finally, the order in which category exemplars are introduced or assimilated could determine whether children treat a concept as richly structured. If a child first considers just the prototypical members of a category (e.g., for *birds*: robins, sparrows, and wrens), the category will be more coherent (see Mervis & Pani, 1980, for an excellent empirical demonstration of this phenomenon). Therefore, the child should be more likely to treat the category as a natural kind. In contrast, if the child is first introduced to all the anomalous and peripheral category members (e.g., parrots, hummingbirds, and flamingoes), the category may seem to lack sufficient coherence to be a natural kind. In this sense, prototypes may have functional utility: Children's notorious difficulty in learning atypical category members (see Mervis & Rosch, 1981, for a review) could help keep categories coherent and so enable children to determine more quickly when they are natural kinds.

Summary

We hypothesize several components, acting in combination, that may contribute to children's expectation that certain words map onto categories that are richly structured and inference-promoting. In the absence of conflict among them, the default is that the category name refers to a richly structured, inference-promoting category (*natural kind assumption* and *linguistic transparency*). However, this default can be overridden if the word fails to map onto a coherent category (*coherence assumption*). Children also gather additional clues from the linguistic form in which a word is embedded, the structure of the input that children hear, and the order in which category instances are introduced or assimilated (with children's presumption of prototypes playing an important role). Although not all the evidence is in, preliminary results support the promise of this framework.

Summary and conclusions

In this chapter we have examined the interrelations between language, concepts, and the world in the developing child. By studying natural kind categories we have provided a test case of the more general question of how language structures thought. Language helps structure children's categories, but the influence is subtle and works within the context of children's nonlinguistic understanding.

We began the chapter by endorsing the claim that the everyday categories of adults, like the most sophisticated categories of scientists, are informed and held together by theories. This is a proposition that has recently received much support and is certainly not our own idea. From there, however, we went on to suggest six properties of theory-laden categories: They have a nonobvious basis, promote inductive inferences, are thought to embody an essence, incorporate anomalous members, observe division of linguistic labor, and are subject to revision. We argued that adults' categories vary in the extent to which they embody these properties and accordingly vary in the degree to which they are theory-laden. Natural kind categories seem to be the best examples of theory-laden categories for adults, embodying all of these properties.

Next, we applied this framework to children's categories, arguing that despite the fact that children lack an extensive knowledge base, their natural kind concepts exhibit many of the properties that characterize adults' natural kinds. Our work, and the work of many others, leads to the conclusion that many of children's categories promote inductive inferences, incorporate nonobvious properties, and reveal psychological essentialism. The jury is still out on the remaining three properties, but to a lesser degree children accept some category anomalies and may observe division of linguistic labor.

In the final section, we sketched how children's categories may come to function as though they were theory-laden despite children's relatively sparse scientific knowledge. We proposed that by preschool age children have three general assumptions about language, concepts, and their interaction, which lead to the construction of natural kind categories. Most importantly, children assume that every object belongs to a natural kind and that common nouns can convey natural kind status (as well as their accompanying properties). Much more work is needed to test this framework, fill in the details, and examine it from a developmental perspective. Nonetheless, the preliminary evidence to date is supportive.

In sum, what does language – in particular, naming – do? Names are the embodiments of our theories. We form theories about the structure of the world, encode these theories in language, and pass them down to children. Language, then, is an extremely powerful tool for passing on the knowledge and beliefs of one's culture. Moreover, names encourage children to make inferences, search for nonobvious similarities, and stretch their knowledge far beyond what they have been taught directly. In this sense, language encourages children to seek out and discover for themselves deeper explanations of their world.

Notes

1. Actual sizes were computed separately for each subject and fell midway between the values the subject had given for the largest quarter and the smallest pizza.
2. Although it is still an open question as to precisely what constitutes a theory, Murphy and Medin (1985) suggest that theories have the following properties: (a) They explain some domain of phenomena, (b) they simplify reality, (c) they fit in with, or at least do not contradict, what we already know, (d) they have a complex internal structure (i.e., properties are interrelated), and (e) they interact with incoming data and ongoing observations. The implication is that concepts cannot be viewed individually, but are understood only within a larger web of interrelated beliefs and other concepts.
3. These studies have also been criticized for task demands that underestimate children's categorization knowledge; see Gelman and Baillargeon (1983) and Markman and Callanan (1984).
4. All of the properties used in this study were ones that in fact generalize to the entire category. Later we discuss children's sensitivity to properties that vary in how readily they promote inferences for adults.

5. Unlike previous studies, this experiment tested children on properties that were already well known for prototypical category members. Thus, the question arises as to whether the children were making inductive or deductive inferences. We believe that children's inferences can be characterized as inductive, because the atypical instances queried were novel (e.g., before entering the experiment the children did not know that dodo birds are birds or that pterodactyls are not birds), thus requiring inferences beyond what the children already knew with certainty. Furthermore, although the children themselves may have constructed more general arguments (e.g., "All birds live in nests") from which deductive inferences could be drawn (e.g., "This [dodo bird] is a bird, so it too lives in a nest"), the construction of the general argument would itself have required an induction from the available evidence. See Gelman and Coley (1990) for more detailed discussion.
6. Note that although both perceptual learning and labeling may yield category change in the absence of theory, they can also induce more far-reaching theory change. That is, they may induce change not only in children's beliefs as to which entities are category members, but also in more fundamental beliefs concerning what is central to the category.
7. We are not proposing that children possess a theory-independent sense of similarity or coherence. Rather, certain properties are assumed to be privileged from an early age (see R. Gelman, 1987; Medin & Wattenmaker, 1987).
8. Ontological constraints may play a large role in determining when to override linguistic transparency (see Keil, 1979).

References

Atran, S. (1987a). Origin of the species and genus concepts: An anthropological perspective. *Journal of the History of Biology, 20,* 195–279.
Atran, S. (1987b). Ordinary constraints on the semantics of living kinds: A commonsense alternative to recent treatments of natural-object terms. *Mind and Language, 2,* 27–63.
Baldwin, D. A., Markman, E. M., & Melartin, R. (1989, April). *Infants' inferential abilities: Evidence from exploratory play.* Paper presented at the biennial meeting of the Society for Research in Child Development, Kansas City, MO.
Barsalou, L. W. (1983). Ad hoc categories. *Memory and Cognition, 11,* 211–227.
Biderman, C. A. (1989, April). *Flexibility of children's animal and artifact categories when judging anomalous objects' possible existence.* Paper presented at the biennial meeting of the Society for Research in Child Development, Kansas City, MO.
Biederman, I., & Shiffrar, M. M. (1987). Sexing day-old chicks: A case study and expert systems analysis of a difficult perceptual-learning task. *Journal of Experiment Psychology: Learning, Memory, and Cognition, 13,* 640–645.
Blewitt, P. (1983). Dog versus collie: Vocabulary in speech to young children. *Developmental Psychology, 19,* 602–609.
Brown, R. W. (1956). Language and categories. Appendix to J. S. Bruner,

J. J. Goodnow, & G. A. Austin, *A study of thinking* (pp. 247–312). New York: Wiley.

Brown, R. W. (1957). Linguistic determinism and the part of speech. *Journal of Abnormal and Social Psychology, 55*, 1–5.

Bruner, J. S., Goodnow, J. J., & Austin, G. A. (1956). *A study of thinking.* New York: Wiley.

Bruner, J. S., Olver, R. R., & Greenfield, P. M. (1967). *Studies in cognitive growth.* New York: Wiley.

Callanan, M. A. (1989). Development of object categories and inclusion relations: Preschoolers' hypotheses about word meanings. *Developmental Psychology, 25*, 207–216.

Carey, S. (1982). Semantic development: The state of the art. In E. Wanner & L. R. Gleitman (Eds.), *Language acquisition: The state of the art* (pp. 347–389). Cambridge University Press.

Carey, S. (1985). *Conceptual change in childhood.* Cambridge, MA: MIT Press.

Chi, M. T., Feltovich, P. J., & Glaser, R. (1981). Categorization and representation of physics problems by experts and novices. *Cognitive Science, 5*, 121–152.

Davidson, N. S., & Gelman, S. A. (1990). Inductions from novel categories: The role of language and conceptual structure. *Cognitive Development, 5*, 151–176.

DeLoache, J. S., & Todd, C. M. (1988, March). *Spatial organization as an early memory strategy.* Paper presented at the Conference on Human Development, Charleston, SC.

Dolgin, K., & Behrend, D. (1984). Children's knowledge about animates and inanimates. *Child Development, 55*, 1646–1650.

Dupré, J. (1981). Natural kinds and biological taxa. *Philosophical Review, 40*, 66–90.

Flavell, J. (1963). *The developmental psychology of Jean Piaget.* New York: Van Nostrand.

Flavell, J. (1977). *Cognitive development.* Englewood Cliffs, NJ: Prentice-Hall.

Gelman, R. (1987, August). *Cognitive development: Principles guide learning and contribute to conceptual coherence.* Paper presented at the meeting of the American Psychological Association, Division 1, New York.

Gelman, R., & Baillargeon, R. (1983). A review of some Piagetian concepts. In J. H. Flavell & E. M. Markman (Eds.), *Cognitive development* (Vol. 3, pp. 167–230, of P. H. Mussen [Gen. Ed.], *Handbook of child psychology*). New York: Wiley.

Gelman, R., Spelke, E. S., & Meck, E. (1983). What preschoolers know about animate and inanimate objects. In D. Rogers & J. A. Sloboda (Eds.), *The acquisition of symbolic skills* (pp. 297–324). New York: Plenum.

Gelman, S. A. (1988). The development of induction within natural kind and artifact categories. *Cognitive Psychology, 20*, 65–95.

Gelman, S. A., & Coley, J. D. (1989, April). *Relations between categorical and perceptual similarity.* Paper presented at the biennial meeting of the Society for Research in Child Development, Kansas City, MO.

Gelman, S. A., & Coley, J. D. (1990). The importance of knowing a dodo is a bird: Categories and inferences in two-year-olds. *Developmental Psychology, 26*, 796–804.

Gelman, S. A., Collman, P., & Maccoby, E. E. (1986). Inferring properties from categories versus inferring categories from properties: The case of gender. *Child Development, 57*, 396–404.

Gelman, S. A., & Markman, E. M. (1985). Implicit contrast in adjectives vs. nouns: Implications for word-learning in preschoolers. *Journal of Child Language, 12,* 125–143.

Gelman, S. A., & Markman, E. M. (1986). Categories and induction in young children. *Cognition, 23,* 183–209.

Gelman, S. A., & Markman, E. M. (1987). Young children's inductions from natural kinds: The role of categories and appearances. *Child Development, 58,* 1532–1541.

Gelman, S. A., & O'Reilly, A. W. (1988). Children's inductive inferences within superordinate categories: The role of language and category structure. *Child Development, 59,* 876–887.

Gelman, S. A., & Taylor, M. (1984). How two-year-old children interpret proper and common names for unfamiliar objects. *Child Development, 55,* 1535–1540.

Gelman, S. A., & Wellman, H. M. (in press). Insides and essences: Early understandings of the non-obvious. *Cognition.*

Gelman, S. A., Wilcox, S. A., & Clark, E. V. (1989). Conceptual and lexical hierarchies in young children. *Cognitive Development, 4,* 309–326.

Ghiselin, M. T. (1969). *The triumph of the Darwinian method.* Chicago: University of Chicago Press.

Goodman, N. (1972). Seven strictures on similarity. In *Problems and projects* (pp. 437–447). Indianapolis, IN: Bobbs-Merrill.

Goosens, W. K. (1977). Underlying trait terms. In S. P. Schwartz (Ed.), *Naming, necessity, and natural kinds* (pp. 133–154). Ithaca, NY: Cornell University Press.

Gordon, P. (1985). Evaluating the semantic categories hypothesis: The case of the count/mass distinction. *Cognition, 20,* 209–242.

Gould, S. J. (1989). *Wonderful life.* New York: Norton.

Holland, J. H., Holyoak, K. J., Nisbett, R. E., & Thagard, P. R. (1986). *Induction: Processes of inferences, learning, and discovery.* Cambridge, MA: MIT Press.

Inagaki, K., & Sugiyama, K. (1988). Attributing human characteristics: Developing changes in over- and underattribution. *Cognitive Development, 3,* 55–70.

Inhelder, B., & Piaget, J. (1964). *The early growth of logic in the child.* New York: Norton.

Jevons, W. S. (1877). *The principles of science* (2nd ed.). New York: Macmillan.

Katz, N., Baker, E., & Macnamara, J. (1974). What's in a name? A study of how children learn common and proper names. *Child Development, 45,* 469–473.

Keil, F. C. (1979). *Semantic and conceptual development.* Cambridge, MA: Harvard University Press.

Keil, F. C. (1986). The acquisition of natural kind and artifact terms. In W. Demopoulos & A. Marras (Eds.), *Language learning and concept acquisition* (pp. 133–153). Norwood, NJ: Ablex.

Keil, F. C. (1987). Conceptual development and category structure. In U. Neisser (Ed.), *Concepts and conceptual development: Ecological and intellectual factors in categorization* (pp. 175–200). Cambridge University Press.

Keil, F. C., & Batterman, N. (1984). A characteristic-to-defining shift in the development of word meaning. *Journal of Verbal Learning and Verbal Behavior, 23,* 221–236.

Kelly, M. H. (1989). *Darwin and psychological theories of classification.* Unpublished manuscript, University of Pennsylvania, Philadelphia.

Knight, D. (1981). *Ordering the world, a history of classifying man.* London: Burnett Books.

Kolstad, V., & Baillargeon, R. (1989). *Context-dependent perceptual and functional categorization in $10\frac{1}{2}$-month-old-infants.* Unpublished manuscript, University of Illinois, Champaign.

Kremer, K. E., & Gelman, S. A. (1989, April). *Children's causal explanations of the origins and structure of natural kinds and artifacts.* Paper presented at the biennial meeting of the Society for Research in Child Development, Kansas City, MO.

Kripke, S. (1971). Identity and necessity. In M. K. Munitz (Ed.), *Identity and individuation* (pp. 135–164). New York: New York University Press.

Kripke, S. (1972). *Naming and necessity.* Cambridge, MA: Harvard University Press.

Kuhn, T. S. (1970). *The structure of scientific revolutions.* Chicago: University of Chicago Press.

Lively, W. J., & Bromley, D. B. (1973). *Person perception in childhood and adolescence.* New York: Wiley.

Locke, J. (1965). *An essay concerning human understanding.* New York: Macmillan. (Originally published in 1706.)

Markman, E. M. (1989). *Categorization and naming in children: Problems of induction.* Cambridge, MA: MIT Press.

Markman, E. M., & Callanan, M. A. (1984). An analysis of hierarchical classification. In R. Sternberg (Ed.), *Advances in the psychology of human intelligence* (Vol. 2, pp. 325–365). Hillsdale, NJ: Erlbaum.

Massey, C. M., & Gelman, R. (1988). Preschooler's ability to decide whether a photographed unfamiliar object can move itself. *Developmental Psychology, 24,* 307–317.

Mayr, E. (1957). Species concepts and definitions. In E. Mayr (Ed.), *The species problem* (Publication No. 50, pp. 1–22). Washington DC: American Association for the Advancement of Science.

Mayr, E. (1988). *Toward a new philosophy of biology: Observations of an evolutionist.* Cambridge, MA: Harvard University Press.

Medin, D. (1989). Concepts and conceptual structure. *American Psychologist, 44,* 1469–1481.

Medin, D., & Ortony, A. (1989). Psychological essentialism. In S. Vosniadou & A. Ortony (Eds.), *Similarity and analogical reasoning* (pp. 179–195). Cambridge University Press.

Medin, D. L., & Wattenmaker, W. D. (1987). Category cohesiveness, theories, and cognitive archeology. In U. Neisser (Ed.), *Concepts and conceptual development: Ecological and intellectual factors in categorization* (pp. 25–62). Cambridge University Press.

Mervis, C. B., & Pani, J. R. (1980). Acquisition of basic object categories. *Cognitive Psychology, 12,* 496–522.

Mervis, C. B., & Rosch, E. (1981). Categorization of natural objects. *Annual Review of Psychology, 32,* 89–115.

Mill, J. S. (1843). *A system of logic, ratiocinative and inductive.* London: Longman Group.

Miller, G. A., & Johnson-Laird, P. W. (1976). *Language and perception.* Cambridge, MA: Harvard University Press.

Morris, B. (1979). Symbolism as ideology: Thoughts around Navaho taxonomy and symbolism. In R. F. Ellen & D. Reason (Eds.), *Classifications in their social context* (pp. 117–138). New York: Academic Press.

Murphy, G. L., & Medin, D. L. (1985). The role of theories in conceptual coherence. *Psychological Review, 92,* 289–316.

Neisser, U. (1987). Introduction: The ecological and intellectual bases of categorization. In U. Neisser (Ed.), *Concepts and conceptual development: Ecological and intellectual factors in categorization* (pp. 1–10). Cambridge University Press.

Nelson, K. (1974). Concept, word, and sentence: Interrelations in acquisition and development. *Psychological Review, 81,* 267–285.

Peevers, B. H., & Secord, P. C. (1973). Developmental changes in attribution of descriptive concepts to children. *Journal of Personality and Social Psychology, 27,* 120–128.

Piaget, J. (1970). Piaget's theory. In P. H. Mussen (Ed.), *Carmichael's manual of child psychology* (pp. 703–732). New York: Wiley.

Putnam, H. (1962). The analytic and the synthetic. In *Minnesota studies in the philosophy of science: Vol. 3.* Minneapolis: University of Minnesota Press.

Putnam, H. (1970). Is semantics possible? In H. E. Kiefer & M. K. Munitz (Eds.), *Language, beliefs, and metaphysics* (pp. 50–63). Albany, NY: State University of New York Press.

Putnam, H. (1973). Meaning and reference. *Journal of Philosophy, 70,* 699–711.

Quine, W. V. (1969). Natural kinds. In W. V. Quine (Ed.), *Ontological relativity and other essays* (pp. 114–138). New York: Columbia University Press.

Quine, W. V. (1974). *The roots of reference.* La Salle, IL: Open Court.

Richards, D. D., & Siegler, R. S. (1984). The effects of task requirements on children's abilities to make life judgments. *Child Development, 55,* 1687–1696.

Richards, D. D., & Siegler, R. S. (1986). Children's understanding of the attributes of life. *Journal of Experimental Child Psychology, 42,* 1–22.

Rips, L. J. (1989). Similarity, typicality, and categorization. In S. Vosniadou & A. Ortony (Eds.), *Similarity and analogical reasoning* (pp. 21–59). Cambridge University Press.

Rosch, E. (1978). Principles of categorization. In E. Rosch & B. B. Lloyd (Eds.), *Cognition and categorization* (pp. 27–48). Hillsdale, NJ: Erlbaum.

Rosch, E., & Mervis, C. B. (1975). Family resemblances: Studies in the internal structure of categories. *Cognitive Psychology, 7,* 573–605.

Ruse, M. (1969). Definitions of species in biology. *British Journal of Philosophy of Science, 20,* 97–119.

Salmon, N. (1981). *Reference and essence.* Princeton, NJ: Princeton University Press.

Schwartz, S. P. (1977). Introduction. In S. P. Schwartz (Ed.), *Naming, necessity, and natural kinds* (pp. 13–41). Ithaca, NY: Cornell University Press.

Schwartz, S. P. (1979). Natural kind terms. *Cognition, 7,* 301–315.

Siegler, R. S. (1989). Commentary. *Human Development, 32,* 104–109.

Skyrms, B. (1975). *Choice and chance: An introduction to inductive logic* (2nd ed.). Encino, CA: Dickenson.

Smiley, S. S., & Brown, A. L. (1979). Conceptual preference for thematic or taxonomic relations: A nonmonotonic age trend from preschool to old age. *Journal of Experimental Child Psychology, 28,* 249–257.

Smith, E. E., & Medin, D. L. (1981). *Categories and concepts.* Cambridge, MA: Harvard University Press.

Smith, L. B., & Kemler, D. G. (1977). Developmental trends in free classification: Evidence for a new conceptualization of perceptual development. *Journal of Experimental Child Psychology, 24,* 279–298.

Sokal, R. R. (1977). Classification: Purposes, principles, progress, prospects. In P. N. Johnson-Laird & P. C. Wason (Eds.), *Thinking: Readings in cognitive science* (pp. 185–198). Cambridge University Press.

Springer, K., & Keil, F. C. (1989). On the development of biologically specific beliefs: The case of inheritance. *Child Development, 60,* 637–648.

Taylor, M., & Gelman, S. A. (1988). Adjectives and nouns: Children's strategies for learning new words. *Child Development, 59,* 411–419.

Taylor, M., & Gelman, S. A. (1989). Incorporating new words into the lexicon: Preliminary evidence for language hierarchies in two-year-old children. *Child Development, 60,* 625–636.

Vygotsky, L. S. (1962). *Thought and language.* New York: Wiley.

Waxman, S. R. (1990). Linguistic biases and the establishment of conceptual hierarchies: Evidence from preschool children. *Cognitive Development, 5,* 123–150.

Wellman, H. M., & Estes, D. (1986). Early understanding of mental entities: A reexamination of childhood realism. *Child Development, 57,* 910–923.

Wellman, H. M., & Gelman, S. A. (1988). Children's understanding of the nonobvious. In R. J. Sternberg (Ed.), *Advances in the psychology of human intelligence* (Vol. 4, pp. 99–135). Hillsdale, NJ: Erlbaum.

Wimmer, H., & Perner, J. (1983). Beliefs about beliefs: Representation and constraining function of wrong beliefs in young children's understanding of deception. *Cognition, 13,* 103–128.

6. Theories, concepts, and the acquisition of word meaning

FRANK C. KEIL

Introduction

A new emphasis has emerged in the literature on concepts and concept acquisition. There is now a strong focus on the role of theories and other explanatory belief systems in structuring concepts and conceptual change. A series of recent studies on adult concepts (e.g., Medin & Wattenmaker, 1987; Murphy and Medin, 1985; Rips, 1989) and a rediscovery of older work, such as Asch (1946), Luchins (1957), and Chapman and Chapman (1969), as well as developmental analyses (e.g., Carey, 1985; Keil, 1986, 1989; Wellman & Gelman, 1988), reveal the vital importance of theorylike beliefs in understanding concept structure and development. At roughly the same time, and for subtly related reasons, there has been a resurgence of interest in domain specificity of knowledge in cognitive development, with the consequence that researchers are now wondering whether the development of knowledge in different theoretical domains might influence concepts in ways that are unique to each domain. This chapter assesses how these two trends link up to help us understand the acquisition of word meaning.

Although the mapping between concept structure and semantic structure is certainly not one to one, as has been clearly illustrated by Clark (1983), neither are the relations random. I will argue that higher structural relations within and across concepts, as well as patterns of conceptual change, can have major and systematic influences on word meanings themselves. In this chapter I explore four aspects of concepts and conceptual change that may be partic-

The preparation of this chapter and some of the research reported herein were supported by NIH Grant 1-R01-HD23922. I thank Susan Gelman and Jim Byrnes for extensive and thoughtful comments on earlier drafts.

ularly relevant to our understanding of semantic development: (a) interdomain differences, (b) causal beliefs versus atheoretical tabulations, (c) differentiation versus sharpening, and (d) the effects of a changing conceptual base on lexical induction. All of these topics are intimately related to issues of the domain specificity and the theory-laden nature of concepts. Because the emphasis on these two issues is relatively recent, by necessity much of this chapter attempts to go beyond limited current empirical findings and suggest likely relations between theories, concepts, and the acquisition of word meaning.

Interdomain differences

Different sorts of kinds (i.e., demarcatable classes of entities) may have different representational formats. If the differences in the structures of kinds are sufficiently dramatic, such differences might well be mirrored in the way they are represented and thereby might result in differences in the way words become attached to such conceptual representations. There has been a long history of claims that the real-world relations responsible for partitioning entities into kinds are not all of the same type (e.g., Aristotle, 1963), which is hardly surprising since such a claim largely amounts to the view that the sorts of regularities that exist in our natural and social worlds are not all structurally equivalent.

One of the clearest contrasts between structural bases for kinds is that between nominal kinds (e.g., triangles, weeks, and islands) and natural kinds (e.g., dogs, gold, and water). Locke (1690/1964) went to considerable lengths in his *Essay Concerning Human Understanding* to lay out the difference between these two kinds and its consequence for their associated mental representations. Locke focused on the question of types of essences associated with kinds, in particular nominal and real essences, and their relations to natural and nominal kinds. His close linkage of perception with knowledge led him to claim that real essences of natural kinds could not be discovered since they could not be perceived. As a consequence, one's only method of representing kinds would involve their nominal essences, which in large part were stipulative definitions agreed to as part of a broader system of social conventions. More informally, the argument seems to be that the deepest principles responsible for natural kinds are unknowable, so the only way to think and talk about such kinds is to agree upon a set of criteria for picking them out; but as shown later, the criteria are not fully arbitrary. Although some (e.g., Dupré, 1981) suggest that the representational format of nominal essences can vary considerably, Locke was quite explicit in choosing to limit it to one specified by singly necessary and jointly sufficient features very much like the "defining features" notion in more current psychological usage (e.g., Smith & Medin, 1981).

Even though natural kinds also have nominal essences, Locke saw them as manifested in different ways than nominal kinds, ways that had potential representational consequences. For triangles and the like, the real essence and the nominal essence are the same; but for natural kinds, they are fundamentally different. Moreover, Locke suggested that the real "insensible" essence is causally responsible for all the perceivable properties that become associated with the nominal essence. Thus, nominal essences for natural kinds are not purely arbitrary assignations of properties to those kinds; they are causal products of real essences, where the real essence and much of the mechanism of causal manifestation may be unknowable. Triangles may also be different from other nominal kinds that are merely stipulative. Thus, many have held that *triangleness* is a preexisting Platonic form that humans have merely apprehended. By contrast, kinds such as *week* may be almost entirely stipulative and a product of social convention. It is in the latter sense that Schwartz (1980) sought to distinguish nominal kinds from natural kinds.

In more recent times, the nominal kind–natural kind contrast has become of increasing interest to psychologists. One related contrast that has received special attention is that between artifacts and natural kinds. Artifacts are often construed as being akin to nominal kinds, because they are rarely thought to have an intrinsic essence (Schwartz, 1980); instead, the intended function of their creator is said to be the primary basis for sorting them into kinds. Since intended function is often driven by social and conventional concerns, there is a similarity to nominal kinds. Lewis (1969), for example, discusses at length how goals and intentions in coordination problems give rise to many conventional structures, including some nominal kinds. Other nominal kinds such as triangles, however, are less dependent on intention and may be discovered abstract entities.

The most relevant psychological claims are that nominal kind concepts have (a) structures that are the same as, or close to, classical definitions consisting of necessary and sufficient features, (b) no representation of an underlying essence that is causally responsible for surface features, and (c) a strong component for all artifacts and many natural kinds that is dependent on human intentions. Thus, there seems to be an "intention as intension" view regarding concepts of artifacts and many nominal kinds, which may be contrasted with concepts that somehow recognize essences for natural kinds. Medin and Ortony (1989) have stressed this idea of an essence that is causally responsible for surface properties, going so far as to suggest that this essentialist bias is an important part of all our concepts. Elsewhere, I have claimed that this bias may be restricted to natural kinds (Keil, 1986). Moreover, Gelman (Gelman, 1988a; Kremer & Gelman, 1989) has shown that even preschoolers make inductions that suggest they assume more shared essential properties for natural kinds than for artifacts. Artifacts here are construed as being on a continuum from natural to nominal kinds, with simple artifacts, such as hammers and rulers, being similar to more intentional nominal kinds, such as bachelors and pets. (This continuum is discussed extensively in Keil, 1989.)

If nominal, natural, and artifact concepts are indeed represented differently because of dissimilar conceptions of the roles of real essence and cause, the consequences for the acquisition of word meanings might be dramatic. For example, for pure nominal kinds, children may come to attach word meanings to the defining features; for artifacts, they might instead finally attach meaning to the intended function of the creator; and for natural kinds, they may ultimately attach lexical meaning to beliefs about hidden essence. Each of these could result in different developmental patterns. The acquisition of nominal kind terms might depend critically on an increasing awareness of a network of social conventions and of the entire idea of stipulative definitions. Accordingly, early on, labels might be largely attached to clusters of typical features and little else. By contrast, with natural kinds, knowledge of social conventions may play a minor role, whereas knowledge of the sorts of causal structures involved in the segregation of entities into such kinds might be critical.

In general, causal relations may be more important in the acquisition of terms for natural kind concepts than those for nominal kinds. With natural kinds, the earliest stages of labeling might be attached either solely to clusters of typical features or, perhaps in a more rudimentary way, also to some beliefs about causal mechanisms responsible for those features. In the case of causal mechanisms, even a young child might regard *dog* as referring to something that not only has all the typical features of dogs but also has nonphenomenal core properties that causally generate the typical ones. Thus, part of the concept *dog* might be the supposition that more essential aspects guide its growth and development into a mature form.

Finally, some awareness of artifacts as being intimately linked to human intentions must come to dominate the meanings of artifact terms; but it is less clear how such an awareness might be involved in the early stages of lexical development. Is there some rudimentary understanding from the earliest ages that the detailed properties of artifacts are ultimately linked to the intentions of their creators, or are they not distinguished from other sorts of kinds? There seems to be increasing evidence that the artifact–natural kinds contrast may be fundamental and emerge very early. For example, in one exploratory study (Keil, 1989), 5-year-olds were fully competent at judging which objects were made by people and which ones occurred on their own, independent of intentional agents. Their performance was especially impressive given that a large percentage of the objects were totally unfamiliar natural kinds and artifacts. Gelman (Gelman, 1988a; Kremer and Gelman, 1989) has found signs of such an awareness in preschoolers as well; and although the links to lexical knowledge are not yet established, these demonstrations support the plausibility of such effects.

There are several ways in which these potential contrasts could be further developed with more elaborate speculations concerning their influence on semantic development, but complexities in making finer distinctions illustrate the need for more empirical work. Consider, for example, distinctions between artifacts and natural kinds. Despite the apparent clarity of the distinction for such things as hammers and herons, there are other members of these kinds with less transparent relations to intention and cause. Plastics, for example, would normally be considered artifacts since they are created by humans, often with particular design principles in mind. Yet their method of construction relies totally on the natural laws of organic and inorganic chemistry, laws that supposedly normally conspire to segregate spontaneously occurring compounds in the world into natural kinds. Moreover, most of their typical salient features are linked causally through well-specified mechanisms to underlying "essences." An even more obvious case would be the synthetic elements such as lawrencium. Although technically artifacts because they are created by humans, they are really "synthetic natural kinds" since they differ from other natural kinds, such as gold, only in terms of being created by humans rather than nature.

There are other cases of natural kinds that take on increasingly artifactlike properties, such as domesticated animals and cultivated plants. Breeding patterns over the centuries have resulted in kinds of animals and plants many of whose most salient properties are direct products of human intentions to enhance, or even create, a certain function in the kind. Hunting dogs, pit bulls, most current livestock, and most commercial produce are good examples.

These exceptions illustrate that the contrasts between natural kinds and artifacts, as well as between these and nominal kinds, are not always simple and easy to draw. Moreover, they suggest that the course of semantic development for their corresponding terms may be different than for most clear-cut cases. There are, nonetheless, strong general tendencies associated with each kind. Natural kinds generally have richer causal structures associated with their features, especially causal structures that are intrinsic to the kinds. To the extent that causal relations are associated with nominal kinds, they tend to be more extrinsic to the kinds and are concerned with explanations of the forces behind their creators' intentions, that is, why people build the artifacts they do and why social, cultural, and ergonomic factors influence such intentions (see Simon, 1981).

Another possible contrast between the kinds may revolve around verbal labels and the causal theory of reference. Putnam (1975) is well known for his statement that for natural kinds, "meaning ain't in the head"; instead, it is a more public phenomenon consisting of appropriate causal chains back to original instances. Putnam makes this point with thought experiments showing that meanings can change when nothing in the head changes and that changes in the head might not change meaning. He discusses nominal kinds in less detail, but seems to leave open the possibility that they do not require such a referential causal chain, such that perhaps their meanings are more in the head.

To be more specific, Putnam shows how John Smith on Earth in 1700 and his doppelgänger on Twin Earth in its 1700 might have identical mental states when saying *water* even though by *water* John Smith means the stuff that is H_2O and his twin means the stuff that has the molecular structure *XYZ*. This is because referential chains back to the initial namings of the two "waters" are linked to their essences, which although not known in 1700 or 1700_{TE}, will prove to be different. By contrast, for things that may not have essences and that are defined more by stipulative meanings, such as a hammer or a triangle, it is more difficult to construct scenarios in which two individuals would have identical mental states but mean different things.

Do any of these potential contrasts have relevance for the way language becomes attached to underlying conceptual structure? Are the semantic representations of nominal kinds fundamentally different because they refer less to causal relations and because they need not ultimately make a referential connection? A better understanding of such questions will require a careful look at the structure of the associated concepts for such kinds and at how those concepts might influence the acquisition and use of language.

In sum, long-standing views on differences between sorts of kinds in the world have in recent years led to increasing speculation that concepts for these kinds may have different sorts of mental structures. To the extent that such conceptual–structural contrasts exist, one would want to examine whether there are corresponding differences in the way their associated word meanings are acquired. These differences could range from whether specific causal links are included in the semantic representations, to whether the earliest representations are like Roschean prototypes, to whether different kinds of feedback are optimal for learning of distinct classes of terms. There are far too many degrees of freedom to speculate here on all the possible outcomes; rather, the point is to suggest there is a reasonable chance that such differences will exist and that they will be an excellent way to explore how concepts and word meanings, though surely not equivalent, are structurally linked.

One particularly intriguing set of future studies may focus on terms that are ambiguous as to whether they refer to natural kinds or nominal kinds and may then examine whether, given biasing contexts of one of the two types, patterns of acquisition and the eventual representations are different. Different biases might result in the same set of surface features being encoded semantically in dramatically different ways. For example, causal relations might be central in one case but intention might be central in another. Thus, will different forms of semantic representation arise as a result of a "contextual set" that implies either artifact or natural kind, but nothing else?

What effects does "cause" have on the lexicon?

Assuming that conceptual knowledge is, in some sense, a vast interconnected set of relations, the question arises as to whether words can be arbitrarily mapped on any aspect of that structure or whether certain kinds of structural configurations can act as "magnets" for semantic labels. Such an account would require either that the internal structure of concepts be heterogeneous, such that different sorts of internal parts could have potentially different effects on word meaning, or that the concepts themselves be of different structural types. One result of the recent work emphasizing the importance of theory in understanding the nature of concept structure has been the realization that a full specification of the structure of at least some concepts, that is, those for natural kinds, will critically involve causal relations. This has raised the broader question of how causal relations should figure in concept structure and, ultimately, how causal relations might influence the manner in which linguistic labels are attached to the underlying concept structure. To be of interest, this question must assume that causal relations can be contrasted with a different facet of concept structure.

Recent empirical research strongly supports the proposal of heterogeneous structure within individual concepts. For example, Medin and Shoben (1988) have shown that high typicality and high centrality do not have an equivalent influence on concept structure. Thus, curvedness, although equally typical of bananas and boomerangs, is causally considered to be much more central to the concept of a boomerang. Consequently, straight boomerangs are considered to be much more marginal members of the boomerang category than straight bananas are of the banana category. Rips (1989) has made a similar argument concerning the contrast between mere typicality and deeper relational structure. Others, such as Gentner (1983), although not explicitly invoking causal relations, argue strongly that concept structure must include a deeper relational structure than is normally observed in typicality distributions.

Finally, in a recent series of studies with Chris Johnson (Johnson & Keil, 1989), we have shown that typicality and theoretical centrality make markedly different contributions to interpretations of novel conceptual combinations. For example, if one independently obtains lists of typical versus central features for each of the two terms in a future combination, one can then show with new subjects that altering theoretically central features of the two constituents has a much more systematic effect on the combined concept's perceived structure than altering the merely typical features.

An analogous account can be made for the acquisition of concepts, where it is exceedingly difficult to model widely observed developmental changes in conceptual structure without reference to changing sets of causal beliefs in which those concepts are embedded. There is little disagreement that some aspects of concept structure and word meaning change with development; and it is becoming increasingly evident that these changes cannot be depicted solely in terms of atheoretical, acausal tabulations of feature frequencies and correlations.

With the rise of prototype theory (Rosch & Mervis, 1975) and other probabilistic models of concepts (see Smith & Medin, 1981), it was a reasonable first hypothesis that concept development might be simply accounted for in terms of shifting weights on the values of features, correlations, exemplars, and the like. Anglin (1977), for example, described some of the most salient phenomena of semantic development, the under- and overextensions of word meanings, in terms of shifting weights in prototype structures and changing threshold criteria for being a member of a category. These sorts of accounts were appealing, because they promised models of conceptual change based on a continuous and very general process operating on a uniformly structured conceptual system.

Despite their appeal, accounts of conceptual change in such simple probabilistic terms have not turned out to be adequate. If attempts are made to model the details of conceptual change, in many cases models based on changing criteria or feature weights are either incorrect or hopelessly ad hoc. Thus, all children between ages 3 and 8 might well have pretty much the same intuitive sense of typicality distributions for the salient features of *uncles,* but they may understand that concept and use its associated term in quite different ways, ways that are not simply explained by assuming that older children have different thresholds beyond which overall feature weights indicate category membership. When one introduces the notion of emerging theories and causal beliefs that can restructure similarity relations, these problems disappear (Keil, 1987, 1989). Of course, such a move creates its own problems of explaining how theories and causal beliefs enter the concept space and how they change.

The new emphasis on causal beliefs and theories does not mean that all aspects of concept and semantic structure must be couched in such terms. Just as models cannot be successful without referring to causal structure, neither can they succeed if they ignore all probabilistic, atheoretical aspects of representations. Demonstrations of the differences between centrality and typicality are also demonstrations that both play an important part in our understanding of concept structure. This heterogeneity of concept structure is hardly a new idea. It has long been speculated that concepts have two qualitatively different parts, one associated with symptoms, typicality, and superficial familiarity, and the other associated with deeper beliefs and theories (e.g., Darwin, 1859; Locke, 1690/1964; Quine, 1977). At the least, then, the contrast between these two facets of concepts must be mentally represented. At the most, the actual representational format of causal beliefs is structured differently than that of more associative forms of knowledge. In this chapter I assume the stronger interpretation of different representational formats.

Causal, explanatory belief systems may be construed as providing an interpretative framework for some subset of a more associative network. We may all be continuously monitoring and tabulating such things as feature frequencies, correlations, and exemplar instances, but often without much of an idea as to why those patterns occur. This mass of information may be too large to reason with without some interpretation provided by an explanatory set of beliefs. The occurrence of such a process is evident in a great many domains. For example, I may daily encounter several instances of furniture and may roughly sort instances into classes, as well as create new classes, on the basis of clusters of features. The amount of information, however, is overwhelming if all possible features are continuously tabulated. We quickly develop certain preconceptions of which features and feature correlations are important and use these preconceptions to bias further data collection. Moreover, these biases usually are based on causal explanatory beliefs. Thus, I may decide that texture and softness are important features for distinguishing furniture types because of my beliefs about the roles that furniture plays in our everyday lives and why people make furniture. I may decide to ignore such features as a piece of furniture's dirtiness or temperature because of a belief that those sorts of properties are irrelevant to my "theory" of furniture kinds.

Theory may guide from the start what sorts of features and correlations one attends to in local domains, and its growth and differentiation may provide more and more guidance with development; but it can never fully explain all patterns of correlations even among those features it preselects for tabulation and analysis. In sorting cars into subcategories, for example, I may disregard the properties of the license plate and age and may focus on shape, wheelbase, number of doors, and so on to yield such categories as sports cars, sedans, and four-wheel-drive vehicles. But even in that narrower class of features, my theory cannot do all the work; thus, my sorting of passenger sedans into different makes (e.g., Ford vs. Dodge) is based solely on typicality/prototype information since I cannot divine any principled or causal reasons for differences in style, shape, and so on within that category. Thus, explanatory belief systems and more automatic tabulations must coexist at all times in concept structure, even though their relative distributions can vary greatly with expertise. One's belief systems allow one to narrow down the class of relevant inputs, to make more powerful inductions about properties, and simply to understand more fully the patterns in the world.

The details of such systems of belief, or theories, still have to be worked out; but some structural patterns are likely to hold:

(1) Some beliefs arise not out of data but out of other beliefs or from the start. This assumption is needed to account for the widespread observation of illusory correlations, where theory drives one to see correlations that do not exist or heavily distorts their values.

(2) Beliefs about causal relations among features are not distributed evenly among all features; they form tight clusters separated by relatively empty spaces. This can be envisioned by imagining all features to be equally distributed in a multidimensional space in which there are not only links between features representing correlations but also ones representing causal relations. Two dimensions of such a space are shown in Figure 6.1a, where curved lines represent mere associations and arrows represent causal relations. It is assumed that both of these types of interfeature relations are not of equal density throughout the space. Kinds are seen as such, because there are real-world mechanisms that cause them to be segregated into entities with shared clusters of features, each of the features tending to support the presence of others (Boyd, 1984). This causal homeostasis in the world is suspected to lead to a comparable representation of clusters of causal

beliefs about the properties associated with kinds. This is shown maximally in Figure 6.1c.

(3)   Although both tabulations of correlations and beliefs of causal relations might show clustering around kinds with reduced density on relations between kinds, there may be a greater gradient of density change for causal relations, since they tend to be driven more by considerations of internal coherence and consistency and because they tend to support each other mutually in ways that mere correlations cannot. Thus, one of the characteristics of beliefs about causal relations may be their tendency to be maximally interconnected into a relatively well bounded domain. For example, there are many strong correlations among features of birds, but also many other strong correlations with properties and instances of nonbirds. Birds make messes on cars, birds fly north in certain flyways and not others, birds have lighter-colored meat than mammals, and so on – correlations with only indirect links to other bird properties. Causal relations can also connect to other kinds, of course, but they may have a greater tendency to loop back into other properties in the bird domain. Wings on birds enable flight; feathers enable light wings, which enable flight; high metabolic rates ensure enough energy for flight; and so on. This difference is currently only a conjecture, but it is open to empirical assessment as to whether mere associative/correlational knowledge and causal knowledge show different gradients of clustering within and between kinds.

Given this view of concept structure as composed of two distinct parts, there may be systematic patterns in the way lexical items become attached to this structure. One pattern in particular merits further exploration: I suspect that lexical items are more likely to be attached to dense clusters than to less dense configurations, and I suspect that causal clusters, when available, play a more important role in guiding lexical assignment than mere tabulations of frequencies and correlations. A preference for causal structure may not always be easy to document, because correlations are often closely linked to causal ones; but as noted earlier there are cases when the two can be different, as in the research of Medin and Shoben (1988). Similarly, studies on nominal kind terms suggest a shift from a heavy reliance on characteristic features to representations that focus on a few central or "defining" features, although frequently for nominal kinds these features may have no causal roles (Keil, 1989; Keil & Batterman, 1984).

Thus, it seems likely that different aspects of concept structure will not be equally well linked to lexical structure. There may be a hierarchy of preferences for which sorts of concept structures attract labels, with less preferred structures being linked to words only in default situations. When no theory is available, children or novices

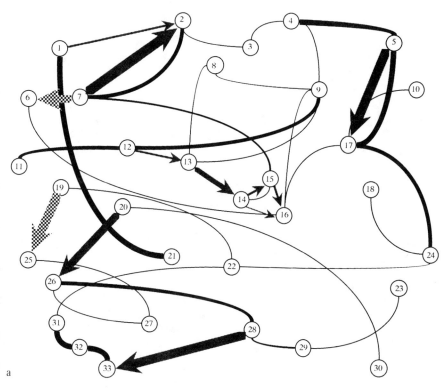

a

Figure 6.1a. The following sequence of three diagrams represents the progressive elaboration of the networks of beliefs and associations linked with a subset of 33 features out of the very much larger total feature space. Arrows represent causal relations, with checkered arrows representing negative causal relations (i.e., *x* cannot have causal influences on *y*). Curved lines represent associative links. The thickness of the lines represents the strength of the causal relation or the association. The progression across the three diagrams depicts the increasing concentration of relations around small sets of nodes, clusters that presumably are partially reflecting homeostatic causal clusters in the real world. When these clusters are sufficiently dense, as in Figure 6.1c, they come to be seen as standing for the class of entities that conform to those relations, or as a part of the concept of a kind. Thus, in Figure 6.1c, the two clusters centering most heavily around features 12 and 28 might be seen as corresponding to two different natural kinds. The proposal that gradients of causal relations might fall off more steeply from such clusters than associative relations is shown by more curved arcs leaving the clusters and linking to isolated features or to those of the other natural kind.

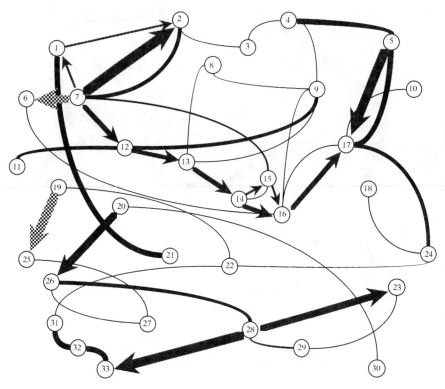

Figure 6.1b.

by necessity attach lexical labels to merely associative clusters; but when presented with a causal cluster alternative, they may always shift toward it, thereby adjusting the associated representations so that they more directly correspond to the causal structure. These sorts of issues must be explored more empirically. For example, one might teach a novel concept, *twutlet*, to adults that includes details about both causal and correlational structure across typical instances. One might then present new deviant cases that either preserve the complete correlational structure but disrupt the causal, or disrupt the correlational while preserving the causal. If told that the label applies to only one of the two new cases, subjects might then show a preference for the one that is causally similar to the original concept. There remains the additional question of whether they will act differently in a task that does not involve labels, such as sorting. Finally, the degree to which labels are attached to causal relations may vary as a function of the kinds involved, perhaps being stronger

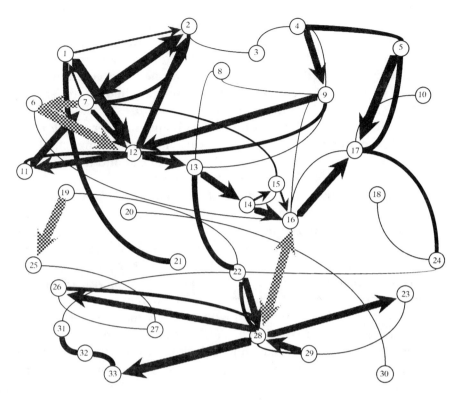

Figure 6.1c.

for natural kinds than nominal kinds. Some of Gelman's (1988a, b) findings concerning inductions about natural kinds and artifacts lend support to this conjecture.

In sum, the causal belief component of concepts may have a unique influence on where in the broader array of concept structure lexical items become most closely affiliated. An assessment of this view will depend critically on further research on the nature of causal beliefs and their relation to the more associative aspects of concept structure.

Conceptual heterogeneity and the differentiation–sharpening conflict

If one examines the literature on the acquisition of word meaning over the past 100 years or so, two pervasive and seemingly contradictory themes emerge, themes, moreover, that are echoed in the more recent research tradition on novice–expert differences (Murphy & Wright, 1984). One theme argues that initially word meanings are represented in terms of too little information; they lack all the details associated with forms. This information is commonly described in terms of features, whereby younger children are said to have a subset of the adult complement of features.

The rationales for this feature impoverishment refer to the more limited experience and/or storage capacities of young children. Children presumably cannot possibly know all the information about instances that adults do and must therefore start out basing word meanings on only some of the features that adults associate with those terms. Development, then, consists of the gradual addition of features until the full adult set is reached. One salient piece of evidence for this pattern is the overextensions of terms observed in young children (Clark, 1973). There have been ample observations of overextensions for more than a century (Darwin, 1877), and these seem to be accounted for by a model wherein younger children have too few features associated with lexical items and gradually acquire more with increasing age. I call this account the *differentiation theme*, the idea being that children's knowledge of lexical items gradually differentiates into a larger and larger set of features and relations.

A contrasting theme, with an equally long history, is that word meanings are initially represented in terms of too much information, resulting in global holistic representations. Children start off tabulating all salient information that is correlated with labeled instances, and only gradually winnow out the central, crucial features from the irrelevant, merely symptomatic ones. Early studies on children's vocabularies (Chambers, 1904), on through Vygotsky (1934/1962) and Werner (1948), revealed a pattern in which younger children were said to be excessively captured by all salient properties of instances, thereby failing to focus on the more critical subset of elements for lexical meaning. Werner's "holistic-to-analytic" shift is perhaps the clearest statement along these lines.

The view remains today, as can be seen in Anglin's (1977, 1985) suggestion, that younger children rely too heavily on prototype structures such that they both overextend and underextend word meanings according to excessive weighting of merely typical features. The characteristic-to-defining shift could also be seen as supporting that pattern, as could Gentner and Toupin's (1986) claim of a developmental shift from organizing entities on the basis of "surface similarity" to organizing them on the basis of "relational similarity." In general, this view sees younger children as headlong "phenomenalists," who only with time learn to home in on information and relations that are central to adult semantic representations. I call this view the *sharpening theme*. With development, children bring into sharper and sharper focus an increasingly smaller set of features and relations.

It would seem that the two themes of differentiation and sharpening are contradictory. Differentiation suggests that children start out with far too few semantic features and then gradually add more and more, whereas sharpening suggests that they start off with far too many and then gradually prune away the unnecessary ones. It may be possible to resolve this contradiction, however, by looking more closely at the concept structure that underlies semantic structure.

As already described, concepts seem to have two parts: a network of merely associative relations and sets of explanatory/causal beliefs. *Associative relations* is meant to be a general term for any atheoretical, probabilistically based tabulation of features, properties, and relations. Explanatory/causal beliefs provide insight and prediction to this atheoretical network, making more efficient representations and reasoning in many tasks. They are beliefs about relations (usually causal) that help explain both feature–feature correlations and feature–overall instance correlations. These two sorts of representational states may be mutually parasitic and thus must always coexist for concepts about all natural phenomena, but the relative balance between the two can change dramatically with development.

It also seems likely that the predominant force behind the change is an expanding set of explanatory/causal beliefs and that the associative network may remain relatively stable. Thus, a 4-year-old and a 44-year-old may have very similar representations of the typicality values of the features of dogs; but they may differ radically in their beliefs about why those frequencies occur and which ones are truly significant. On this view, concept development may often consist primarily of theory change and, in particular, of differentiation of sets of explanatory/causal beliefs.

Thus, it would seem that there is a model for the differentiation view of semantic development. The primary conceptual change is an ever-expanding network of explanatory beliefs about frequencies and correlations. An overall interconnectedness can be constantly increasing, which is one form of a representational change from having a few elements to having a much larger number. If, early on, words can be attached to only a few theoretical relations (assuming they are where word meanings gravitate as described earlier), then to increasingly larger sets, it would appear that at least one version of the traditional overextension/feature addition view of semantic development is supported.

There is also, however, a different way of looking at conceptual change that has different implications for word meaning. As beliefs become more and more elaborated, they also tend to converge in clusters such that they highlight certain features and relations. Thus, through this emerging and steadily increasing web of belief (Quine & Ullian, 1973), there is a simultaneous narrowing down of the number of features or relations that are perceived as central to the concept. This in turn means that word meanings are seen as most closely associated with an ever-shrinking set of features and properties.

These simultaneously occurring patterns are illustrated in Figures 6.1a–c. In Figure 6.1a there is a network of associations (shown by curved lines with differing widths corresponding to differing associative strengths) overlaid by a set of causal beliefs (shown by arrows, where thicker arrows stand for stronger causal relationships). Checkered arrows stand for negative causal relations, meaning that a particular causal relation is believed not to be possible. Note that in Figure 6.1a there is no strong highlighting of some features over others. There is some tendency for clusters of associative relations around features 16, 17, and 24 and some causal clusterings around features 2, 15, and 16; but neither pattern is strong or compelling. As beliefs expand, however, there is an increased tendency toward clustering, such that features 7, 28, and 16 start to emerge as important.

The increasing network of causal beliefs therefore narrows down the domain of theoretically interesting features and relations. This is even more evident in Figure 6.1c, where features 7, 28, and 16 remain central, but feature 12 has emerged as perhaps most central of all. In addition, several causal links have increased in strength and/or become bidirectional, in particular those that seem to support a coherent homeostatic system. Moreover, new beliefs in anticausal relations (e.g., 28, 16) have emerged that help contrast clusters. Contrary to Quine (1977), I doubt that the initial state in a child is ever completely associative structure uninfiltrated by belief. For most natural concepts, there may well be initial biases to prefer some kinds of causal patterns over others, biases that may be specific to such domains as a naïve physics or psychology. Whether such biases have the status of explicit beliefs or are closer to channels that directly yield such beliefs is an open question, but some sort of "preparedness" for certain causal patterns may be an essential component of an emerging conceptual system from the start; without this causal preparedness, merely associative representations would flounder in a sea of unlimited possibilities, dooming the child to inductive bankruptcy.

This pattern of growth thereby contains elements of both differentiation and sharpening patterns. There is a gradual and steady differentiation of causal beliefs, but at the same time this differentiation provides a basis for sharpening and narrowing down onto a smaller set of core features. It is crucial that not just any pattern of differentiation would produce this effect. Thus, a random growth of increased causal links between features would work in the opposite direction, raising the potential relevance of more and more features. There can be a narrowing down to a smaller set of features only if the emerging causal/explanatory beliefs cluster in the appropriate sorts of patterns. They also might form well-bounded chains where no one feature is emphasized but where the group forms a stable unit; the 12:13:14:16:17 chain might be such an example.

In the sequence in Figure 6.1, the associative links and strengths change only a little, for the reasons already suggested. Some changes are possible, however, such as when theories suggest looking more carefully for a link such as the one that is "discovered" between elements 28 and 22.

In this system, one can imagine a younger child being "holistic" because she does not have adequately differentiated causal beliefs that highlight critical features. She might also be observed to over- and underextend, when in an effort to attach labels she defaults and uses associative clusters with instances. In doubt of which node is the critical one, she is more likely to hedge her bets, thereby attaching a label to a broader network of associative relations. In the example shown here, one might imagine that two very different and independent patterns of causal relations are associated with the labeled instances, those that cluster around feature 12 versus those that cluster around 28, but that this duality is not realized by the younger child. Examples of such changes abound in young children, who might, for example, confuse biological and psychological causal relations in learning about kinship terms (Keil, 1989).

In sum, if conceptual structure is organized in the twofold manner suggested, and if the development involves some kind of clustering of the sort shown, quite specific reasons can be plausibly attributed to changing word meanings. In addition, there might be subtle differences in the way such changes occur as a function of the kind involved.

The conceptual base and the interpretation of new lexical information

I have discussed at some length how changing concept structure might result in different structures onto which lexical items can be attached, thus causing changes in word meaning over time. A related issue concerns how existing concept structure guides inferences about novel lexical items. More broadly, it is becoming increasingly clear that different conceptual biases or "sets" can result in very different patterns of induction over the same inputs. For example, Vera and Keil (1988) have shown that either preschoolers' inductions about what properties go with what animals can seem very similar to Carey's (1985) results whereby children referred to a conceptual base of social relations, or their inductions can be patterned very differently and apparently on a biological base. For example, a child who is told that a given animal eats might nonetheless come up with very different inferences about what sorts of other things eat as a function of the explanatory context in which eating is introduced. If it is described in a social causal context (eating together helps enhance friendships), the property will be attributed to a different class of entities than it will if it is described in a biological causal context (eating gives the body essential things to keep it from starving). This suggests that even when given the same initial information, a child might make very different inferences about word meanings if different contexts are also invoked.

The clearest case of this phenomenon involves the explicit teaching of a new word meaning, as often happens in school and occasionally in other settings. Most real "definitions" of word meaning are a mix of what are roughly characteristic and defining features. Thus, even standard reference dictionaries use many phrases indicating typical properties and instances. Consider the following excerpt from the definition of *fertilizer* in *Webster's New World Dictionary*, second college edition (1970): ". . . any material, as manure, chemicals, etc. put on or in the soil to improve the quality or quantity of plant growth. . . ." Or consider part of the same dictionary's definition of *fruit*: ". . . a sweet and edible plant structure consisting of a fruit (sense 6)[1] or false fruit of a flowering plant, usually eaten raw or as a dessert. . . ."

In many instances children at all ages are able to remember all of the information that is presented to them in association with a new word meaning, but they may differ radically in how they weight that information. In particular, their weightings might differ in two ways:

(1) Children may refer to a different theoretical system, either because they lack the one that older children use or simply because they find it less compelling. In either case, they will pick a different set of features as central because different sets are central to the two theories. For example, younger children may interpret *uncle* predominantly in social or behavioral terms, whereas older ones may interpret it predominantly in biological terms, resulting in different uses of the word in certain contexts. Moreover, these sorts of differences should be systematically related to the domain of knowledge that the child is using; other kinship terms should show the same sorts of changing patterns of usage with age. Some preliminary studies examining the teaching of new terms to children lend support to such a prediction (Keil, 1989).
(2) Children may not see the relevance of any theoretical system, or their available theory may be so undifferentiated as to provide little guidance in feature selection. In such instances, they fall back on a more global weighting of all salient features based on how typically they are associated with new information.

The primary point here is that exactly the same patterns of input concerning word meanings might end up being represented in different ways as a function of dissimilarities in the underlying conceptual systems. For example, it is possible to show that although parents may give precisely the same definitions of words such as *appetizer* and *luggage* to 3-year-olds and 7-year-olds, the children encode those items very differently (Keil, 1989). These differences in encoding should be predictable from prior assessments of those conceptual structures. Clearly, research along these lines should have an impact on instruction in more applied settings. A teacher interested in teaching the meaning of a new term must realize that precisely the same definition will not end up being represented in the same manner by all students. Since definitions generally contain a mix of the characteristic and the more critical features, they all require the learner to make some decisions about which aspects are most central. Armed with such knowledge, the teacher has several possible options, including (a) trying to point out explicitly the central features and why they are central and discounting the others and (b) trying to make another conceptual system more dominant and/or more highly differentiated.

Conclusions

I have suggested that the organization of conceptual knowledge into distinct theoretical domains can have a dramatic impact on the acquisition of word meaning, and I have placed particular emphasis on two themes: (a) variations in concept structure across different kinds may have powerful and quite predictable influences on patterns of semantic development, and (b) an assumption of a heterogeneous internal structure consisting of associativelike tabulations and causal/explanatory beliefs enables one to make a number of specific predictions about how aspects of concept structure become attached to word meaning, how both differentiation and sharpening can occur simultaneously, and how explicit instruction in word meaning is likely to interact with developing conceptual systems. It is equally important, however, to note that the link between concept structure and semantic structure is complex and subtle. The notion of concepts as being embedded in networks of associations and beliefs makes it clear that there is no simple one-to-one mapping between lexical items and corresponding items in concept structure; concept structure is somewhat more continuous and many conceptual distinctions are not reflected in the lexicon.

Despite the need for caution in trying to make direct mappings from concept structure to lexical structure, it is the intent of this chapter to suggest that systematic relations between the two do exist and that we will be in a much better position to understand many of the phenomena of semantic development if we can build up more detailed characterizations of concepts, theories, and conceptual change.

Note

1. Sense 6 is a more strictly biological definition.

References

Anglin, J. M. (1977). *Word, object, and conceptual development.* New York: Norton.
Anglin, J. M. (1985). The child's expressible knowledge of word concepts: What preschoolers can say about the meanings of some nouns and verbs. In K. E. Nelson (Ed.), *Children's language* (Vol. 5, pp. 77–127). Hillsdale, NJ: Erlbaum.
Aristotle. (1963). *Categories* (J. L. Ackrill, Ed. and Trans.). Oxford: Oxford University Press.
Asch, S. E. (1946). Forming impressions of personality. *Journal of Abnormal and Social Psychology, 41,* 258–290.
Boyd, R. (1984, November). *Natural kinds homeostasis and the limits of essentialism.* Paper presented at Cornell University, Ithaca, NY.
Carey, S. (1985). *Conceptual change in childhood.* Cambridge, MA: MIT Press.
Chambers, W. G. (1904). How words get meaning. *Pedagogical Seminary, 11,* 30–50.
Chapman, L. J., & Chapman, J. P. (1969). Illusory correlation as an obstacle to the use of valid psycho-diagnostic signs. *Journal of Abnormal Psychology, 74,* 272–280.
Clark, E. V. (1973). What's in a word? On the child's acquisition of semantics in his first language. In T. E. Moore (Ed.), *Cognitive development and the acquisition of language* (pp. 65–110). New York: Academic Press.
Clark, E. V. (1983). Meanings and concepts. In P. Mussen (Ed.), *Handbook of child psychology* (Vol. 3, pp. 787–840). New York: Wiley.
Darwin, C. (1859). *On the origin of species by means of natural selection, or the preservation of favoured races in the struggle for life.* London: Murray.
Darwin, C. (1877). A biographical sketch of an infant. *Mind, 2,* 286–294.
Dupré, J. (1981). Biological taxa as natural kinds. *Philosophical Review, 90,* 66–90.
Gelman, S. A. (1988a). The development of induction within natural kind and artifact categories. *Cognitive Psychology, 20,* 65–95.
Gelman, S. A. (1988b). Children's expectations concerning natural kind categories. *Human Development, 31,* 28–34.
Gentner, D. (1983). Structure-mapping: A theoretical framework for analogy. *Cognitive Science, 7,* 155–170.
Gentner, D., & Toupin, C. (1986). Systematicity and surface similarity in the development of analogy. *Cognitive Science, 10,* 277–300.
Johnson, C., & Keil, F. C. (1989, November). *Theoretical centrality vs. typicality in conceptual combinations.* Paper presented at the 30th annual meeting of the Psychonomic Society, Atlanta, GA.
Keil, F. C. (1986). Semantic fields and the acquisition of metaphor. *Cognitive Development, 1,* 73–96.
Keil, F. C. (1987). Conceptual development and category structure. In U. Neisser (Ed.), *Concepts and conceptual development: Ecological and intellec-*

tual factors in categorization (pp. 175–200). Cambridge University Press.

Keil, F. C. (1989). *Concepts, kinds, and cognitive development.* Cambridge, MA: MIT Press.

Keil, F. C., & Batterman, N. (1984). A characteristic-to-defining shift in the development of word meaning. *Journal of Verbal Learning and Verbal Behavior, 23,* 221–236.

Kremer, K. E., & Gelman, S. A. (1989, April). *Children's causal explanations of the origins and structure of natural kinds and artifacts.* Paper presented at the biennial meeting of the Society for Research in Child Development, Kansas City, MO.

Lewis, D. (1969). *Convention.* Cambridge, MA: Harvard University Press.

Locke, J. (1964). *An essay concerning human understanding* (A. D. Woozley, Ed.). London: Collins. (Original work published 1690.)

Luchins, A. S. (1957). Experimental effects to minimize the impact of first impressions. In C. I. Hovland (Ed.), *The order of presentation in persuasion* (pp. 148–181). New Haven, CT: Yale University Press.

Medin, D., & Ortony, A. (1989). Psychological essentialism. In S. Vosniadou & A. Ortony (Eds.), *Similarity and analogical reasoning* (pp. 179–195). Cambridge University Press.

Medin, D. L., & Shoben, E. (1988). Context and structure in conceptual combination. *Cognitive Psychology, 20,* 158–190.

Medin, D. L., & Wattenmaker, W. D. (1987). Category cohesiveness, theories, and cognitive archeology. In U. Neisser (Ed.), *Concepts and conceptual development: Ecological and intellectual factors in categorization* (pp. 25–62). Cambridge University Press.

Murphy, G., & Medin, D. (1985). The role of theories in conceptual coherence. *Psychological Review, 92,* 289–316.

Murphy, G. L., & Wright, J. C. (1984). Changes in conceptual structure with expertise: Differences between real-world experts and novices. *Journal of Experimental Psychology: Learning, Memory, and Cognition, 10,* 144–155.

Putnam, H. (1975). The meaning of meaning. In H. Putnam (Ed.), *Mind, language and reality* (Vol. 2, pp. 215–221). Cambridge University Press.

Quine, W. V. O. (1977). Natural kinds. In S. P. Schwartz (Ed.), *Naming, necessity, and natural kinds* (pp. 155–175). Ithaca, NY: Cornell University Press.

Quine, W. V. O., & Ullian, J. S. (1973). *The web of belief.* New York: Random House.

Rips, L. J. (1989). Similarity, typicality, and categorization. In S. Vosniadou & A. Ortony (Eds.), *Similarity and analogical reasoning* (pp. 155–175). Cambridge University Press.

Rosch, E., & Mervis, C. B. (1975). Family resemblances: Studies in the internal structure of categories. *Cognitive Psychology, 7,* 573–605.

Schwartz, S. (1980). Natural kinds and nominal kinds. *Mind, 83,* 182–195.

Simon, H. A. (1981). *The sciences of the artificial* (2nd ed.). Cambridge, MA: MIT Press.

Smith, E. E., & Medin, D. L. (1981). *Categories and concepts.* Cambridge, MA: Harvard University Press.

Vera, A. H., & Keil, F. C. (1988, November). *The development of inductions about biological kinds: The nature of the conceptual base.* Paper presented at the 29th meeting of the Psychonomic Society, Chicago.

Vygotsky, L. S. (1962). *Thought and language* (E. Hanfmann & G. Vakar, Trans.). Cambridge, MA: MIT Press. (Original work published 1934.)

Wellman, H., & Gelman, S. A. (1988). Children's understanding of the non-obvious. In R. J. Sternberg (Ed.), *Advances in the psychology of human intelligence* (Vol. 4, pp. 99–135.) Hillsdale, NJ: Erlbaum.

Werner, H. (1948). *Comparative psychology of mental development* (2nd ed.). New York: International Universities Press.

III. Logical, causal, and temporal expressions

7. Language and the career of similarity

DEDRE GENTNER AND MARY JO RATTERMANN

It is probable . . . that man's *superior association by similarity* has much to do with those discriminations of character on which his higher flights of reasoning are based.

William James (1890, p. 345)

The brute irrationality of our sense of similarity, its irrelevance to anything in logic and mathematics, offers little reason to expect that this sense is somehow in tune with the world.

Quine (1969, pp. 125–126)

Similarity has been cast both as hero and as villain in theories of cognitive processing, and the same is true for cognitive development. On the positive side, Rosch and her colleagues have suggested that similarity is an initial organizing principle in the development of categorization (e.g., Rosch, Mervis, Gray, Johnson, & Boyes-Braem, 1976), and Carey (1985) implicates a similarity mechanism in children's learning of the biological domain. It has also been suggested that similarity may play a role in word acquisition (Anglin, 1970; Bowerman, 1973, 1976; E. V. Clark, 1973; Davidson & Gelman, 1990; Gentner, 1982c). Others have taken a more pessimistic view, according to which similarity is either a misleading or at best an inferior strategy used as a last resort. Keil (1989), for example, posits that children begin with theories of the world and that

The theoretical work described in this chapter was supported by the Office of Naval Research under Contract N00014-89-J-1272 and the National Science Foundation under Grant BNS 87-20301. The developmental research was supported by the National Institute of Education under Contract 400-31-0031 awarded to the Center for the Study of Reading and the National Institute of Mental Health under Training Grant HD 07205.

We thank Renee Baillargeon, Cindy Fisher, Judy DeLoache, Linda Smith, Becki Campbell, Usha Goswami, Susan Gelman, and Jim Byrnes for their helpful comments on this chapter; Jennifer Glenn and Terry Sturdyvin for their help in preparing the manuscript; and Robert Dufour for his translations of Piaget.

similarity functions merely as a fallback strategy to be resorted to when theory fails.

A related issue is the course of development of similarity. Many researchers have suggested that children's use of similarity changes from an early and naïve form to a later, more enlightened form. Quine (1969) puts this view eloquently, describing the "career of the similarity notion" as "starting in its innate phase, developing over the years in the light of accumulated experience, passing then from the intuitive phase into theoretical similarity, and finally disappearing altogether" (Quine, 1969, p. 138). According to this view, there are different kinds of similarity, and the kinds of similarity children can use change with development. If this is true, then a further question is, what causes this development? Although Quine's description suggests a maturational change in the ability to perceive similarity, this is not the only possibility. In particular, we wish to explore the possibility that changes in similarity use might result from increases in children's knowledge rather than from changes in their intellectual competence.

Our plan in this chapter is as follows: First, we describe the development of similarity processes and give evidence for shifts in the kinds of similarity children use. Second, we consider the underlying causes of this evolution: whether developmental shifts in the processing of similarity result from global changes in intellectual competence or from the accretion of knowledge. Finally, we consider interactions with language, especially its possible role in the development of analogical similarity.

Distinguishing classes of similarity

Before beginning our survey, it is useful to distinguish three subclasses of similarity: analogy, mere appearance, and literal similarity. *Analogy* can be defined as similarity in relational structure, independently of the objects in which those relations are embedded (Gentner, 1982a, 1983, 1989). *Mere-appearance* matches are the complement of analogy: They are matches based primarily on common object descriptions. *Literal similarity* involves a greater degree of commonality: Both relational structure and object descriptions are shared.

There is considerable evidence that this distinction between relational similarity and object-based similarity is psychologically real (Clement & Gentner, 1988, 1991; Gentner, 1988; Gentner & Clement, 1988; Gentner & Landers, 1985; Gentner & Rattermann, 1990; Goldstone, Medin, & Gentner, 1991; Medin, Goldstone, & Gentner, 1990; Schumacher & Gentner, 1990). For example, in similarity-based retrieval tasks, adults recalled more matches that shared object attributes than matches that shared relational structure. Yet when asked to rate inferential soundness (described as "the degree to which an assertion that is true for one situation would hold in the other"), the same subjects rated matches sharing relational structure as both more sound and more similar than those sharing object attributes (Gentner & Rattermann, 1990). This dissociation between the kind of similarity that best promotes memory access and the kind that (at least subjectively) best supports inferences suggests a psychological distinction among different similarity types. In other research we have found that subjects judging perceptual similarity behave as though attributional commonalities and relational commonalities function as two different psychological pools (Goldstone, Gentner, & Medin, 1989; Goldstone et al., 1991; Medin et al., 1990).

The career of similarity

Given this set of distinctions, we now ask about the development of similarity. Gentner (1988) proposed that there is a *relational shift* in the development of analogy and metaphor: Young children focus on common object descriptions, whereas older children and adults focus on common relations. In this chapter we seek to test this proposal and to extend it in three ways. First, we wish to explore its generality across different tasks and domains. Second, we wish to extend our account of the career of similarity to encompass early development as well as later development. Third, we wish to investigate the causes of developmental change in similarity processing. In particular, we want to ask whether changes in children's similarity processing can be accounted for by acquisition of domain knowledge rather than by changes in intellectual competence. Our extended account of the career of similarity draws on three proposals:

(1) The differentiation hypothesis proposed by E. J. Gibson (1969) and elaborated by Shepp, Kemler, and Smith and their colleagues (e.g., Shepp, 1978; Smith, 1989; Smith & Kemler, 1977), which postulates

that early similarity is holistic and global and that the ability to process various kinds of partial similarity – such as similarity of color or of shape – develops later.

(2)   The relational-shift hypothesis, which postulates that the ability to process object-based commonalities precedes the ability to process relational commonalities (Gentner, 1988).

(3)   The further proposal that the ability to process first-order relational commonalities precedes the ability to process higher-order relational commonalities.

The third hypothesis was originally proposed by Piaget (Inhelder & Piaget, 1958) and has been developed by Halford (1987) and by Sternberg and his colleagues (Sternberg & Downing, 1982; Sternberg & Nigro, 1980; Sternberg & Rifkin, 1979). We depart somewhat from these approaches in that Piaget and Sternberg focused on only one higher-order relation, namely, identity of first-order relations.[1] In our account and in Halford's account, other higher-order relations are included. A more important difference is that the consensus among the other researchers is that the shift is due to changes in cognitive competence: specifically, the advent of formal operations (e.g., Inhelder & Piaget, 1958; Piaget, Montangero, & Billeter, 1977). We emphasize instead the logical dependency of higher-order predicates on prior possession of their lower-order arguments. We therefore leave open the possibility that the progression may be governed by the degree of knowledge rather than by the child's stage of cognitive competence (e.g., Brown, 1989; Ortony, Reynolds, & Arter, 1978).

Combining these three hypotheses, we arrive at the following account of the career of similarity. The early use of similarity is characterized by a reliance on highly conservative holistic similarity matches: exact or nearly exact matches between all aspects of the two situations (e.g., the commonality between an *apple on the table* and another *apple on the table*). Early development is characterized by a gradual lessening of the closeness of the match required to perceive similarity. Thus, various kinds of partial matches become possible. Objects and other separable components of situations can be matched even when the rest of the situation does not match (e.g., an *apple on the table* can match an *apple in a tree*). Next, object attributes can be matched even when the other qualities of the objects do not match (e.g., a RED *apple* can match to a RED *block*), and it also becomes possible to respond to purely relational commonalities (e.g., the first-order relational commonality that an *apple* FALLING FROM *a tree* is similar to a *book* FALLING FROM *a shelf* [Gentner, 1988]).

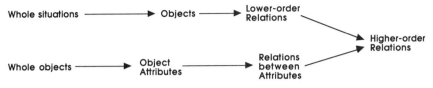

Figure 7.1. The career of similarity.

On the basis of Smith's (1989) discussion, we suggest that the first purely relational match that children can reliably extract is that of identity between whole objects (e.g., the commonality between *two identical apples* and *two identical books*). Identities between parts and along dimensions are extracted later (e.g., the *identical-color* commonality between *a red apple near a red book* and *a green lime near a green ball*), as are identities based on other first-order relations. Finally, children acquire the ability to match situations based on common higher-order relations (e.g., the similarity between *an apple falling from a tree*, PERMITTING *a cow to reach it* and *a book falling from a shelf*, PERMITTING *a child to reach it*) (Gentner, 1988; Halford, 1987). As we will discuss, throughout this developmental sequence there is often tension between perceiving object-based similarity and perceiving relational similarity. We do not wish to propose a strict ordering in which all object–attribute comparisons enter before all relational comparisons; as shown in Figure 7.1, these are not logically dependent on one another.

Thus, we follow Quine in hypothesizing a development from a naïve to a more sophisticated use of similarity. Also like Quine, we leave open the possibility that adults continue to experience original "brute similarity" even after acquiring the use of theoretical similarity. Our account of the career of similarity also draws on prior psychological theories that have suggested a shift from holistic, unanalyzed, concrete concepts to more highly differentiated and/or more abstract concepts, notably E. J. Gibson's (1969) notion of differentiation and Bruner's proposed shift from reliance on perceptual information to reliance on functional information (Bruner, Olver, & Greenfield, 1966). However, we differ from most prior theorists in an important respect. Rather than seek to explain the development of similarity in terms of global stages of competence, we will ask whether a weaker explanation will suffice, namely, accretion of knowledge (Brown, 1989; Brown & Campione, 1984; Gentner,

1977a, b; Ortony et al., 1978). We will return to comparisons with other views after elaborating our position.

The relational shift

The relational-shift hypothesis is that the ability to process similarity based on object commonalities precedes the ability to process similarity based on relational commonalities. To support this hypothesis, Gentner (1988) cited several findings. For example, when asked to interpret a figurative comparison,[2] such as "A cloud is like a sponge," 5-year-olds produced object-attributional commonalities, such as "They're both round and fluffy," whereas adults mentioned relational commonalities, such as "They both store water and later give it back to you." Nine-year-olds produced a mixture of the two response types. Thus, the younger children responded mainly on the basis of object similarity, whereas the adults responded on the basis of relational similarity. Similar findings were reported by Billow (1975). He asked 5- to 13-year-old children to interpret a series of verbally presented metaphors, which embodied either object similarity (e.g., "Hair is spaghetti") or "proportional" (relational) similarity (e.g., "My head is an apple without any core"). He found that the ability to interpret metaphors based on relational similarity developed later than the ability to interpret metaphors based on object similarity. A possibly related development from naïve to sophisticated patterns in metaphor interpretation has also been observed by Gardner and Winner and their colleagues (Gardner, Kircher, Winner, & Perkins, 1975; Gardner & Winner, 1982). Finally, patterns consistent with the relational shift have also been observed in metaphor production. Winner (1979) analyzed the metaphoric productions of a child (Adam) from the time he was 2,3 years old to the time he was 4,10 years old. She found that shape-based metaphors (e.g., metaphors based on common contour, such as "A pencil is a big needle") were predominant (65%) and that relationally based metaphors (e.g., metaphors based on configuration, such as "Adam sleeping on Daddy" when putting a small alphabet letter on a larger one) were quite rare (12%).

Before interpreting this change in performance as due to an increase in children's facility with relation similarity, we must ask whether it could instead be explained simply as an increase in knowledge of metaphoric aesthetics. Perhaps it is not children's fundamental apprehension of similarity that is changing, but rather their sense of what is considered clever or apt in discourse. The possibility is vitiated by the results of another task: an analogical mapping task conducted by Gentner and Toupin (1986), in which children had to map a plot structure from one set of actors to another. Two factors were varied: (a) the degree to which corresponding actors resembled one another (*transparency*) and (b) whether children were given an explicit summary of the higher-order relational structure (i.e., the social or causal moral that governed the plot) (*systematicity*). The plots themselves were identical across conditions. The performance of 6-year-olds was affected only by the transparency of the object correspondences; for example, they could accurately retell the story when *squirrel* mapped onto *chipmunk*, but not when it mapped onto *moose*. The presence of a higher-order relational structure had no effect on them. In contrast, 9-year-olds were affected by both variables. Without a systematic representation, their performance, like that of the 6-year-olds, was governed by object transparency. However, in the systematic condition they were able to transfer the story accurately regardless of the transparency of the correspondences. In summary, the younger children relied on object matches, whereas the older group, given explicit relational structure, could carry out an analogical mapping despite difficult object correspondences. Other studies of analogical transfer have found similar effects. For instance, Holyoak, Junn, and Billman (1984) found that 5-year-old children transferred a problem solution more successfully when object similarity was consistent with the correct solution strategy.

The finding of a relational shift in transfer tasks is a crucial addition to the findings of metaphor interpretation and production tasks. It means that developmental changes in the aesthetics of figurative language, though they may occur, cannot account for the whole phenomenon. However, there remain several possible explanations for the results obtained. First, the shift could reflect a *global change* in basic cognitive competence. As discussed earlier, Piaget posited that the ability to process analogical similarity is associated with formal operations (Inhelder & Piaget, 1958). Indeed, Billow (1975) interpreted his findings in this light and suggested that the performance of the children in his experiment was closely aligned with their Piagetian stage. This possibility is especially relevant here since the studies reviewed so far, as well as many others, have shown a shift during an age range roughly compatible with the onset of formal operations (see Goswami, 1991, for a review). Second, the relational shift could reflect the *acquisition of domain knowledge*[3] (Brown, 1989; Brown & Campione, 1984; Brown & DeLoache, 1978; Chi, Feltovich, & Glaser, 1981; Gentner, 1977a, b; Larkin & Simon, 1981; Ortony et al., 1978). On this account, young children's inability to perform relational mappings results from a lack of knowledge about the requisite domain relations (Brown, 1989; Goswami & Brown, 1989). There is a third possibility, namely, that the relational shift reflects the accretion of *learned mapping strategies*, in the spirit of Carey's (1984) discussion of acquired intellectual tools. That is, even given the basic intellectual competence and requisite domain knowledge to carry out an analogy, there might still be differences in performance due to the amount of practice (and, hence, the degree of acquired fluency) in the processes of carrying out a relational mapping.

These three classes of explanation make different predictions. The maturational-stage view predicts global changes in intellectual competence. The domain-knowledge view predicts that the relational shift will occur at different ages across different domains. The learned-strategy view is not as clear in its predictions, but roughly predicts an intermediate pattern of results. As in the domain-knowledge account, the relational shift should appear earliest in the simplest and most familiar domains; but as in the maturational-stage view, there should be some cross-domain linkage to the extent that the mapping strategies learned in one domain can be transferred to other domains. Although the learned-strategy view is appealing, its compatibility with a wide range of results makes it difficult to test. Therefore, we will concentrate chiefly on the other two explanations, which make very different predictions. Our method will be to survey research on the development of similarity across different domains. If the ability to perceive relational similarity develops at approximately the same age across different domains, this will constitute evidence for the maturational-stage view and against the domain-knowledge view. If shifts in similarity processing occur earlier for domains that are highly familiar to young children, this will be evidence for the domain-knowledge explanation and against the maturational-stage explanation. We begin by surveying children's performance on tasks utilizing familiar causal situations.

Tasks set in familiar causal domains

If the domain-knowledge hypothesis is correct, children's performance on similarity tasks should be better in familiar domains. Ann Brown and her colleagues have carried out many insightful studies that support this claim. Crisafi and Brown (1986) found that children's performance on a complex problem improved substantially when the objects and events used in the problem were made more familiar. Brown and Kane (1988) gave children a simple transfer task in which they had to carry across familiar relations such as *stacking*, *pulling*, and *swinging*. They found that even 3-year-olds were quite good at transferring solutions across situations when their task conditions promoted thinking about relational similarity. Brown (1989) used an especially simple task, in which children had to use a tool to reach for a desired toy. She found that even 24-month-old children were able to chose a correct pulling tool from a transfer set after initial experience with a similar tool that could be used in the same way. In another analogy task, Gentner (1977a, b) showed that young children can perform a spatial analogy between a human body – which is a highly familiar domain, even for preschoolers – and simple pictured objects, such as trees and mountains. She showed children simple pictures, such as a picture of a tree, and asked, "If a tree had a knee, where would it be?" Even 4-year-olds (as well as 6- and 8-year-olds) were able to perform the mapping of the human body to the tree. They were as accurate as adults, even when the orientation of the tree changed or when confusing surface attributes were added to the picture.

We have seen evidence that young children perform well on similarity-based tasks involving familiar domains, consistent with the domain-knowledge interpretation of the relational shift. However, in many of these tasks there was at least a partial correlation between relational similarity and object similarity. We need to know whether children can respond relationally when relational similarity is uncorrelated with, or even pitted against, object similarity. In a study aimed in part at testing the relational-shift hypothesis, Goswami and Brown (1989) manipulated relational similarity and object similarity independently. They presented children aged 3, 4, and 6 years with a set of pictures that formed the first three terms of a simple $A:B::C:D$ analogy and asked the children to pick the fourth. Other research on analogical transfer using similar $A:B::C:D$

analogies had found poor performance in grade school children
(Sternberg & Nigro, 1980; Sternberg & Rifkin, 1979). However, previous research by Goswami (1989) had shown that when the relations in an analogy were made sufficiently accessible, it was possible
for children to map relations. She presented 4- to 7-year-old children
with analogies based on simple relations such as shape, color, and
pattern and found that children as young as 6 years were able to
solve the analogies. Goswami and Brown drew on this methodology
in their studies of causal analogies. They attempted to control for
the effects of domain knowledge and relational complexity by using
familiar causal transformations such as *cut*, *burned*, and *dirtied*. They
also pretested the children's knowledge of these relations to ensure
that they understood the nature of the transformations. The children were then shown pictures forming the first three terms of an
analogy ($A:B::C:?$) and were asked to choose which of several pictures correctly completed the analogy. Included in these choices were
the correct object with the right transformation (the correct answer),
the correct object with the wrong transformation, the wrong object
with the right transformation, an object that shared a few object
attributes with the C term of the analogy,[4] and other alternatives.
Goswami and Brown found that all of their subjects, even the 3-
year-olds, performed well in this task, selecting the correct alternative 52% of the time and choosing the same-attributes choice only
8% of the time. Four-year-olds performed even better: 88% correct
and 1% attribute choices. The authors concluded that even 3-year-
olds can resist object similarity and respond relationally when given
simple causal relations to map.

The Goswami and Brown study admirably addressed the effects
of familiar domains and relations on children's ability to carry out
analogical mappings. However, we suspect that object similarity may
have played a considerable role in the results. We obtained adult
ratings of similarity for the stimuli used in this study.[5] The subjects
were shown the stimulus pictures used by Goswami and Brown and
were asked to rate the perceptual similarity of each possible response when compared with the C term of the analogy. In all cases,
the correct answer was rated as more similar to the C term than the
attribute match. Thus, these results do not tell us whether children
can respond to purely relational similarity, particularly if pitted against
object similarity.

In summary, the results of tasks set in simple familiar domains provide evidence of transfer ability in young children. However, it is difficult to isolate relational similarity from object similarity in most of these tasks. Thus, in many of the tasks the relational structure was supported by various kinds of correlated object similarities. (In fact, had this not been the case, the tasks might have been quite unnatural, defeating the effort to simplify the domains.) Thus, although tasks involving simple causal situations have provided suggestive evidence, it is not yet possible to draw strong conclusions regarding children's ability to use purely relational similarity.

Similarity in perceptual domains

We now turn from studies involving causal relations to those involving perceptual relations – for example, first-order relations such as BIGGER (X, Y), SAME COLOR (X, Y), and ABOVE (X, Y) and higher-order relations such as *identity* and *symmetry*. Although tasks based on perceptual similarity lack the dynamic interest of tasks based on causal similarity, they have several advantages for our purposes. First, perceptual relations can be inferred directly from the stimuli, whereas the inferring of causal relations typically requires additional background assumptions. Second, perceptual relations have a wide latitude of application relative to causal relations.[6] Thus, in studies of perceptual similarity it is possible to vary objects and relations independently, permitting one to test different kinds of matches. Finally, since children are exposed from birth to spatial configurations of objects, even infants have some familiarity with perceptual relations. This allows us to extend our survey of similarity development to a much earlier age.

Very early similarity use. Assessing the similarity perceptions of young infants poses something of a challenge. One method that has proved successful is that of sequential touching, in which the order of spontaneous manipulations of objects is observed (Nelson, 1973a; Ricciuti, 1965; Starkey, 1981). Infants as young as 12 months will sequentially touch or group identical objects. For example, Sugarman (1982) presented children aged 12 to 36 months with a collection containing two identity classes – for example, four plates and four square blocks. One object from each class was placed on the table, and the child was allowed to place the other six objects. As in comparable studies, all age groups engaged in some similarity-based grouping behavior (Nelson, 1973a; Ricciuti, 1965; Starkey, 1981), with younger infants producing simple one-class groupings (e.g., making a row of plates while ignoring the blocks) and older infants often producing two-class groupings (e.g., making a row of plates and a row of blocks), a process that requires comparing items to determine similarity and difference.

Thus, very young infants can respond to identities among objects. Other research suggests that close similarity among objects may be sufficient. Mandler and Bauer (1988) used object manipulation and sequential touching as the dependent measure in a study with 12-, 15-, and 20-month-old subjects. They presented the infants with objects from two different basic-level categories (e.g., *dogs* and *cars*), two superordinate categories (e.g., *animals* and *vehicles*), or two contextual categories (e.g., *bathroom things* and *kitchen things*). The objects in the superordinate and contextual categories were physically quite dissimilar. By using these different sets of objects Mandler and Bauer hoped to determine whether categories with a high degree of within-category similarity (e.g., basic level) are easier to form than categories with a low degree of within-category similarity (e.g., superordinate and contextual categories). They found that at all ages the infants tended to touch objects sequentially from the same basic-level category (50% of the 12-month-olds did so) and, to a lesser extent, objects from the same superordinate (25%) and contextual (35%) categories. Mandler and Bauer also found that the infants' propensity to respond to superordinate categories increased with age. Here, too, similarity influenced the infants' performance: Mandler and Bauer reported that "children find it easier to differentiate sets of objects from two superordinate classes when the objects look alike than when the sets are physically less similar."

Young infants appear to be guided by object identity or very close similarity in sequential exploration of collections of objects. This is consistent with our suggestion that the first stage in the career of similarity is marked by the use of massive overall similarity matches. We now turn to an insightful and revealing set of studies by Baillargeon and her colleagues (Baillargeon, 1987, 1990, 1991, in press; Baillargeon, Spelke, & Wasserman, 1985) that (a) reinforces the claim that very early similarity is highly conservative and (b) suggests that a shift toward the ability to process partial matches begins very early. This study uses a different paradigm than the previous studies, and

Habituation Event

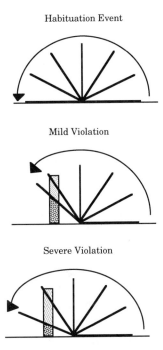

Mild Violation

Severe Violation

Figure 7.2. Apparatus from moving-screen study. (Adapted from Baillargeon, in press.)

the reasoning is rather subtle. Therefore, we begin by laying out the basic task.

Baillargeon habituated $4\frac{1}{2}$- and $6\frac{1}{2}$-month-old infants to a screen that rotated back and forth through a 180-degree arc from a position flat on the table at one end of the arc to the same position at the other end of the arc. After the infant had become habituated to the movement, a 25-cm-tall box was placed 12.5 cm behind the screen, and the infant saw one of two events. In the *possible* event, the screen rotated until it hit the box (112 degrees). In the *impossible* event, the screen rotated 135 degrees, seemingly passing through the top 50% of the box (a mild violation), or 157 degrees, seemingly passing through the top 80% of the box (a severe violation), or 180 degrees, seemingly passing through the entire space occupied by the box (an extreme violation) (Figure 7.2).

The question was whether the infants in the impossible-event condition would look reliably longer at the display than the infants in the possible-event condition. If so, they were assumed to have detected the violation. The younger infants ($4\frac{1}{2}$-month-olds) showed such a pattern only for the extreme violation, when the screen passed entirely through the box. The $6\frac{1}{2}$-month-olds could detect the violation when the screen passed through the top 80% of the box. (They readily accepted the milder 50% violation.)

In a subsequent study, Baillargeon (1991) again presented $4\frac{1}{2}$- and $6\frac{1}{2}$-month-olds with the occluded-box task. However, this time an identical box was placed beside the first box out of the screen's path; this second box remained visible through the test trials. When the visible box was in place, (a) the $4\frac{1}{2}$-month-old infants detected both the mild (50%) and severe (80%) violations and (b) the $6\frac{1}{2}$-month-old infants detected the mild (50%) violation. The infants seemed to use the visible box as a standard on which to base expectations regarding the target box behind the screen. If so, this would constitute a kind of mapping from the visible box – its size and position – to the invisible box. Having shown that the infants used an identical visible box as a standard, Baillargeon (in press) went on to manipulate the degree of similarity between the visible box (which was always a red box with white dots) and the target box. In the *high-similarity* condition the target box was also red but with green dots. In the *moderate-similarity* condition the target box was yellow with green dots, and in the *low-similarity* condition the target box was yellow and decorated with a clown face (Figure 7.3). When Baillargeon presented infants with the mild violation (the screen passing through 50% of the box) under these three levels of similarity-of-standard, she found an interesting pattern of performance. Only in the high-similarity condition were the younger infants ($4\frac{1}{2}$-month-olds) surprised. In the low- and medium-similarity conditions they failed to detect the violation. The older infants ($6\frac{1}{2}$-month-olds), in contrast, detected the violation in both the high-similarity and the moderate-similarity conditions, but not in the low-similarity condition.

These results suggest two fascinating possibilities. First, young infants may be able to map inferences from a visible object to an occluded object; that is, they can carry out an early form of analogical mapping. Second, this inferential process is extremely conservative. It requires massive overall similarity between the standard and the target. Younger infants ($4\frac{1}{2}$ months) are highly reliant on object similarity; anything less than a perfect match between the two stimuli

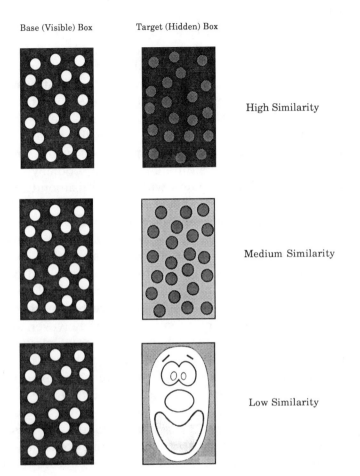

Figure 7.3. Stimuli from moving-screen study. (Adapted from Bail-largeon, in press.)

diminishes the infants' ability to transfer. By $6\frac{1}{2}$ months there is slightly less reliance on massive similarity, although the infants' transfer is still quite restricted.

So far we have discussed evidence for an early reliance on close object similarity, with a gradually developing ability to use less complete similarity matches. We now discuss an intriguing study that suggests something akin to a relational shift occurring in the first year of life. Kolstad and Baillargeon (1990) familiarized $5\frac{1}{2}$-, $8\frac{1}{2}$-, and $10\frac{1}{2}$-month-old infants to an event in which a silver-gloved hand held a yellow cylindrical container decorated with red hearts upright in the center of a display. Then, as the infant watched, the hand rotated the container forward, so that the infant could see the opening, and backward, so that the infant could see the bottom of the container. After the container was returned to an upright position, it was moved to the back of the display, where there was a tap. The infant watched as salt poured from the tap and filled the container. The hand then moved the container to a hole in the center of the display and poured out the salt. This sequence of events was repeated two more times with two different, but perceptually similar containers (a blue cylinder decorated with purple diamonds and a pink cylinder decorated with black dots).

After these three familiarization events, the infant was shown two test events. The test events were identical to the familiarization events except that different containers were used. In the *box* test the container was a rectangular box covered with white paper and pastel flowers. In the *tube* test the container (a yellow cylinder decorated with black diamonds) was similar in appearance to the cylinders used in the three previous familiarization events; however, it appeared to have no bottom (in fact it had a transparent plastic bottom). If the infants watching these test events were basing their inferences of containment on surface similarity, one would expect that they would be surprised when the perceptually different box contained salt. If, in contrast, the infants were basing their inferences on the relationally relevant feature of having a bottom, they would be surprised when the (bottomless) cylindrical tube contained salt. Baillargeon found that $5\frac{1}{2}$- and $8\frac{1}{2}$-month-old infants looked reliably longer at the box event, suggesting that they were surprised that an object that differed in appearance from the original cylinder events could hold salt. In contrast, the $10\frac{1}{2}$-month-old infants looked reliably longer at the cylindrical-tube event, suggesting that they were surprised that an object that had no bottom could contain salt. This research suggests that a shift from a focus on overall object similarity to a focus on relational similarity begins to occur even in the first year of life, at least for some very familiar relations such as containment.

Now we turn to research by DeLoache (1989, 1990) on preschoolers' ability to map between entire situations. DeLoache's task utilized relations and objects likely to be highly familiar to preschool children, namely, dolls, dollhouses, and an ordinary room. Children aged 31 months and 38 months watched as a large Snoopy doll was hidden in the regular-sized room. Then the children were told that a miniature Snoopy was hiding in the same place in a small scale-model room. The children's task was to find little Snoopy in the model room. When given this task, 38-month-old children could find little Snoopy in the model room (about 80% correct retrieval); however, 31-month-old children were virtually unable to perform the task (about 15% correct retrieval). (Yet, like the older children, they were able to retrieve the large doll from the original room 80% of the time, showing that they had no trouble remembering the locaton of the original doll.) What makes these findings remarkable is that the two rooms were nearly identical except for size – they contained the same furniture in the same arrangement. Moreover, before the task began, all of the children were shown both the original room and the model room and the correspondences were pointed out (e.g., "This is big Snoopy's couch; this is little Snoopy's couch").

Since both object similarity (in that the pieces of furniture were alike except for size) and relational similarity (in that the relative locations of the furniture were alike) were present, this task can be viewed as a literal similarity mapping from the large room to the small room.[7] Indeed, for adults this seems to be such a strong case of literal similarity that it is difficult to grasp that a 2-year-old might fail. Yet even under what seem to be conditions of very strong overall similarity, we see a marked difference from the performance of 31-month-olds, who generally failed the mapping task when there was a difference in size, to the performance of 38-month-olds, who seemingly shared the adult sense that a simple change in scale does not greatly diminish similarity.

In another study, DeLoache tested the older children's abilities by manipulating the object similarity – that is, the similarity of furniture – between the original room and the model. In the high-object-similarity condition the furniture in the model was highly similar to the furniture in the room (as in the previous task). In the low-object-similarity condition each piece of furniture in the model room shared the same basic shape and size (and relative location) as the corresponding object in the original room, but was otherwise dissimilar in appearance. Performance was markedly lower in this low-object-similarity condition. The 38-month-olds could perform the mapping in the high-similarity condition (70% correct) but performed badly in the low-similarity condition (20% correct). (Not surprisingly, this similarity manipulation had little effect on the 31-month-olds, who were already performing badly even in the highest-similarity condition.)[8] Thus, the results indicate a strong dependence on literal similarity: For 38-month-olds, changing the appearance of the objects is disruptive.

As in the research discussed in the preceding section on familiar domains, the objects and relations in the DeLoache studies have been perfectly correlated. Consequently, there remains the question of the relative contributions of common objects and common relational structure to the children's performance. DeLoache performed a further study that addressed this question. In this task the object similarity between the furniture pieces was high, but the model was rearranged so that the spatial relations between the furniture in the original room and the model were different. There were two conditions: (a) the toy was hidden behind the corresponding piece of furniture (*same object*), or (b) the toy was hidden in the same relative position in the two rooms (e.g., both toys were hidden in the southwest corners of the rooms) (*same spatial relation*).

Before experiencing this rearranged model, the 3-year-olds in both conditions of the study were first run in the standard retrieval task. One day later, they were given the rearranged search task under one of the two experimental conditions. The Day 1 results replicated those found for 3-year-olds in Experiment 1: The rate of correct retrievals was approximately 80%. The results when the furniture was rearranged on Day 2 were quite striking: The children performed well in the same-object condition (approximately 80% correct retrieval) but very badly in the same-spatial-relation condition (approximately 5% correct retrieval). Thus, the children could perform a mapping based on object similarities, but not a mapping based solely on common relations. This rules out the possibility that the children in DeLoache's task were using a purely relational mapping.

We might ask whether the reverse possibility is true: that performance on the tasks described so far might have been based entirely on object matches. There is evidence, however, that this was not the case. In the study just discussed, the children received the normal mapping task (in which model and room had the same arrangement of furniture) before performing the rearranged mapping task. When DeLoache gave 3-year-olds the rearranged mapping task as their initial task, they performed very badly, even in the similar-object condition (20 to 30% correct performance, as opposed to 80%

correct performance when the task was preceded by the normal mapping task). The fact that their performance on the object-mapping version of the different-configuration mapping task was so much better after they had experience with the standard-configuration mapping task suggests that the children may have required an initial literal-similarity match encompassing the entire situation. They apparently used both object similarity and relational similarity in their initial detection of the correspondence between model and room. However, these results also suggest that one outcome of making this initial mapping was that the children then went on to extract a partial match, namely, one based on object similarity.

The results of this series of studies suggest a striking degree of conservatism in young children's similarity matches; the children seemed to rely on an exact match between the two situations, even in the very simple mapping task. Indeed, for 31-month-olds, similarity in shape, color, texture, and category was not sufficient; similarity in size was also necessary. Children's ability to carry out similarity mappings appears to be sensitive to both relational commonalities and object commonalities.

Attributes and dimensional relations. Much of the early research on attributes and dimensions was based on Garner's investigations of stimulus structure and its effects on classification and memory (Garner, 1974). Before discussing this work, we need a bit of terminology. Our distinction between attributes and dimensions follows that of Garner (1978). An *attribute* is a component property of a stimulus, such as color, size, or form, that helps to define the object but is not equivalent to it. A *dimension* is a set of mutually exclusive attributes, or, as Palmer (1978) puts it, a set of mutually exclusive relations between an object and a value. For example, "three feet tall" can be an attribute of an object, but it is clearly a *dimensional* attribute since "three feet tall" precludes "four feet tall" or any other member of the same dimensional class. Gibson (1969) further noted that dimensions are often continuous and ordered sets of attributes. For our purposes, it is important to note that for children to perceive a set of attributes as a dimension[9] they require some knowledge of the relations between those attributes (mutual exclusivity, ordering, etc.).

Garner and Felfody (1970) hypothesized that pairs of dimensions differ in their combinatorial properties (as perceived by adults). Integral dimensions, such as hue and brightness, are perceived as one combined dimension, whereas separable dimensions, such as size and shape, are seen as two perceptually distinct components. Shepp and his colleagues reported a developmental progression whereby some combinations of dimensions that are seen as separable by adults are perceived as integral by young children (Shepp, 1978; Shepp & Swartz, 1976). For example, 5-year-olds show a redundancy gain in a speeded sorting task when color and form are correlated. This redundancy gain is taken as an indication of integral processing and suggests that color and form are perceived integrally by young children, though separably by adults (Garner & Felfody, 1970). Similarly, young children classify stimuli varying in size and brightness according to overall similarity, again treating as integral two dimensions that for adults are separable. On the basis of these findings, Shepp (1978) proposed a developmental trend from perceived overall similarity to perceived dimensional structure.[10]

Smith and Kemler (1977) provided further evidence for a developmental trend from holistic similarity processing in young children to analytic similarity processing based on common dimensions in older children and adults. Smith (1989) has amplified and extended this proposal into an admirably specific framework. Of particular importance here is her suggestion of a progression in children's similarity processing from overall similarity to object identity to common values on a particular dimension to common dimensional relations. For example, Smith (1984) used a follow-the-leader task to investigate 2-, 3-, and 4-year-old children's ability to process similarity defined in terms of object identity, common attributes, common identity relations, or common dimensional relations. Two experimenters chose objects from sets of toys that shared one of the following:

(1) *Object identity* – for example, both experimenters chose green planes, so that the child had only to match $X1$ and $X1$; the correct response was another green plane.
(2) *Identity relation* – for example, Experimenter 1 (E1) chose two red cars and E2 chose two white daisies, so that the child had to match IDENTICAL $(X1, X2)$ and IDENTICAL $(Y1, Y2)$; the correct response was two cars of the same color (but not necessarily white or red).
(3) *Common attributes* – for example, both experimenters chose red objects, so that the child had to match RED (X) and RED (Y); the correct response was another red object.
(4) *Common dimensional relations* – for example, E1 chose two green objects and E2 chose two yellow objects, so that the child had to match IDENTICAL (color, $(X1)$, color $(X2)$) and IDENTICAL (color, $(Y1)$, color $(Y2)$); the correct response was (e.g.) two red objects.

All of the children performed extremely well on the object-identity trials (all of the 2-year-olds achieved criterion of 75% correct), as well as on the identity relations trials (90% of the 2-year-olds achieved criterion). They also performed well on the common-attribute trials; 70% of the 2-year-olds achieved criterion on color and 80% on size. However, performance dropped sharply on the trials involving common dimensional relations; in fact, none of the 2-year-olds reached criterion for either color or size. In this and in other studies, the order of emergence seems to be matching *identical objects* – which Smith (1989) suggests has a special place in the development of similarity – followed by matching the *identity relation* and then by matching simple *object attributes.* Still later, attributes become organized into dimensions such as color and size, and children can match *relations between attributes* along the same dimension.

Comparing the effects of object similarity and relational similarity

As discussed earlier, an advantage of perceptual domain is that it is possible to decompose relational similarity and object similarity. In collaboration with Judy DeLoache, we investigated the performance of 3- and 4-year-olds on a perceptual mapping task in which relational similarity was pitted against object similarity (Rattermann & Gentner, 1990; Rattermann, Gentner, & DeLoache, 1987, 1989). In this task, the child and the experimenter each had a set of three objects (clay pots or blue plastic boxes), which displayed *monotonic increase* in size. That is, the objects increased in size along a continuum from left to right. The child watched while a sticker was placed under one of the objects in the experimenter's set and then searched for the sticker under one of the objects in the child's set.[11] The task was designed so that the relational response was always correct; that is, the correct response was always based on relative size (e.g., largest object to largest object).[12] The child was always shown the correct answer and, if correct, was allowed to keep the sticker.

We introduced a tension between object similarity and relational similarity by staggering the sizes of the two triads. For example, if the experimenter's set contained objects of size 1, 2, and 3, the child's set contained objects of size 2, 3, and 4. This arrangement created a cross-mapping between the two triads: If the experimenter chose object 3 in her triad, the child should choose object 4 (the object of the same relative size) in his triad, resisting the perfect object match between the experimenter's object 3 and the child's object 3. Thus,

Stimulus Sets

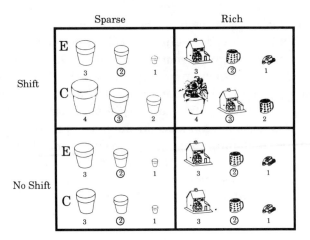

Figure 7.4. Stimulus sets from Rattermann, Gentner, and DeLoache (1987, 1989).

the logic of this task was to pit object similarity against relational similarity and observe whether the child would carry out the relational mapping between the two structures.

To carry this logic further, if indeed the tension between object-based and relation-based similarity in the cross-mapping condition hampers children's performance, then this disrupting effect should vary with the degree of similarity. To test this, we compared the simple stimuli discussed so far with complex, distinctive objects such as a large red flower, a medium brown wooden house, and a small green and pink coffee mug (Figure 7.4). This manipulation should enable us to address the issue of effects of object similarity more precisely, for the richer an object (i.e., the greater the number of features it possesses) the greater should be its similarity to an identical object (Tversky, 1977). Therefore, the disruptive effects of the object matches in the cross-mapping condition should be greater with the richer stimuli. The results of the richness manipulation were as predicted. The children performed worse with the rich than with the sparse stimuli (33 vs. 54% for the 3-year-olds and 38 vs. 63% for the 4-year-olds). Consistent with the competing-similarity account, we also found significantly more object identity responses with the rich stimuli than with the sparse stimuli. Performance was disrupted when object similarity was in conflict with the correct relational similarity, and this decrement was worse with richer stimuli and for younger children.

As an additional check on the consistency of the predictions, we ran a literal-similarity condition, in which object similarity was correlated with relational similarity. To accomplish this we restructured the experimenter's set and the child's set such that both contained objects of size 1, 2, and 3. Thus, the experimenter's choice (e.g., the object of size 3) could be mapped onto the child's correct choice (also size 3) on the basis of relational similarity, object similarity (the objects were identical), or both. As expected, children performed extremely well in this condition. The 4-year-olds performed virtually perfectly with both rich and sparse stimuli. In contrast, the 3-year-olds performed well only with the rich stimuli (86% correct, as opposed to 55% correct with sparse stimuli). The 3-year-olds appeared to benefit from the additional similarity conferred by a rich object match. These two tasks present a consistent picture: In a task that requires attention to relational similarity, 3-year-olds benefit from rich object similarity when object similarity and relational similarity are correlated and are distracted by it when the two are in competition. Four-year-olds show greater ability to extract purely relational similarity when necessary, though they too find the task easier when both relational and object similarity point in the same direction.

The shift from lower-order relations to higher-order relations. The last step in our proposed career of similarity is the shift to the ability to perceive similarity solely on the basis of common higher-order relations. Kotovsky and Gentner (1990a, b) studied children's ability to perceive similarity based on perceptual higher-order relations such as monotonicity and symmetry. They gave 4-, 6-, and 8-year-old children a forced-choice triads task in which they were shown a standard embodying some relational structure – say, symmetry (e.g., XoX) – and asked to say which of two other figures it was most similar to: another instance of symmetry (HiH) or a second figure that lacked the symmetry relation (iHH). Four-year-olds chose randomly, whereas 6- and 8-year-olds were progressively more likely to select the figure with the common higher-order relations. Additional evidence is provided by Chipman and Mendelson (1979), who presented 5-, 7-, 9-, and 11-year-old children with pairs of patterned displays and asked them to judge relative complexity. They found an age-related increase in the effect of structure on these complexity judgments. The older children judged stimuli that contained higher-order visual structure as relatively less complex than did the younger children. Similarly, Halford and Wilson (1980) found that 4-year-old children were able to learn mappings based on first-order relations but not those based on higher-order relations, whereas children over 5 years of age were able to learn both.

Taken together, these results suggest that in perceptual similarity (a) there is a shift toward greater perception of common higher-order relations and (b) some higher-order relational commonalities are perceived well before the advent of formal operations. Recently, Kotovsky and Gentner (1990b) have found that even 4-year-olds can be taught to choose on the basis of higher-order relations with training. The fact that higher-order commonalities can be taught to young children is further evidence for an experiential, rather than a solely maturational, basis for this progression.

Summary and comparison with other views

In our summary of the development of similarity in causal domains, we found a progression from the ability to perceive overall similarity between two situations to the ability to perceive various kinds of partial matches: matches between particular objects, matches between object attributes and between first-order relations, and finally matches between higher-order relations. A similar, though more detailed, developmental sequence appears to hold in perceptual domains. The ability to perceive overall similarity between scenes is gradually augmented, first by the ability to perceive identity matches between objects, then by the ability to perceive matches between object attributes and first-order relations (including identity relations between objects and, later, dimensional relations between object attributes), and finally by the ability to perceive matches between higher-order relations such as symmetry. In both perceptual and causal domains, this evolution is cumulative, so that later abilities supplement prior abilities rather than replacing them. Further, the evidence suggests that the shift in similarity use is not based on age. As can be seen in Figure 7.5, the shift from objects to relations and from conservative literal similarity to partial matches can be seen at several different ages. The fact that similar shifts occur at different

	INFANCY		EARLY CHILDHOOD		LATE CHILDHOOD	
	5 months	10 months	(early)	(late)		
Kolstad and Ballargeon Infants habituate to a cylindrical container then see a square container or a cylindrical non-container	Dishabituate to square container but not to cylindrical non-container (object-similarity inference)	Dishabuate to cylindrical non-container but not to square container (relational inference)				
Baillargeon Infants watch frame pass through object (impossible event); A similar object is available as standard	4 months Can use highly similar standard to make inferences about possible events	6 months Can use moderately similar standard to make inferences about possible events				
DeLoache Children see a toy hidden in a room and must find a miniature toy in a model room			31 months Cannot find the toy in the model room	38 months Can find toy when similarity is high between room and model		
Rattermann, Gentner & DeLoache Children must use relational similarity to select correct object. A Ⓑ C initial set B Ⓒ D target set			41 months Succeed with sparse stimuli; fail (i.e., make object identity error) with rich stimuli	54 months Succeed with (i.e., transfer relations) with both rich and sparse stimuli		
Gentner Verbal interpretations of metaphors such as "A cloud is a sponge"					5-7 years Mainly attributional responses: "Both are round and fluffy"	7-9 years Many relational responses: "Both can hold water"
Gentner & Toupin Retell a story (with or w/o explicit causal structure) using new characters. original: A B C high sim: A' B' C' X-mapped: B' C' A'					5-7 years Performance depends only on object similarity; hi sim >> X-mapped	8-10 years Performance depends on both object similarity and presence of causal structure

Figure 7.5. A sampler of research on the career of similarity, showing shifts occurring at different ages in different domains.

ages from infancy to late childhood[13] suggests that it is not maturation but increases in a child's knowledge that drives the evolution of similarity.

This view of a developmental course from a naïve to sophisticated use of similarity is not new. In addition to Quine's characterization discussed earlier, it draws upon prior theories of development. An important influence on this framework, as already discussed, is E. J. Gibson's (1969) differentiation hypothesis. We have incorporated her view that the environment is rich in stimulus information and that the main task of the perceiver is to make sense of the information. Young children perceive this input in an undifferentiated fashion, whereas older children and adults analyze stimuli into their constituent features and dimensions. Our position has much in common with Bruner's proposal that children shift from a reliance on perceptual-configural information to a reliance on functional information, since the function of an object is one aspect of its relational structure (Bruner et al., 1966). Thus, both accounts predict that children will acquire the ability to utilize functional relations later than the ability to utilize perceptual attributes of an object. The accounts differ, however, in that for Bruner the cut is between perceptual and functional information, whereas for us the most important theoretical cut is between objects and relations, with perceptual versus functional (causal) information being a lesser issue. A more fundamental difference between our view and many of these prior views concerns the *cause of the shift*. The evidence presented here indicates that shifts in similarity processing occur at very different times in different domains. Therefore, we depart from prior theorists who have proposed maturational-stage accounts of the shift in similarity. We suggest instead that changes in the kinds of similarity a child can perceive are driven largely by the accretion and gentrification (as discussed later) of knowledge of the world.

A theoretical perspective that shares Gibson's emphasis on the role of the environment in learning and development is that of *situated cognition* (e.g., Brown, Collins, & Duguid, 1989). According to this view, the environment in which learning occurs has a marked effect on what is learned and how well it can be transferred. Our view of the initial conservative use of similarity is akin to the claim that initial learning is contextually situated. We stress, however, that part of learning is the "desituating" of cognition, that is, an increase in the ability to extract and use partial matches. This is compatible with the suggestion that the use of multiple contexts of learning can lead to more abstract, generalizable knowledge (Collins, Brown, & Newman, 1989). One process by which the initial conservative use of overall similarity might give way to selective matches is the abstraction process whereby the result of a similarity comparison is a slightly more abstract data structure, as discussed by Ross (1989) and others (Elio & Anderson, 1981; Forbus & Gentner, 1986; Gick & Holyoak, 1983; Hayes-Roth & McDermott, 1978; Medin & Ross, 1989). These accounts imply a role for conservative literal-similarity comparisons, since these are likely to be noticed initially and can gradually lead to more abstract matches.

There are also positions that differ markedly from our own. For instance, Bryant (1974) proposes that children are able to use relational information developmentally before they are able to use absolute information (object attributes). He offers as evidence results from many tasks in which children are more adept at using relations such as *bigger* than at using an absolute attribute such as *six inches tall*. A partial resolution between Bryant's position and our own is that the evolutionary shift we postulate is between objects and relations, not object attributes and relations. (As will be remembered from the section on perceptual development, making object matches precedes making either attribute matches or relational matches.) In most of the tasks Bryant considers, the objects were quite sparse; in fact, they typically differed along only one dimension (i.e., in one attribute). Thus, a possible rapprochement is as follows: Object matches are made before relational matches (as stipulated in the present hypothesis), except when the objects are so sparse as to reduce to single-attribute comparison (as in some of the transposition studies considered by Bryant). As we have seen with the Rattermann, Gentner, and DeLoache search task, the effects of object identity may vary with the richness of the objects being matched.

Another contrasting position is that of Frank Keil (1989). He proposes that children are natively endowed with rich theoretical structures that guide much of their behavior and suggests that they fall back on their sense of similarity only when their theory of a domain fails them. He points out that adults display behavior similar to that of children when they are placed in domains in which they do not have knowledge of the true mechanisms. We agree with many of Keil's insights, including the observation that reliance on naïve similarity varies inversely with knowledge of the correct domain theory.

However, Keil's theory and our *career of similarity* hypothesis differ in their account of the causal relationship between similarity and theory building. For Keil, the use of similarity not only is unsophisticated but is a relatively unimportant aspect of development; it is merely a strategy to fall back on when theories fail. In contrast, we see similarity as contributing to the development of theories. Children's similarity comparisons allow them to extract commonalities, which can then be the grist for theory building. Conversely, as children gain theoretical insight into a given domain, their representations of situations in the domain will begin to incorporate the relations sanctioned by the theory, so that subsequent similarity comparisons come to be more illuminating. A compelling example of this process is provided by Carey's (1985) studies of children acquiring biological knowledge. Carey found that children's attribution of biological attributes to animals was based in part on their similarity to humans (possibly because children's knowledge about humans is rich enough to serve as a kind of prototype). An even more striking use of humans as a universal base is Inagaki and Hatano's (1987) finding that preschool children base inferences about how plants take nourishment on a mapping from humans. With development, children become more selective and theory-guided in their use of similarity. Carey attributes this change in performance to changes in the nature and organization of their domain knowledge.

Language and the career of similarity

So far, we have discussed the relational shift as a purely conceptual phenomenon. Now we turn to its interactions with language acquisition: specifically, with the acquisition of word meaning. At least three directions of influence are possible. First, we might expect similarity processing to influence word meaning. To the degree that children's word meanings are based on the commonalities they perceive when they hear a word applied to several exemplars, the kinds of similarities children can extract in a given domain will influence the word meanings they will derive. Second, there could be influences from language to similarity. Perhaps, in a variant of the Whorfian hypothesis, the possession of certain words (e.g., relational terms) confers a greater ability to extract certain kinds of similarities, or perhaps practice with language confers the habit of extraction. Third, there may be parallels between the development of meaning and

the development of similarity caused by their both being constrained by a third factor, such as the child's current cognitive stage
or current domain representations. For example, it has been suggested that the acquisition of early relational expressions, such as
allgone, coincides with the child's stage of understanding of object
permanence (Gopnik & Meltzoff, 1984; Tomasello & Farrar, 1984).
We will consider the evidence in the following order: (a) general
developmental parallels; (b) influences from similarity to language;
and (c) influences from language to similarity.

General developmental parallels

Order of vocabulary acquisition. If we apply the patterns we have found
for the development of similarity to the development of meaning,
several predictions follow. First, we might expect an early holistic
stage in word acquisition before object meanings are extracted. Second, we would expect words for objects to enter children's vocabulary before words for attributes and especially before words for
relations. Finally, words for higher-order relations should be acquired later than words for first-order relations.[14]

There is evidence that children do not immediately catch on to
the notion of reference. Several investigators have reported an early
stage at which they use a kind of prereferential vocalization between
babbling and true words.[15] Prewords often appear to be contextually
embedded parts of routines rather than true referential symbols. For
example, Gillis (1986, 1987) observed the early form *brrrm-brrrm,* at
first uttered only when the child was pushing a certain toy car. A
common next step is for the child to experience a spurt in vocabulary at around $1\frac{1}{2}$ to 2 years. This vocabulary spurt consists chiefly
of concrete nouns (both common and proper) and has been called
the "nominal insight" (Macnamara, 1982).[16] Stern (1914) refers to
this as the "greatest discovery of the child's life" – that "*each* thing
has its name" (Stern, 1914, p. 108; quoted in Vygotsky, 1962, p. 43).
Thus, the child's first truly semantic achievement is to extract and
name objects separately from their contexts. This suggests another
parallel with the development of similarity: Words for objects should
be acquired before words for relations. Indeed, this appears to be
the case. Concrete nouns (including both proper and common nouns)
outnumber verbs and other relational terms by a large margin in
children's early production vocabularies (Dromi, 1982; Gentner, 1982c;

Huttenlocher & Smiley, 1987; Macnamara, 1982; Nelson, 1973b) as well as in their comprehension vocabularies (Goldin-Meadow, Seligman, & Gelman, 1976).[17] Gentner (1982c) used cross-linguistic vocabulary evidence to establish the generality of this early noun advantage and to rule out various explanations specific to English, such as SVO (subject–verb–object) word order and the greater morphological variability of verbs as compared with nouns, both of which are presumably disadvantageous to verbs in acquisition. Even stronger evidence for the generality of the noun advantage comes from studies by Schwartz, Camarata, and Leonard in which children were presented with novel words, either as nouns or as verbs, and then tested for the production of these words. Even when stress, frequency, phonological makeup, and word order are equated, children are more likely to produce words experienced as nouns than as verbs (Camarata & Leonard, 1986; Camarata & Schwartz, 1985; Schwartz & Terrell, 1983). Thus, it appears that the reasons for the early noun advantage are conceptual or semantic factors. We suggest that part of the explanation is that objects are easier to extract from the stream of experience than are relations.

Even after relational terms have entered the vocabulary, children are slow to acquire their full meanings (Berman, 1980; Bowerman, 1978a, b; Gentner, 1982c). The correct usage of common verbs such as *come* and *go* (Clark & Garnica, 1974), *buy* and *sell* (Gentner, 1975), *mix, beat,* and *stir* (Gentner, 1978), and *pour* and *fill* (Bowerman, 1982; see also Pinker, 1984, pp. 309–312) is not fully mastered until rather late (5 or 6 years of age and, in some cases, as late as 8 years or older). Relational adjectives, such as *high/low, more/less,* and *big/ little,* are also slow to be fully mastered. For example, children about 4 or 5 years old sometimes interchange opposite members of dimensional pairs (H. H. Clark, 1970; Donaldson & Wales, 1970; Wales & Campbell, 1970).

More to the point, relational adjectives are sometimes used attributionally at first, as though they referred to properties of objects instead of to relations between objects. The clearest cases of this kind of usage occur with dimensional terms, as reported by Smith and her colleagues (Sera & Smith, 1987; Smith, Rattermann, & Sera, 1988). For example, Smith, Rattermann, and Sera asked 3- and 4-year-olds to judge which of two butterflies was "higher" or "lower," given pairs of butterflies placed at various heights. The 4-year-olds correctly responded according to the spatial relations between the butterflies. In contrast, the 3-year-olds responded as though "higher" and "lower" were object attributes meaning "high" and "low," respectively; that is, they might call both butterflies "higher" if they were more than three feet from the floor and otherwise "lower."

In summary, there appear to be parallels between the order of vocabulary acquisition and the developmental progression found for similarity. As Macnamara (1972, p. 4) states:

> Children learn names for colors, shapes, and sizes only after they have learned names for many objects. . . . A further hypothesis is that the child will not learn the name for states or activities until he has firmly grasped the name for at least some entities which exemplify such states and activities. Thus the order of learning would be as follows: names for entities, names for their variable states and actions, and names for more permanent attributes such as color.

This order differs slightly from the order we have suggested, but it still roughly parallels the order of extraction of partial similarities that we postulated in the first part of this chapter.

Mutual influence between similarity-based categories and word-based categories. One factor that affects whether a set of objects receives the psychological status of a category is the degree of similarity among the objects. Another is whether they receive the same linguistic label. Thus, there is a constant potential for interaction between similarity acting as a bottom-up influence and word reference acting as a top-down influence. In this section we first consider evidence that early in acquisition children rely heavily on physical similarity to determine the extensions of words. We then consider evidence that later in acquisition, category labels may prompt children to look beyond overall physical similarity.

Applying words to new instances: Do young children expect the referents of a word to be similar to one another? In a highly influential paper, E. V. Clark (1973) reviewed diary studies of early vocabularies and showed that early overextensions typically involved perceptual commonalities, notably shape (e.g., "mooi" [moon] for cakes, round marks on a window, round shapes on books, tooling on leather book covers, postmarks, and the letter *O*). She suggested that an important aspect of early word meanings is the child's expectation that the referents of a term will be perceptually similar to one another.

Many subsequent studies have corroborated this pattern: Children's early overextensions of nominal terms appear to be based primarily on perceptual commonalities, especially shape (Anglin, 1977; Bowerman, 1976, 1978a). This suggests that young children may be operating under the assumption that the extensions of object names are based on physical similarity.

Other evidence that young children bring an assumption of physical similarity to the learning of word meanings comes from a study by Gentner (1982b). Children were taught names for two objects with different forms and functions: a "jiggy," a yellow box with a face that wiggled its eyebrows when the child pulled its lever, and a "zimbo," a red candy machine that dispensed jelly beans when the child pulled its lever. The two toys were simply presented as toys left in various rooms of the experimental suite, and their names were taught in a naturalistic manner. (Whoever came by would refer to them by saying, "Have you played with the jiggy? See how it works?") When the children could produce both words spontaneously, they were shown a new object that looked like the jiggy, but that (to their astonishment) dispensed jellybeans when they pulled its lever. When asked to name this new object, the preschoolers (aged 2 to 5 years) were governed by physical similarity. More than 80% called it a "jiggy," despite the fact that it shared a highly salient function with the zimbo. Children aged 5 to 9 years gave more function-based responses (about 60% "zimbo").[18] An interesting feature of these results is that the zimbo's function of dispensing jelly beans was quite salient to the children, especially to the preschoolers. Indeed, we informally noticed that preschoolers learned the term "zimbo" more quickly than the term "jiggy" and used it much more often. Yet in choosing which term to extend to the new object, they chose on the basis of form, even though that meant using the "less preferred" term. As Gentner (1982b) noted, this suggests that children impose implicit selection criteria as to which aspects of objects enter into word reference. In this initial stage, it appears that perceptual information predominates in their implicit theory of reference.[19]

Another early-word-learning task was that of Tomikawa and Dodd (1980), who taught 2- to 4-year-olds names for categories that were based either on common shape or on common function. They used a 3 (shapes) × 3 (functions) matrix of objects. Each child was taught three words, each applying to three objects, in a storytelling format.

The key variable was whether the three objects had a common shape (e.g., "mep" applied to a rectangular magnet, a rectangular box that could be opened and closed, and a rectangular rattle) or a common function (e.g., "mep" applied to a rectangular magnet, a circular magnet, and an L-shaped magnet). After hearing the story, in which the nine objects were named and their functions demonstrated, the child was given a comprehension test. Three of the objects, each differing in shape and in function from the other two, were held up in turn and their functions demonstrated again. Then they were placed before the child, who was asked to point to the "mep." The child was then shown two more triads of objects in the same pattern, each with a different word (thus receiving one test on each of the three words learned). Corrective feedback was given on each trial. Then the story was retold and the child retested, up to six times or until the child could pick out all three objects.

The results were quite striking. The children readily learned names for the common-shape categories but performed dismally on the common-function categories. Combining the results of two experiments (Experiments 3 and 4), 10 of 12 children in the common-shape condition could correctly identify the referents of the names they had learned, and none of the 12 children in the common-function condition were able to do so. It is interesting that when children of the same age (2 to 4 years) were asked simply to group the objects without linguistic labels, their groupings, though still dominated by physical similarity, were more mixed: 72–76% common-shape and 15–13% common-function groupings (in Experiments 1 and 2, respectively).[20] Consistent with the results of the previous study, it appears that the use of words increased young children's (already high) focus on physical similarity. Tomikawa and Dodd concluded that perceptual similarity is a strong determinant of early word reference.

A growing body of research, much of it by Markman, Waxman, Gelman, and their colleagues, has explored the ways in which the use of common nouns as linguistic labels can influence children's categorization choices. For example, Markman and Hutchinson (1984) contrasted children's categorization patterns with and without linguistic labels. They gave 2- to 3-year-olds a triad sorting task, for example, putting a police car where it belongs, either with another car (same category, and also highly similar) or with a policeman (thematically related). The children shifted from roughly chance sorting (59% categorical sorting) to predominantly categorical sorting (83%) when a novel object name was used. ("This is a dax. Put it with the other dax.") It is important that the children did not have to know in advance what the word meant in order to show this shift. They apparently believed that words pick out categories of like (rather than thematically related) objects. An interesting question is whether the scope of this effect varies with age, as might be predicted from what we have said so far. For 2- and 3-year-olds, the effect has been demonstrated only for highly similar objects (members of the same basic-level class, such as *birthday cake* and *chocolate cake*). Four-year-olds were tested on a broader range of stimuli and showed the switch to category-based responding even when the named object did not resemble its fellow category member.[21] For example, given a car to group with either a bicycle or a car tire, they would put the car with the tire in a nonlabeling task but put it with the bicycle in a labeling task. It remains to be seen whether the younger children would show the labeling effects without the benefit of strong object similarity.

A study by Taylor and Gelman (1989) provides further evidence for the role of similarity in early word meanings. Taylor and Gelman were interested in the way children learn subordinate categories. First they taught $1\frac{1}{2}$- to $2\frac{1}{2}$-year-old children a novel word for an object; for example, they referred several times to a large green beach ball as a "tiv." (Because the study concerns subordinate categories, they used objects such as dogs and balls that already had generic names in the child's lexicon.) They then asked the child to "put the tiv in the box," choosing from the original object and another possible "tiv" exemplar as well as other objects. The other possible "tiv" could be either quite similar to the original "tiv" (e.g., a red beach ball) or very dissimilar (e.g., an orange and black soccer ball). The results showed striking effects of similarity. When the new possible exemplar was highly similar to the original one, the children distributed their "tiv" responses across both exemplars. But when the new exemplar was dissimilar, most of the children chose only the original named toy. These results suggest that children $1\frac{1}{2}$ to $2\frac{1}{2}$ years of age are able to form a subordinate category and to extend it to other instances but that this ability may be limited to conditions of strong physical similarity.

Finally, research that directly addressed the effects of language on children's classification abilities was performed by Waxman and

Gelman (1986). They presented 3- and 4-year-olds with a free classification task in which the children were placed in one of three conditions: (a) the *label* condition, in which superordinate category labels were provided, (b) the *instance* condition, in which common instances of the category were provided, and (c) the *group* condition, in which common instances of the category were provided and the children were instructed to consider the instances as a group. Waxman and Gelman found that the 4-year-olds classified virtually perfectly in all three conditions (approximately 98% correct classifications). The 3-year-olds, in contrast, classified perfectly only in the label condition (approximately 95% correct classifications as opposed to approximately 80% in the group condition and 74% in the instance condition). In a further study Waxman and Gelman found that the young children classified equally well with known English or novel Japanese labels. The children's performance with the Japanese labels shows that children's categorizing behavior is based not on particular word meanings but on a general understanding of what words do. This research suggests a relationship between children's linguistic competence and their ability to form taxonomic structures.

More precise information on how words focus children's attention was contributed by Landau, Smith, and Jones (1988). They found that the use of a nominal label prompts young children to pay attention to the common shape of objects. Their results suggest that young children very early on have specific opinions concerning *which aspects* of the referent enter into word meanings, at least for object names. Their first guesses as to the meanings of object terms are perceptual similarity, particularly shape.

Words taken as signals of nonapparent commonalities. Other studies have shown that children can overcome the effects of object similarity when they are given the same category label for dissimilar objects. Gelman and Markman (1987) investigated the role of similarity and common word labels in determining whether 3- and 4-year-old children would extrapolate characteristics from one object to others. They showed children a picture of a standard – for example, a bluebird – and told them a new fact about it – for example, "This bird feeds its babies mashed-up food." The children were then asked whether this property would apply to each of four new objects: a bluebird (highly similar to standard and same category as standard), a blackbird (low similarity, same category), a blue butterfly (high similarity, different category), and a dog (low similarity, different category). In one condition, the *picture-only* condition, the children were told, "This one feeds its babies mashed-up food" when shown the standard, and asked of each of the test pictures, "Does this one feed its babies mashed-up food?" In the *word-and-picture* condition, the children were given labels for all the objects – for example, "This bird feeds its babies mashed-up food," and "Does this bird/butterfly/dog feed its babies mashed-up food?" As would be expected, children in the picture-only condition were more likely to base their inferences on the degree of similarity between the standard and the new item (53% similarity-based responses) than the children in the word-and-picture condition (29% similarity-based responses). In contrast, when labels were added, the children's inferences were strongly influenced by the category information provided by the label; they attributed the characteristic "feeds its baby mashed-up food" to the items given the same label as the example (63.5% category-based responses in the word-and-picture condition vs. 46% category-based responses in the picture-only condition).[22] Yet even in the labeling condition object similarity did have an effect. Within a category the children drew more inferences from one picture to another when their appearances were similar.

Taken together, these findings suggest that children initially expect that words apply to sets of physically *similar* objects, as evidenced by the fact that they (a) spontaneously extend words to other similar objects; (b) find it easier to learn new words that apply to sets of physically similar objects than to learn new words for sets of functionally similar objects; and (c) choose a physically similar object when asked to find another instance of a new word. However, if an established category label is applied to a *dissimilar* item, the child (at least by 3 or 4 years of age) may accept this extension of the category and base further inferences on it. For older children, a word can function as a promissory note, signaling subtle commonalities that the child does not yet perceive (Gelman & Coley, Chapter 5, this volume). In either case, children strongly assume that the objects labeled by a common word will be similar. Early in the career of similarity, children are limited to overall physical similarity, with perhaps an early emergence of similarity of shape. Later in the career of similarity, although overall similarity within labeled categories remains the initial presumption, children can set aside this assumption when it fails and seek other kinds of similarity, such as relational commonalities.

Effects of language on the relational shift

We have considered influences from conceptual development to language acquisition. We turn now to the reverse question, the perennially intriguing Whorfian issue of whether the acquisition of language changes children's cognitive processing – in this case, their perception of similarity. Vygotsky proposed that "thought development is determined by language, i.e., by the linguistic tools of thought and by the sociocultural experience of the child. . . . The child's intellectual growth is contingent on his mastering the social means of thought, that is, language" (1962, p. 51). He postulated a developmental progression from social speech to egocentric speech and then to inner speech. Once inner speech is available, he suggested, the course of cognitive development is fundamentally altered.

Returning to our specific focus, we may then ask whether the acquisition of language influences the kinds of similarity a child can use. One affirmative speculation comes from Kuenne (1946). Working within the Hull–Spence tradition, she invoked language to explain children's capacity to learn relational responses in a transposition task, despite their assumed bias for absolute stimulus–response learning. However, clear evidence for such an influence is hard to find, since it requires comparing children with and without language. Fortunately, some insightful inquiries have been conducted with nonhuman subjects. We turn now to Premack's research on teaching chimpanzees an artifical language.[23]

Premack's investigations of nonhuman primates. Premack (1983) found an intriguing relation between analogy and language in his research on teaching artificial languages to chimpanzees. Seven chimpanzees that were closely reared and trained by humans – three that were exposed to language training, four that were not – were tested on various kinds of cognitive tasks, such as reasoning, map reading, conservation, and match-to-sample. Premack found that the two groups were comparable in their performance on most tasks, with the nonlanguage group perhaps slightly superior. However, there was evidence that language training may have conferred benefits on certain kinds of similarity tasks and, in particular, analogy tasks.

We begin with the analogy tasks. Unfortunately, these tasks were given to only one member of the language-trained group, Sarah, who may have been an unusually intelligent animal. However, as discussed later, some corroborating evidence has been found using new populations. One task was a matching-proportion test utilizing cut-up fruit and partly filled containers (Woodruff & Premack, 1981). All the chimps successfully solved a literal-similarity match; for example, they passed a test given one-quarter apple as the sample, with one-quarter apple and three-quarters apple as alternatives. However, only the language-trained chimp, Sarah, could solve an analogical proportion problem – for example, a half-filled container as sample, with half apple and three-quarters apple as alternatives. The difference in performance was sharp: All four non-language-trained animals failed, whereas Sarah passed the analogical problems from the beginning. A further test of the ability to perform relational matches was a match-to-sample task using pairs of items – for example, *XX* goes with *YY* or *CD*, or *XY* goes with *BB* or *CD*. Whereas Sarah was 100% correct on both same–same trials and different – different trials, the non-language-trained chimpanzees performed at chance level and showed no progress, even after 15 sessions of 12 trials with corrective feedback.

As already discussed, one difficulty with the tasks is that only one language-trained chimp (Sarah) was tested, leaving open the possibility that the differences were the result of higher than average intelligence rather than of language training. However, this possibility is vitiated somewhat by two further results. First, all seven chimpanzees were tested on another relational task. In this task, each chimp was shown two samples and had to indicate whether they were same or different – for example, apple/apple (same) or apple/banana (different). Though this task might seem simple, Premack argues that explicitly *labeling* similarity and difference involves another level of difficulty than simply *responding* to sameness, as in match-to-sample tasks. Even after 900 training trials, the four non-language-trained chimpanzees failed to learn the use of the *same/different* labels. In contrast, all three language-trained animals readily learned the task. Finally, Premack (1988) trained four new animals, utilizing a lag procedure so that all the animals received the same training at different times. Premack gave the animals four kinds of language training: (a) learning a lexicon, (b) learning sentences, (c) learning the terms *same* and *different,* and (d) learning the interrogative construction. He then tested their performance on analogy tasks similar to those already described. Their performance was markedly improved by language training. Further, the gain appeared to be specifically related to learning the terms *same* and *different.*[24]

These results suggest that some aspects of language training can lead to improvement in analogical ability. In particular, learning to use the labels *same* and *different* appears to be important. Premack (1983) suggests two other ways in which language training may lead to cognitive benefits. First, it can teach the idea that one thing can stand for another. But noting that this would not be sufficient to account for the improvement in analogical ability, Premack goes on to suggest, second, that language training "appears to change the animal's unit of computation, moving it upward from an element to a relation, thus from a relation between elements to a relation between relations" (Premack, 1983, p. 160).

Spontaneous speech about similarity. We return now to studies of infants' sequential touching patterns to consider the language children spontaneously use during this task. Although this line of study properly belongs to the category of "parallel development" (since there is no telling which direction of influence applies) we have included it here because, like Premack's work, it bears on the relation between language *about similarity* and similarity processing. As discussed earlier, in the sequential touching task infants are given objects drawn from two identity classes, and their spontaneous touching and grouping patterns are observed (Nelson, 1973a; Ricciuti, 1965; Starkey, 1981).

Sugarman (1982) found that 12-month-olds tended to group objects to form one identity group, while 24- to 36-month-olds tended to form two identity groups. However, within this second group, the 24-month-olds formed groups sequentially (e.g., by forming a set of boats followed by a set of dolls); 30- to 36-month-olds formed these two groups by alternating the placement of objects between them (e.g., by placing a boat, then a doll, then a boat, etc.), suggesting that they could compare the two similarity classes. Sugarman further noticed that many of the older children spontaneously engaged in discussion of similarity and difference. The children's language use also showed a progression with age: (a) no reference;

(b) isolated reference: for example, "boat" while grasping a boat (dominant in 18-month-olds); (c) iterative reference to one or both classes: that is, repeated reference to one class sometimes followed by repeated reference to the other class, as in *"lady, lady, lady . . . boat, boat, boat"*; (d) coordinated reference to two classes: as in *"lady, boat, lady, boat."* Children used iterative reference from 24 months on, but only the 30- and 36-month-olds used the more sophisticated coordinated reference. These parallels between language and grouping behavior suggest a relation between them, although, as Sugarman points out, they do not tell us about the direction of influence.

Can relational labels help children focus on relational similarity? So far we have considered the effects of using words on children's use of object similarity. Now we ask whether the use of labels can help a child to extract relational similarity. To test this question, we conducted a follow-up study to the mapping task described earlier (Rattermann, Gentner, & DeLoache, 1987, 1990). Recall that 3-year-olds performed at chance level in the original task, which required children to use a relational rule ("same relative size") to map from one triad of objects to another to find a hidden sticker. They were unable to map relative size when a competing object similarity was present. We wondered whether the use of relational labels could improve their performance. We taught 3-year-olds to apply the words *Daddy*, *Mommy*, and *Baby* to the objects in each triad (large, medium, and small, respectively). We also used the following labels in our questions: "My sticker is under my mommy. Where do you think your sticker is?" Under these conditions, the children correctly performed a relational mapping despite a tempting object foil. Thus, the use of explicit common labels for the relational roles of the objects appears to have highlighted the relational similarity between the triads and permitted an earlier appreciation of relational likeness.

There is also evidence that the choice of relational labels can affect children's performance on a metaphor interpretation task. Vosniadou, Ortony, Reynolds, and Wilson (1984) asked preschool, first-grade, and third-grade children to act out short stories. These stories ended in metaphorical sentences describing an action of one of the characters in the story. The key manipulation was whether the verb in the metaphoric completion sentence was *general* or *specific*. For example, in a story describing how a boy (Paul) became frightened, the *general-verb* version of the final sentence was "Paul was a rabbit *running* to his hole," and the *specific-verb* version was "Paul was a rabbit *hopping* to his hole."[25] The metaphors were designed so that the general verbs could apply naturally in the target domain (Paul's actions) and therefore could be interpreted literally. In contrast, the *specific* verb was inappropriate if interpreted literally. The specificity of the verb affected the younger but not the older children. Younger children were likely to act out the metaphor incorrectly when the verb was specific; for example, they would make Billy hop to his bedroom. In contrast, older children were able to reinterpret the verb in the metaphorically correct manner: Given either verb, they simply made Billy run to his room. Thus, for younger children, the ability to extract the common relation was sensitive to the word used to describe it.

Re-representation. We now discuss a process that we think may be important in learning, which we call *re-representation* (Gentner, 1989). To explain this notion, we consider the mapping process necessary in the Vosniadou et al. task. For simplicity, we suppose that the child already knows (from the story) that Paul is running to his room. To understand this metaphor, the child must map her representation of the rabbit scenario onto her representation of what Paul is doing. Let us assume that she can guess that *rabbit* should map onto *Paul* and *hole* onto *room*. If the verb *running* is used, the alignment is straightforward. But when *hopping* is used in the base, the direct result of the mapping is not quite right, since Paul is not hopping.[26] To align the two representations, the child must drop the *manner* of motion, retaining only *rapid movement by foot*. This requires *re-representing* the verb in a more abstract form. Depending on theoretical preferences, we could describe this as decomposing the verb *hop* and stripping away some of its predicates (e.g., Burstein, 1986) or as moving up an abstraction hierarchy (Falkenhainer's "minimal ascension principle," 1988) or as extracting a common schema (Gick & Holyoak, 1980, 1983; Hayes-Roth & McDermott, 1978).

We conjecture that re-representation induced by trying to align partially similar situations may be one way that children gradually come to an appreciation of abstract commonalities. We further speculate that re-representational efforts may serve gradually to increase the uniformity of children's internal representations. This is because the representation derived from the effort to align two situations is likely to be less idiosyncratic than the representations of either of the prior situations. An arena where this suggestion may be especially workable is the learning of dimensional relations, as discussed by Smith (1989). If the child somehow succeeds in aligning "*A* bigger than *B*" with "*X* louder than *Y*" (perhaps by trying to understand a metaphor such as "a big voice"), it is possible that this results in more uniform representations – for example, "GREATER-THAN (size (*A*), size (*B*))" and "GREATER-THAN (loudness (*X*), loudness (*Y*))."[27] In many cases the impetus to make such an alignment will be common language labels, as in the the earlier example. This leads us to suggest a bootstrapping interaction between the acquisition of meaning and the processing of similarity in a given domain. To the degree that a child has learned words that denote relations, he may be better able to match situations containing these relations. Conversely, to the degree that a child has uniform representations of two situations, he can learn the meaning of a new word applied to both situations. We can imagine that each successful alignment leads to a slightly more uniform representation, which in turn increases the probability that the next two situations can be aligned, and so on. We could think of this gradual process as a kind of *gentrification of knowledge*, by analogy with the regularization of formerly complex, idiosyncratic local domains.

Conclusions

We set out in this chapter to characterize the development of similarity and to inquire about its causes. We found evidence that early similarity is highly conservative and that later development is characterized by an increasing ability to extract partial matches, including matches based only on common relations. Our theme throughout has been one of extraction. Paradoxically, it appears that children progress from complex to simple matches, rather than the reverse. Even infants can achieve matches based on massive overlap between two situations; what expertise confers is an increasing ability to extract sparse, abstract matches. However, despite the manifest differences, we see a continuum between massive global similarity matches and elegant relational isomorphisms. Thus, we find support for Quine's "career of similarity" from brute similarity to theoretical similarity.

Turning to the causes of the changes in similarity processing, we found no evidence for the claim that the shift to relational and higher-order relational similarity depends on reaching the formal operations stage. Very young children – even infants – can apprehend relational similarity when given materials whose relational structure is fully available to them. We cannot rule out maturational effects, but our survey suggests that knowledge is a more important determinant of similarity use. We then turned to another experiential factor: the acquisition of language. We drew on the research of Premack, along with some promising current investigations, to suggest that the possession of names for relations, including *same* and *different*, may be important for the appreciation of analogical similarity. This in turn suggests that the changes in knowledge that drive changes in similarity do not simply consist of accretion of domain facts, but also include the deepening and systematization of the knowledge base.

Notes

1. That is, they focused on analogies of the form $A:B::C:D$, in which the implicit assertion is of a (higher-order) identity between the relation (A, B) and the relation (C, D).
2. For present purposes, we consider metaphors and analogies together as nonliteral similarity comparisons.
3. One widely acknowledged difficulty here is that the concept of a domain is ill-defined. In this discussion we will roughly characterize a domain as a cluster of mutually interrelated concepts around a common topic.
4. This was termed the *mere-appearance* choice; however, in general these items were not similar enough to the C term to qualify as mere-appearance matches in the sense defined in the text. For example, the mere-appearance match to a girl with long brown hair was the fringe on a purple scarf.
5. We thank Usha Goswami for kindly providing us with the stimulus materials.
6. Causal relations are typically quite constrained as to the kinds of objects they can apply to, whereas perceptual relations can apply to a wide variety of objects. For example, the relation $BURN(x, y)$ requires y to be a combustible object, but the relation $ABOVE(x, y)$ can accept practically any pair of concrete objects.
7. The results did not depend on direction: Large-to-small and small-to-large were equally difficult for 31-month-olds. We will discuss only the large-to-small mapping for clarity of exposition.
8. DeLoache also manipulated the similarity of the surrounding walls of the rooms, but this manipulation had no significant effects. The percentage of correct retrieval is collapsed over this factor.
9. In our computer simulation of similarity processing, we represent dimensions as *functions*.

10. Shepp did not propose that dimensional structure ever entirely supplants overall similarity, noting that the work of Rosch and her colleagues indicates that many natural concepts may be structured by overall similarity rather than by a few criterial features or dimensions (Rosch & Mervis, 1975).

11. During a training phase it was explained to the child that the hiding place of the experimenter's sticker in her set could be used as a clue to where the child's sticker was hidden in his set.

12. Relative size and relative position were perfectly correlated, so the child actually had two relational cues to the correct response.

13. Indeed, the work of Chi, Feltovich, and Glaser (1981) comparing novices and experts in physics suggests that similar shifts from object-based to relation-based sorting can occur in adulthood.

14. Because word frequency differences and other differences confound this comparison, we cannot address this prediction adequately.

15. These vocalizations have been called "phonetically consistent forms" (Dore, Franklin, Miller, & Ramer, 1976), "indexical signs" (Dore, 1986), "sensorimotor morphemes" (Carter, 1979), "protowords" (Halliday, 1975; Menn, 1976; Menyuk & Menn, 1979), and "quasiwords" (Stoel-Gammon & Cooper, 1984).

16. Gillis (1984) has argued that the nominal shift is a gradual emergence rather than a sudden insight; but this does not alter the main point here.

17. Gopnik and Meltzoff (1986) appear to disagree with this claim, but the disagreement seems to be more apparent than real. They report the predicted pattern of more object words than relational words in their corpus of early language (Gopnik, 1980, 1981), but note that more *tokens* of each type occurred for the relational terms, a pattern that Gentner (1982c) also noted. Thus, there seems to be agreement that object-reference types outnumber relational types. This is all the more noteworthy because Gopnik and Meltzoff utilize a broad construal of the notion *relational term*. Along with terms that are generally agreed to be relational, such as *off, down,* and *more,* they include many terms that are commonly classified as social-interactional terms or as indeterminates, such as *there, hooray, no,* and *bye-bye.* The latter terms were counted as relational when the context was judged to warrant a relational interpretation (A. Meltzoff, personal communication, January 1991).

18. Adults typically produced combinations like "jiggy–zimbo," but chose on the basis of physical similarity if forced to select one term (75% "jiggy").

19. This suggests a resolution to the form–function debate in early language (E. V. Clark, 1973; Gopnik & Meltzoff, 1986; Nelson, 1973a, 1988). It may be that "function determines *which* [word meanings are learned] while form determines *what* [information is stored in early word meaning]" (Gentner, 1982b, p. 142).

20. Since all nine objects were of the same color and approximate size, the common-shape objects were perceptually quite similar.

21. Markman and Hutchinson (1984) describe this shift in terms of whether the objects are related at the basic level or at the superordinate level.

22. To be sure that the children's responses were based solely on either object similarity or category information, we computed these means

based on the children's responses to the *same category/different appearance* stimuli and the *different category/similar appearance* stimuli.

23. Following Bickerton (1983), we are less interested in the question of whether Premack's system was a true language than in considering the effects of the language-constitutive properties that it did have, that is, whether the use of symbols to refer to objects, properties, relations, and relations between relations has implications for other cognitive activities. It can be argued that Premack's chimps were simply given exercises in the use of relations. However, this kind of exercise is certainly a component of natural language use as well. Therefore, any benefits conferred by this kind of practice are of interest in theorizing about the effects of language on cognition.

24. As Premack notes, because the four tasks were always given in the same order, it is not possible to separate the effects of task (c) from the cumulative effects of tasks (a), (b), and (c).

25. Vosniadou et al. used the terms *literal* and *nonliteral*, whereas we have used the terms *general* and *specific*.

26. Note that in simplifying the situation we are avoiding one alternative explanation of the Vosniadou et al. age differences, namely, that the results were due to age differences in children's subjective plausibility for "Paul hopping to his room" rather than to differences in re-representational fluency.

27. Note that this representation separates out the dimensions *size* and *loudness* and allows them to be put into correspondence, permitting one to preserve abstract commonalities such as transitive dimensional structure (Gentner, 1989; Smith, 1989).

References

Anglin, J. M. (1970). *The growth of word meaning.* Cambridge, MA: MIT Press.
Anglin, J. M. (1977). *Word, object, and conceptual development.* New York: Norton.
Baillargeon, R. (1987). Object permanence in 3.5- and 4.5-month-old infants. *Developmental Psychology, 23,* 655–664.
Baillargeon, R. (1990). *The role of similarity in infants' use of visible objects as cues for hidden objects.* Unpublished manuscript.
Baillargeon, R. (1991). Reasoning about the height and location of a hidden object in 4.5- and 6.5-month-old infants. *Cognition, 38,* 13–42.
Baillargeon, R. (in press). The object concept revisited: New directions in the investigation of infants' physical knowledge. In C. E. Granrud (Ed.), *Visual perception and cognition in infancy* (Vol. 23). Hillsdale, NJ: Erlbaum.
Baillargeon, R., Spelke, E. S., & Wasserman, S. (1985). Object permanence in five-month-old infants. *Cognition, 20,* 191–208.
Berman, R. (1980). Child language as evidence for grammatical description: Preschoolers' construal of transitivity in the Hebrew verb system. *Linguistics, 18,* 677–701.
Bickerton, D. (1983). Creole languages. *Scientific American, 249*(1), 116–122.
Billow, R. M. (1975). A cognitive developmental study of metaphor comprehension. *Developmental Psychology, 11,* 415–423.
Bowerman, M. (1973). Structural relationships in children's utterances:

Syntactic or semantic? In T. E. Moore (Ed.), *Cognitive development and the acquisition of language* (pp. 197–213). New York: Academic Press.

Bowerman, M. (1976). Semantic factors in the acquisition of rules for word use and sentence construction. In D. M. Morehead & A. E. Morehead (Eds.), *Normal and deficient child language* (pp. 99–179). Baltimore: University Park Press.

Bowerman, M. (1978a). The acquisition of word meaning: An investigation into some current conflicts. In N. Waterson & C. Snow (Eds.), *The development of communication* (pp. 263–287). New York: Wiley.

Bowerman, M. (1978b). Systematizing semantic knowledge: Changes over time in the child's organization of word meaning. *Child Development, 49,* 977–987.

Bowerman, M. (1982). Reorganizational processes in lexical and syntactic development. In E. Wanner & L. R. Gleitman (Eds.), *Language acquisition: The state of the art* (pp. 319–346). Cambridge University Press.

Brown, A. L. (1989). Analogical learning and transfer: What develops? In S. Vosniadou & A. Ortony (Eds.), *Similarity and analogical reasoning* (pp. 369–412). Cambridge University Press.

Brown, A. L., & Campione, J. C. (1984). Three faces of transfer: Implications for early competence, individual differences, and instruction. In M. E. Lamb, A. L. Brown, & B. Rogoff (Eds.), *Advances in developmental psychology* (Vol. 3, pp. 143–192). Hillsdale, NJ: Erlbaum.

Brown, A. L., & DeLoache, J. S. (1978). Skills, plans, and self-regulation. In R. Siegler (Ed.), *Children's thinking: What develops?* (pp. 3–35). Hillsdale, NJ: Erlbaum.

Brown, A. L., & Kane, M. J. (1988). Preschool children can learn to transfer: Learning to learn and learning from example. *Cognitive Psychology, 20,* 493–523.

Brown, J. S., Collins, A., & Duguid, P. (1989). *Situated cognition and the culture of learning* (Tech. Rep. No. 481). Champaign: University of Illinois, Center for the Study of Reading.

Bruner, J. S., Olver, R. R., & Greenfield, P. M. (1966). *Studies in cognitive growth.* New York: Wiley.

Bryant, P. (1974). *Perception and understanding in young children: An experimental approach.* New York: Basic Books.

Burstein, M. H. (1986). Concept formation by incremental analogical reasoning and debugging. In R. S. Michalski, J. G. Carbonell, & T. M. Mitchell (Eds.), *Machine learning: An artificial intelligence approach* (Vol. 2, pp. 351–369). Los Altos, CA: Kaufmann.

Camarata, S., & Leonard, L. B. (1986). Young children pronounce object words more accurately than action words. *Journal of Child Language, 13,* 51–65.

Camarata, S., & Schwartz, R. G. (1985). Production of object words and action words: Evidence for a relationship between phonology and semantics. *Journal of Speech and Hearing Research, 28,* 323–330.

Carey, S. (1984). Are children fundamentally different kinds of thinkers and learners than adults? In S. Chipman, J. W. Segal, & R. Glaser (Eds.), *Thinking and learning skills: Current research and open questions* (Vol. 2, pp. 485–517). Hillsdale, NJ: Erlbaum.

Carey, S. (1985). *Conceptual change in childhood.* Cambridge, MA: MIT Press.

Carter, A. L. (1979). The disappearance schema: Case study of a second-year communicative behavior. In E. Ochs & B. B. Schieffelin (Eds.), *Developmental pragmatics* (pp. 131–156). New York: Academic Press.

Chi, M. T. H., Feltovich, P. J., & Glaser, R. (1981). Categorization and representation of physics problems by experts and novices. *Cognitive Science, 5,* 121–152.

Chipman, S. F., & Mendelson, M. J. (1979). Influence of six types of visual structure on complexity judgments in children and adults. *Journal of Experimental Psychology: Human Perception and Performance, 5,* 356–378.

Clark, E. V. (1973). What's in a word? On the child's acquisition of semantics in his first language. In T. E. Moore (Ed.), *Cognitive development and the acquisition of language* (pp. 65–110). New York: Academic Press.

Clark, E. V., & Garnica, O. K. (1974). Is he coming or going? On the acquisition of deictic verbs. *Journal of Verbal Learning and Verbal Behavior, 13,* 559–572.

Clark, H. H. (1970). The primitive nature of children's relational concepts. In J. R. Hayes (Ed.), *Cognition and the development of language* (pp. 269–278). New York: Wiley.

Clement, C., & Gentner, D. (1988). Systematicity as a selection constraint in analogical mapping. In *Proceedings of the Tenth Annual Conference of the Cognitive Science Society* (pp. 412–418). Hillsdale, NJ: Erlbaum.

Clement, C., & Gentner, D. (1991). Systematicity as a selection constraint in analogical mapping. *Cognitive Science, 15,* 89–132.

Collins, A., Brown, J. S., & Newman S. (1989). Cognitive apprenticeship: Teaching the craft of reading, writing, and mathematics. In L. B. Resnick (Ed.), *Knowing, learning, and instruction: Essays in honor of Robert Glaser* (pp. 453–494). Hillsdale, NJ: Erlbaum.

Crisafi, M. A., & Brown, A. L. (1986). Analogical transfer in very young children: Combining two separately learned solutions to reach a goal. *Child Development, 57,* 953–968.

Davidson, N. S., & Gelman, S. A. (1990). Inductions from novel categories: The role of language and conceptual structure. *Cognitive Development, 5,* 151–176.

DeLoache, J. S. (1989). The development of representation in young children. In H. W. Reese (Ed.), *Advances in child development and behavior* (Vol. 22, pp. 1–39). New York: Academic Press.

DeLoache, J. S. (1990). Young children's understanding of models. In R. Fivush & J. Hudson (Eds.), *What children remember and why* (pp. 94–126). Cambridge University Press.

Donaldson, M., & Wales, R. (1970). On the acquisition of some relational terms. In J. R. Hayes (Ed.), *Cognition and the development of language* (pp. 235–268). New York: Wiley.

Dore, J. (1986). The development of conversational competence. In R. L. Schiefelbusch (Ed.), *Language competence: Assessment and intervention* (pp. 3–60). San Diego, CA: College-Hill Press.

Dore, J., Franklin, M. B., Miller, R. T., & Ramer, A. L. H. (1976). Transitional phenomena in early language acquisition. *Journal of Child Language, 3,* 13–28.

Dromi, E. (1982). *In pursuit of meaningful words: A case study analysis of early lexical development.* Unpublished doctoral dissertation, McGill University, Montreal.

Elio, R., & Anderson, J. R. (1981). The effects of category generalizations and instance similarity on schema abstraction. *Journal of Experimental Psychology: Human Learning and Memory, 7,* 397–417.

Falkenhainer, B. (1988). *Learning from physical analogies: A study in analogy and the explanation process* (Tech. Rep. UIUCDCS-R-88-1479). Urbana: University of Illinois, Department of Computer Science.

Forbus, K. D., & Gentner, D. (1986). Learning physical domains: Toward a theoretical framework. In R. S. Michalski, J. G. Carbonell, & T. M. Mitchell (Eds.), *Machine learning: An artificial intelligence approach* (Vol. 2, pp. 311–348). Los Altos, CA: Kaufmann.

Gardner, H., Kircher, M., Winner, E., & Perkins, D. (1975). Children's metaphoric productions and preferences. *Journal of Child Language, 2*, 125–141.

Gardner, H., & Winner, E. (1982). First intimations of artistry. In S. Strauss (Ed.), *U-Shaped behavioral growth* (pp. 147–168). New York: Academic Press.

Garner, W. R. (1974). *The processing of information and structure.* Hillsdale, NJ: Erlbaum.

Garner, W. R. (1978). Aspects of a stimulus: Features, dimensions, and configurations. In E. Rosch & B. B. Lloyd (Eds.), *Cognition and categorization* (pp. 99–133). Hillsdale, NJ: Erlbaum.

Garner, W. R., & Felfody, G. L. (1970). Integrality of stimulus dimensions in various types of information processing. *Cognitive Psychology, 1*, 225–241.

Gelman, S. A., & Markman, E. M. (1987). Young children's inductions from natural kinds: The role of categories and appearances. *Child Development, 58*, 1532–1541.

Gentner, D. (1975). Evidence for the psychological reality of semantic components: The verbs of possession. In D. A. Norman & D. E. Rumelhart (Eds.), *Explorations in cognition* (pp. 211–246). San Francisco: Freeman.

Gentner, D. (1977a). Children's performance on a spatial analogies task. *Child Development, 48*, 1034–1039.

Gentner, D. (1977b). If a tree had a knee, where would it be? Children's performance on simple spatial metaphors. *Papers and Reports on Child Language Development, 13*, 157–164.

Gentner, D. (1978). On relational meaning: The acquisition of verb meaning. *Child Development, 49*, 988–998.

Gentner, D. (1982a). Are scientific analogies metaphors? In D. S. Miall (Ed.), *Metaphors: Problems and perspectives* (pp. 106–132). Brighton: Harvester Press.

Gentner, D. (1982b). A study of early word meaning using artificial objects: What looks like a jiggy but acts like a zimbo? In J. Gardner (Ed.), *Readings in developmental psychology* (2d ed., pp. 137–142). Boston: Little, Brown.

Gentner, D. (1982c). Why nouns are learned before verbs: Linguistic relativity versus natural partitioning. In S. A. Kuczaj (Ed.), *Language development: Vol. 2. Language, thought, and culture* (pp. 301–334). Hillsdale, NJ: Erlbaum.

Gentner, D. (1983). Structure-mapping: A theoretical framework for analogy. *Cognitive Science, 7*, 155–170.

Gentner, D. (1988). Metaphor as structure mapping: The relational shift. *Child Development, 59*, 47–59.

Gentner, D. (1989). The mechanisms of analogical learning. In S. Vosniadou & A. Ortony (Eds.), *Similarity and analogical reasoning* (pp. 199–241). Cambridge University Press.

Gentner, D., & Clement, C. (1988). Evidence for relational selectivity in the interpretation of analogy and metaphor. In G. H. Bower (Ed.), *The psychology of learning and motivation* (Vol. 22, pp. 307–358). New York: Academic Press.

Gentner, D., & Landers, R. (1985). Analogical reminding: A good match is hard to find. In *Proceedings of the International Conference on Systems, Man and Cybernetics* (pp. 607–613). Tucson, AZ.

Gentner, D., & Rattermann, M. J. (1990). *The roles of similarity in transfer: Determinants of similarity-based reminding and mapping.* Unpublished manuscript.

Gentner D., & Toupin, C. (1986). Systematicity and surface similarity in the development of analogy. *Cognitive Science, 10,* 277–300.

Gibson, E. J. (1969). *Principles of perceptual learning and development.* New York: Appleton-Century-Crofts.

Gick, M. L., & Holyoak, K. J. (1980). Analogical problem solving. *Cognitive Psychology, 12,* 306–355.

Gick, M. L., & Holyoak, K. J. (1983). Schema induction and analogical transfer. *Cognitive Psychology, 15,* 1–38.

Gillis, S. (1984). *De verwerving van talige referentie.* Unpublished doctoral dissertation, University of Antwerp, Belgium.

Gillis, S. (1986). This child's nominal insight is actually a process: The plateau-stage and the vocabulary spurt in early lexical development. *Antwerp Papers in Linguistics, 45.*

Gillis, S. (1987). Words and categories at the onset of language acquisiton: Product versus process. In A. De Houwer & S. Gillis (Eds.), *Perspectives on child language* (pp. 37–53). Brussels: Université de Bruxelles.

Goldin-Meadow, S., Seligman, M. E. P., & Gelman, R. (1976). Language in the two-year old. *Cognition, 4,* 189–202.

Goldstone, R. L., Gentner, D., & Medin, D. L. (1989). Relations relating relations. In *Proceedings of the Eleventh Annual Conference of the Cognitive Science Society* (pp. 131–138). Hillsdale, NJ: Erlbaum.

Goldstone, R. L., Medin, D. L., & Gentner, D. (1991). Relational similarity and the non-independence of features in similarity judgments. *Cognitive Psychology 23,* 222–262.

Gopnik, A. (1980). *The development of non-nominal expressions in one to two year old children.* Unpublished doctoral dissertation, Oxford University, Oxford.

Gopnik, A. (1981). The development of non-nominal expressions in 12–24-month-olds. In P. S. Dale & D. Ingram (Eds.), *Child language: An international perspective* (pp. 93–104). Baltimore: University Park Press.

Gopnik, A., & Meltzoff, A. N. (1984). Semantic and cognitive development in 15- to 21-month-old children. *Journal of Child Language, 11,* 495–513.

Gopnik, A., & Meltzoff, A. N. (1986). Words, plans, things, and locations: Interactions between semantic and cognitive development in the one-word stage. In S. A. Kuczaj and M. D. Barrett (Eds.), *The development of word meaning: Progress in cognitive development research* (pp. 199–223). Berlin: Springer.

Goswami, U. (1989). Relational complexity and the development of analogical reasoning. *Cognitive Development, 4,* 251–268.

Goswami, U. (1991). Analogical reasoning: What develops? A review of research and theory. *Child Development, 62,* 1–22.

Goswami, U., & Brown, A. L. (1989). Melting chocolate and melting snowmen: Analogical reasoning and causal relations. *Cognition, 35,* 69–95.

Halford, G. S. (1987). *A structure-mapping definition of conceptual complexity: Implications for cognitive development* (Tech. Rep. No. 87/1). St. Lucia, Australia: University of Queensland, Centre for Human Information Processing and Problem-Solving.

Halford, G. S., & Wilson, W. H. (1980). A category theory approach to cognitive development. *Cognitive Psychology, 12,* 356–411.

Halliday, M. A. K. (1975). *Learning how to mean: Explorations in the development of language.* London: Arnold.

Hayes-Roth, F., & McDermott, J. (1978). An interference matching technique for inducing abstractions. *Communications of the ACM, 21,* 401–411.

Holyoak, K. J., Junn, E. N., & Billman, D. O. (1984). Development of analogical problem-solving skill. *Child Development, 55,* 2042–2055.

Huttenlocher, J., & Smiley, P. (1987). Early word meanings: The case of object names. *Cognitive Psychology, 19,* 63–89.

Inagaki, K., & Hatano, G. (1987). Young children's spontaneous personification as analogy. *Child Development, 58,* 1013–1020.

Inhelder, B., & Piaget, J. (1958). *The growth of logical thinking from childhood to adolescence.* New York: Basic Books.

James, W. (1890). *The principles of psychology* (Vol. 2). New York: Dover.

Keil, F. C. (1989). *Concepts, kinds, and cognitive development.* Cambridge, MA: MIT Press.

Kolstad, V. T., & Baillargeon, R. (1990). *Context-dependent perceptual and functional categorization in 10.5-month-old infants.* Unpublished manuscript.

Kotovsky, L., & Gentner, D. (1990a, March). Pack light: You will go farther. In D. Gentner (Chair), *Similarity as structural alignment.* Symposium conducted at the 2nd Midwest Artificial Intelligence and Cognitive Science Conference, Carbondale, IL.

Kotovsky, L., & Gentner, D. (1990b). *Relational similarity: To see or not to see.* Unpublished manuscript.

Kuenne, M. R. (1946). Experimental investigation of the relation of language to transposition behavior in young children. *Journal of Experimental Psychology, 36,* 471–490.

Landau, B., Smith, L. B., & Jones, S. S. (1988). The importance of shape in early lexical learning. *Cognitive Development, 3,* 299–321.

Larkin, J. H., & Simon, H. A. (1981). Learning through growth of skill in mental modeling. In *Proceedings of the Third Annual Conference of the Cognitive Science Society* (pp. 106–111). Hillsdale, NJ: Erlbaum.

Macnamara, J. (1972). Cognitive basis of language learning in infants. *Psychological Review, 79,* 1–13.

Macnamara, J. (1982). *Names for things: A study of human learning.* Cambridge, MA: MIT Press.

Mandler, J. M., & Bauer, P. J. (1988). The cradle of categorization: Is the basic level basic? *Cognitive Development, 3,* 247–264.

Markman, E. M., & Hutchinson, J. E. (1984). Children's sensitivity to constraints on word meaning: Taxonomic versus thematic relations. *Cognitive Psychology, 16,* 1–27.

Medin, D. L., Goldstone, R. L., & Gentner, D. (1990). Similarity involving attributes and relations: Judgments of similarity and difference are not inverses. *Psychological Science, 1,* 64–69.

Medin, D. L., & Ross, B. H. (1989). The specific character of abstract thought: Categorization, problem-solving, and induction. In R. J. Sternberg (Ed.), *Advances in the psychology of human intelligence* (Vol. 5, pp. 189–223). Hillsdale, NJ: Erlbaum.

Menn, L. (1976). *Pattern, control, and contrast in beginning speech: A case study in the development of word form and word function.* Unpublished doctoral dissertation, University of Illinois at Urbana-Champaign.

Menyuk, P., & Menn, L. (1979). Early strategies for the perception and production of words and sounds. In P. Fletcher & M. Garman (Eds.), *Language acquisition: Studies in first language development* (pp. 49–70). Cambridge University Press.

Nelson, K. (1973a). Some evidence for the cognitive primacy of categorization and its functional basis. *Merrill-Palmer Quarterly, 19,* 21–39.

Nelson, K. (1973b). Structure and strategy in learning to talk. *Monographs of the Society for Research in Child Development, 38* (1–2, Serial No. 149).

Nelson, K. (1988). Constraints on word learning? *Cognitive Development, 3,* 221–246.

Ortony, A., Reynolds, R. E., & Arter, J. A. (1978). Metaphor: Theoretical and empirical research. *Psychological Bulletin, 85,* 919–943.

Palmer, S. E. (1978). Fundamental aspects of cognitive representation. In E. Rosch & B. B. Lloyd (Eds.), *Cognition and categorization* (pp. 259–303). Hillsdale, NJ: Erlbaum.

Piaget, J., Montangero, J., & Billeter, J. (1977). La formation des correlats. In J. Piaget (Ed.), *L'Abstraction reflechissante* (pp. 115–129). Paris: Presses Universitaires de France.

Pinker, S. (1984). *Language learnability and language development.* Cambridge, MA: Harvard University Press.

Premack, D. (1983). The codes of man and beasts. *Behavioral and Brain Sciences, 6,* 125–167.

Premack, D. (1988). Minds with and without language. In L. Weiskrantz (Ed.), *Thought without language* (pp. 46–55). Oxford: Oxford University Press.

Quine, W. V. (1969). *Ontological relativity and other essays.* New York: Columbia University Press.

Rattermann, M. J., & Gentner, D. (1990, March). The development of similarity use: It's what you know, not how you know it. In D. Gentner (Chair), *Similarity as structural alignment.* Symposium conducted at the 2nd Midwest Artificial Intelligence and Cognitive Science Conference, Carbondale, IL.

Rattermann, M. J., Gentner, D., & DeLoache, J. (1987 April). *Young children's use of relational similarity in a transfer task.* Poster presented at the biennial meeting of the Society for Research in Child Development, Baltimore, MD.

Rattermann, M. J., Gentner, D., & DeLoache, J. (1989, April). *Effects of competing surface similarity on children's performance in an analogical task.* Poster presented at the biennial meeting of the Society for Research in Child Development, Kansas City, MO.

Rattermann, M. J., Gentner, D., & DeLoache, J. (1990). *Effects of relational and object similarity on children's performance in a mapping task.* Unpublished manuscript.

Ricciuti, H. N. (1965). Object grouping and selective ordering behavior in infants 12 to 24 months old. *Merrill-Palmer Quarterly, 11,* 129–148.

Rosch, E., & Mervis, C. B. (1975). Family resemblances: Studies in the internal structure of categories. *Cognitive Psychology, 7,* 573–605.

Rosch, E., Mervis, C. B., Gray, W. D., Johnson, D. M., & Boyes-Braem, P. (1976). Basic objects in natural categories. *Cognitive Psychology, 8,* 382–439.

Ross, B. H. (1989). Remindings in learning and instruction. In S. Vosniadou & A. Ortony (Eds.), *Similarity and analogical reasoning* (pp. 438–469). Cambridge University Press.

Schumacher, R. M., Jr., & Gentner, D. (1990). *Analogical access: Effects of repetition, competition, and instruction.* Unpublished manuscript.

Schwartz, R. G., & Terrell, B. Y. (1983). The role of input frequency in lexical acquisition. *Journal of Child Language, 10,* 57–64.

Sera, M., & Smith, L. B. (1987). *Big* and *little:* "Nominal" and relative uses. *Cognitive Development, 2,* 89–111.

Shepp, B. E. (1978). From perceived similarity to dimensional structure: A new hypothesis about perceptual development. In E. Rosch & B. B. Lloyd (Eds.), *Cognition and categorization* (pp. 135–167). Hillsdale, NJ: Erlbaum.

Shepp, B. E., & Swartz, K. B. (1976). Selective attention and the processing of integral and nonintegral dimensions: A developmental study. *Journal of Experimental Child Psychology, 22,* 73–85.

Smith, L. B. (1984). Young children's understanding of attributes and dimensions: A comparison of conceptual and linguistic measures. *Child Development, 55,* 363–380.

Smith, L. B. (1989). From global similarities to kinds of similarities: The construction of dimensions in development. In S. Vosniadou & A. Ortony (Eds.), *Similarity and analogical reasoning* (pp. 146–178). Cambridge University Press.

Smith, L. B., & Kemler, D. G. (1977). Developmental trends in free classification: Evidence for a new conceptualization of perceptual development. *Journal of Experimental Child Psychology, 24,* 279–298.

Smith, L. B., Rattermann, M. J., & Sera, M. (1988). "Higher" and "lower": Comparative and categorical interpretations by children. *Cognitive Development, 3,* 341–357.

Starkey, D. (1981). The origins of concept formation: Object sorting and object preference in early infancy. *Child Development, 52,* 489–497.

Stern, W. (1914). *Psychologie der fruehen kindheit.* Leipzig: Quelle & Meyer.

Sternberg, R. J., & Downing, C. J. (1982). The development of higher-order reasoning in adolescence. *Child Development, 53,* 209–221.

Sternberg, R. J., & Nigro, G. (1980). Developmental patterns in the solution of verbal analogies. *Child Development, 51,* 27–38.

Sternberg, R. J., & Rifkin, B. (1979). The development of analogical reasoning processes. *Journal of Experimental Child Psychology, 27,* 195–232.

Stoel-Gammon, C., & Cooper, J. A. (1984). Patterns of early lexical and phonological development. *Journal of Child Language, 11,* 247–271.

Sugarman, S. (1982). Developmental change in early representational intelligence: Evidence from spatial classification strategies and related verbal expressions. *Cognitive Psychology, 14,* 410–449.

Taylor, M., & Gelman, S. A. (1989). Incorporating new words into the lexicon: Preliminary evidence for language hierarchies in two-year-old children. *Child Development, 60,* 625–636.

Tomasello, M., & Farrar, M. J. (1984). Cognitive bases of lexical development: Object permanence and relational words. *Journal of Child Language, 11,* 477–493.

Tomikawa, S. A., & Dodd, D. H. (1980). Early word meanings: Perceptually or functionally based? *Child Development, 51,* 1103–1109.

Tversky, A. (1977). Features of similarity. *Psychological Review, 84,* 327–352.

Vosniadou, S., Ortony, A., Reynolds, R. E., & Wilson, P. T. (1984). Sources of difficulty in the young child's understanding of metaphorical language. *Child Development, 55,* 1588–1606.

Vygotsky, L. S. (1962). *Thought and language.* Cambridge, MA: MIT Press. (Original work published 1934.)

Wales, R., & Campbell, R. (1970). On the development of comparison and the comparison of development. In G. B. Flores d'Arcais & W. J. M. Levelt (Eds.), *Advances in psycholinguistics* (pp. 373–396). Amsterdam: North-Holland.

Waxman, S., & Gelman, R. (1986). Preschoolers' use of superordinate relations in classification and language. *Cognitive Development, 1,* 139–156.

Winner, E. (1979). New names for old things: The emergence of metaphoric language. *Journal of Child Language, 6,* 469–491.

Woodruff, G., & Premack, D. (1981). Primative mathematical concepts in the chimpanzee: Proportionality and numerosity. *Nature, 293,* 568–570.

8. The matter of time: Interdependencies between language and thought in development

KATHERINE NELSON

As the chapters in this book testify, the relation between language and thought in development has been conceptualized in many different ways. As the question of how children acquire language has come into focus in the past 25 years, theorists have argued either that language depends on cognition or the opposite – that cognition depends on language. This argument has taken many forms (for some of the forms and their ramifications see Cromer, 1988; Johnston, 1985). The classical views are reviewed elsewhere in this volume. In order to put my own conception of this relation into perspective it is revealing to consider briefly the many variations that are implicit in current psychological and linguistic models.

First, there is the strong cognitive determinism position attributed to Piaget – that acquiring and using language depends on the prior acquisition of supportive cognitive structures. Despite many efforts to find empirical support for this general proposition, there is little hard evidence that specific cognitive achievements are prerequisites of the acquisition of specific linguistic developments. Second, in the linguistic determinism position (known as the Sapir–Whorf hypothesis), thought, in its final forms, is held to be a function of the particular system of language that an individual has learned to use. Although both weak and strong forms of this position have been generally discredited in the recent past, a revival of sorts is under way (see Lakoff, 1987; Lucy, 1985; Silverstein, 1985). Third, the position that cognition *is* language – that the two are functionally equivalent – was implied in Watsonian behaviorism, which held thought to be covert verbalization. In a strangely related stance, Fodor (1975, 1981) has elaborated the claim that language forms (words) are mapped onto an underlying system of concepts that constitute the "language of thought." This is a translation paradigm in which

278

there is an equivalence but not an identity of language and thought. Note that according to this view the more basic system – the conceptual – is held to be innate, not learned: The superficial surface forms of the particular language serve only to "trigger" the appropriate underlying concepts.

Another possibility is that language and cognition constitute two parallel streams. A popular version of this position is that language and cognition tend to develop along similar courses because of deeper developmental mechanisms that determine both. For example, the complexity of symbolic play and that of sentences increase at approximately the same rate, not because one determines the other, but because both are propelled by the same force (Shore, O'Connell, & Bates, 1984).

A variation on this scheme is the classical Vygotskian (1986) claim that language and cognition are initially separate (but not necessarily parallel) but that they converge at a point in development where language first differentiates into social and nonsocial speech and is finally internalized as inner speech. Through this mechanism thought becomes socialized and organized in the direction laid out by adult language speakers, especially teachers.

Of all these positions only Whorf's and Vygotsky's have taken seriously the central role of language in the development of thought in the human child. Vygotsky's "higher mental functions" all depend on the use of language for their acquisition and their subsequent development. It seems ironic that for all the extraordinary attention that has been given to language *acquisition* and development in the past 25 years the importance of language in human thought and culture has been neglected in developmental psychology. Language has tended to be viewed from a linguistic perspective as an end in itself, an autonomous system buffered from "mere" cognition, as though one could exist without the other. Or, as in some current hypotheses, linguistic constraints are meant to restrict – rather than expand – the possibilities of the more open cognitive system (see Markman, Chapter 3, Waxman, Chapter 4, and Callanan, Chapter 12, this volume; see Nelson, 1988a, for a critique). And from the developmental psychologist's perspective, the focus on cognitive skills (number, classification, memory) and logical concepts (space, causality, conservation) has made it possible for most theorists of cognitive development to ignore the role of language, except for its role in communicating instructions and coding responses on cognitive tasks. The resulting positions seem to me to be untenable, both with respect to the way the child acquires language and with respect to essential conditions for cognitive development.

I will argue here for a transactional or dialectical model in which cognition and language are *interdependent* throughout development. Language cannot begin to be acquired without a cognitive, that is, a conceptual, base, but as soon as first language forms appear, the conceptual base becomes transformed. The transformation continues throughout the course of language development, which does not end in early to middle childhood as commonly supposed, but continues throughout the life span. Language continuously enters into and changes prior conceptions. Language neither replaces nor becomes identical with cognition; rather, the two continuously interact. A vitally important factor driving this interactive system is the condition that language is a social construction. This brief statement will be fleshed out in the discussion to follow.

In this discussion I will refer to two levels of representation – the *conceptual* and the *semantic* (primarily lexical, i.e., concerned with word meanings). In many discussions the semantic is considered equivalent to the conceptual, but I think it important to keep the two separate, both for expository reasons and because it is necessary for an interactive system that there be at least two components to interact (cf. E. V. Clark, 1983). At some points and in some parts, lexical representations may be indistinguishable from conceptual representations, but this unity should not be taken as definitive or inevitable. The relation between the two may, and I believe does, change with development (Nelson, 1985). Thus, to equate word meanings and concepts is to conflate what needs to be explained.

It should also be noted that I will refer to *event knowledge* and *event representations*. These are to be considered part of the conceptual level of knowledge representation (not the semantic). It is assumed on theoretical grounds that they embed concepts and verbal forms within larger organized structures representing real-world experience (see Nelson, 1986, for further explication and evidence).

In this chapter I will first lay out some general considerations with respect to theories of the acquisition of meaning by first language learners, pointing out problems with some current approaches and presenting reasons for developing a different approach. I will then take up the case of the acquisition of concepts related to time and time language, to exemplify the problem in all its complexity. Next I will relate this level of knowledge to the child's event knowledge system and to the use of both in discourse transactions. Finally, I will draw some general implications for the study of the acquisition of meaning for abstract language terms and for the general relation of language and thought in development.

The acquisition of meaning: General considerations

To learn a word is to learn to produce (or simply to recognize) a word form (phonemic or graphemic) and to associate it with a meaning. We ordinarily take the first of these for granted; it is the meaning part that causes theoretical difficulties. For what does it mean to acquire the meaning of the word? Is meaning a linguistic or a cognitive problem? In this section I consider some basic issues related to these questions.

The object–word relation: From Augustine to the present

"When they [my elders] named any thing, and as they spoke turned towards it, I saw and remembered that they called what they would point out, by the name they uttered" (Augustine, 397/1950, p. 9). This model of word learning as set forth by Augustine has been accepted with very little variation by authors as various as Brown (1958), Macnamara (1982), Quine (1960), and more recently Markman (1987) and a number of others who have employed it in an experimental paradigm. This model, called *ostensive learning*, basically involves a tutor who points to an object and names it for the learner, who then forms a hypothesis about what the word refers to and, on the basis of further experience with the word, tests and confirms or disconfirms this hypothesis. In other words, the word is mapped onto something in the learner's head that causes him to assume that it can be used generally to refer to things of a certain sort. The learner's meaning of the word in this model is whatever forms his hypotheses. We then have to ask what lies behind those hypotheses, and here we run into interesting possibilities.

In one view, the learner maps the word onto a set of semantic features, which constitute the meaning of the word, although the particular set picked out may not be that defined by the language community (E. V. Clark, 1973). The set of all possible semantic features, however, is innately determined by the language module (Bierwisch, 1970). Other versions of the ostensive learning model appear to claim only that the word is mapped onto an object percept. Of course, the percept cannot take the child very far toward a generalized meaning; at the least, one would have to know what perceptual attributes are crucial to recognizing a particular object or object class. In many other views the word is mapped onto an already formed object concept; but this raises the issue of where the concept came from. In Fodor's (1981) view the word–object pair triggers an innate concept. According to a number of others, the child forms concepts on the basis of prelinguistic experience (e.g., Nelson, 1974). A critical limitation in deciding among these views is that the only way we can gain insight into what meaning the child may attach to the word is by observing how she uses the word, because at least in the first stages we cannot ask the child what she thinks it means.

A vast array of ingenious experiments have been carried out recently to try to determine what kinds of hypotheses children have when they hear a word in an ostensive learning situation, by testing how they extend the word to new items (e.g., Au & Markman, 1987; Carey, 1978; Dickinson, 1988; Heibeck & Markman, 1987; Landau, Smith, & Jones, 1988; Markman & Hutchinson, 1984; Soja & Carey, 1986). But as E. V. Clark (1988) has emphasized, it is impossible to be certain what the child's meaning is from observing how the word is used. (To be sure, she has not posed this argument against these experiments, but it is applicable here as well.) There are thus reasons to doubt that these studies can tell us much that is definitive about meaning, although they may tell us a good deal about the use of strategies in ostensive learning situations (Nelson, 1988a).

Moreover, the case can be made that the ostensive learning paradigm is inadequate to deal with the problem of the child's acquisition of word meaning, simply because ostensive learning is not typical of lexical acquisition. I have elsewhere discussed this problem at length (Nelson, 1988a) and will not review the argument in detail here. Briefly, ostensive learning is most typical of very early word learning, specifically of learning a few names for objects. But after a first vocabulary (50 or so words) is acquired, the typical situation for learning object names is for the *child* to ask for a word for something that is of interest (for which assumedly he has a concept), reflected in the oft-heard "What's that?" of the 18- to 20-month-old. Alternatively, children may acquire words from an ongoing discourse context or from an adult's explanation (as described later). Pointing and naming are simply not the paradigmatic way of teaching or learning word meanings after the age of $1\frac{1}{2}$ to 2 years. Further, the child is faced very early on, as I will show, with learning meanings for words that *cannot* be learned ostensively.

Before proceeding, it is helpful to keep in mind that four components are involved in the acquisition of a new word: (a) acquisition of the phonological form of the word; (b) acquisition of its extension to referents or its use in discourse; (c) acquisition (by inference or through explication) of its semantics – the meaning it conveys; (d) understanding of its relation to other forms in the lexicon (including possible paraphrases). These processes do not necessarily occur in any particular order for any class of words or at any given stage of development. For example, some meaning may be grasped before the child has acquired productive use of the form or its full extension in the adult language. (This seems to be the case for many early object names.) In the case of terms involved in the temporal lexicon, we may find that steps (a) and (b) precede steps (c) and (d) sometimes by several years.

Philosophical and linguistic theories of meaning seek to explain what words mean independent of any particular speaker or context, a goal that even some philosophers (e.g., Putnam, 1975, 1988) and linguists (e.g., Sampson, 1980) have argued is impossible to achieve. A psychological theory, in contrast, must explain what and how speakers mean in context (where "speaker" may also be interpreted as communicating with self, i.e., using words in thought). A subset of the psychological problem is how children come to learn to use words to convey meanings to others. To address these problems it is not necessary to assume that any given word *has a* meaning that is the same for all speakers. It is only necessary to assume that a word acquires a potential to mean for a speaker in particular contexts. A particular speaker may not even be aware of its canonical meaning in the language community (as formulated perhaps in Webster's dictionary).

In the light of this distinction, it can be seen that much of the work that has taken place investigating the developmental psychology of word meaning is based on the linguistic, not the psychological, model. The problem has usually been stated in terms of specifying the conditions under which children will acquire the right, or true, meaning, or full semantic representation of the word. To formulate the psychological problem more appropriately, the following points must be considered:

(1)   Meaning is holistic, a proposition asserted by Quine (1960, 1977) and endorsed by Putnam (1988). This means that words do not mean in isolation, but rather as part of a system. What one word can mean is constrained by what other related words mean, the lexical system forming a whole within which each word has its place. This does not imply that the meaning of the word is deterministic, however; rather, it implies that a word's meaning for an individual may shift with the meanings of other words in the system.

(2)   Moreover, there is not one system but millions of idiosystems, each individual having acquired a particular set of related meanings; thus, each individual's potential meanings of words will differ from every other's.[1]

(3)   Further, each individual's meanings will change over time as new words are acquired. Meaning develops and changes within a person and within a culture or language community. An obvious example of such change (due to Sampson, 1980) is the meaning of the word *atom*, which originally meant indivisible into smaller elements; but in the course of scientific investigation those things called atoms were discovered to consist of more elementary particles. Thus, the meaning of the word *atom* changed for most users of the term; it no longer contrasted with other terms along the dimension of divisibility. This general situation is, of course, very familiar, not only in science, but in everyday life, particularly within subgroups that develop their own jargon. Meanings, even for individual adults, do not stay the same over time.

(4)   Also, meanings are not stable across contexts. Labov (1973) demonstrated that the words *cup, glass, vase,* and *bowl,* terms that form a more or less definable subsystem within the lexicon of English speakers, were applied differently by the same speaker to the same form depending on the context of use (see also Anderson & Ortony, 1975). For example, a tall cylindrical form might be designated a glass if it was described as containing a cold drink, but referred to as a vase if it was said to hold flowers. No single set of features (e.g., one or two handles) could be found to distinguish *cup* from *bowl,* or *glass* from *vase.* Rather, adults were flexible in their application of the terms. Again, this situation is familiar; we use words in a flexible way, depending on our hearers to interpret our meanings in context. But this again undermines the notion that there is *a* meaning even for a single individual for any given word, much less a meaning that is common to all speakers.

(5)   Finally, meanings are social constructions. It might seem that the emphasis on individual lexicons just insisted upon would argue against this proposition, but on the contrary, it is essential to the argument that word meanings are learned from and used with others in social contexts. (This line of argument derives in a general way from Wittgenstein, 1958, as well as from Vygotsky, 1986.) Children may form concepts on their own, but they cannot construct meanings on their own: They need to know how words are used by others in order to

derive a meaning system that is workable in the language community in which they live. Idiosyncratic uses of words, if they are too far removed from standard uses, are generally met with incomprehension, and thus will lead the user to question and revise her understanding of the way the term is used. Thus, meanings are necessarily derived from use in social contexts. But use is not necessarily reference, as will be emphasized later.

Word–concept relations

Even though we may want to keep concepts and word meanings separate both theoretically and empirically, virtually every discussion of meaning refers to concepts in some way. There are at least three discernible relations between the two.

Words may express concepts. In some cases a word may fit an existing concept so exactly that the word is, in effect, mapped onto it. But words may also express concepts very loosely; the fit is not exact, and the speaker may seek a more exact expression through a multiword construction or may make up a nonce word to fit the wanted meaning (E. V. Clark, 1982). In the early stages of language development children do not seem to distinguish between their concepts and the words they find that seem to fit them. "Overextension" of early words (such as *dog* applied to both dogs and cats) as well as "underextension" result. Only later do they seem to take into account that there is not a one-to-one match between the way words are used by others and the concepts that they may have in mind. They may then differentiate previous concepts to fit new words or generalize an old word to new instances.

The opposite case comes about when a concept is derived from the word's use. In this case the child (or adult) hears a word used, and not having an available concept to map it onto, constructs a concept that seems to fit the way the word is used. Frequently parents or others explain the meaning of the new word to the child: "See, it's a Dalmatian; a Dalmatian is a big dog with spots" (Adams & Bullock, 1986). This provides the information that the child needs to locate the word appropriately within the system of lexical relations (e.g., in terms of superordinates and subordinates) and to use known concepts (e.g., *dog*) to construct a subsidiary concept of a type of dog. In other cases the concept is not explained so explicitly and the child (or adult) must rely more on inference based on the context and apparent reference of the word's use.

Finally, and most important for my purposes here, there are concepts that are not just derived from the use of words but are dependent on the use of words because they are in fact constituted through language. Dalmatians, like other natural kinds and human artifacts, exist in the world, and given time the child might observe and form concepts about them independently of the language. But much of our cultural armamentarium is not about things that exist in the world independently of the way we talk about them. Some examples that young children are inevitably exposed to include number; concepts like *work*; manners and customs; taxonomies of objects and events (e.g., "What counts as an animal? a party?"); behavioral roles and rules (e.g., "Big girls don't cry"); character traits such as courage and dishonesty; moral and religious values; geographical and political constructs such as towns, cities, states, and countries; and, of particular interest here, concepts of time. Of course, it might be objected that there is a reality to all of these things – that children are exposed to them independently of language. Of course, there are overt objective signs: Children encounter numbers in many ways, for example. Without language children might form many concepts about the signs of these cultural systems, but they would never understand the significance of the signs within the community. To know what a church looks like tells children nothing about the religion that it symbolizes. That can be conveyed only through words and other meaningful symbols. Thus, a very large number of the word meanings that even young children know are actually constituted through language.

To get a rough idea of the prevalence of different types of words and related concepts, the 211 nouns among the 500 most frequent words in the Thorndike–Lorge (1944) Word Count were dichotomized into those that may refer to concrete objects (those susceptible to ostensive learning) and those that clearly do not (those explicable only in language or derivable from discourse contexts).[2] This count revealed that the majority (63%) were of the latter type. These are not esoteric words, but ones that children hear frequently (e.g., *family, friend, help, home*), and they include all of the most frequently used nouns that refer to time concepts (e.g., *day, morning, week*). Children's acquisition of time concepts and time language may thus be seen to exemplify a frequent type of word acquisition.

Consider, then, how words that bear these different relations to concepts may be learned. Words referring to concepts of objects that a child may already have formed may be learned through pointing and naming. Concepts may be constructed in response to words that adults explain in a sentence or two. But much word learning takes place because the words are embedded in discourse that is concerned with the meanings of large segments of cultural reality. Even that small segment of culture that a child inhabits exhibits whole networks of cultural concepts that are displayed unsystematically and in an intertwined manner so that it is not easy to grasp the parts separately from the whole. This kind of learning of meaning requires going beyond the word or the sentence to examine discourse as a framework for meaning.

The matter of time

Time concepts

Time is a basic component of our experience of reality that has obvious relevance to children as well as adults. However, unlike aspects of space that can be pointed to or explained through gestures – for example, size, shape, and location – concepts of time are abstract, not concrete. In this respect time is like number. It may be represented in imaginal or symbolic form, but it cannot be seen, heard, or touched. Time may be perceived, but it is not directly sensed.

What is it that we conceptualize as time? What can chldren be expected to know of time? The standard Western view of time is one-dimensional, a time line along which either time moves from the future to the past, or ego moves from the past through present into the future. These two perspectives on time provide different metaphors (e.g., "coming up in the weeks ahead" vs. "we're approaching the end of the year"; see H. Clark, 1973; Lakoff & Johnson, 1980) with different implications. The standard view emphasizes the temporal dynamic, in which the present is always moving into the past, a view that necessitates defining the boundaries of a stable but ever-changing "specious present" (James, 1890/1950). *Now* as distinguished from past and future is one of the concepts that children must come to understand very early. Whether *now* is an unlearned (implicit, inherent, or innate) concept is not clear. If Fraser (1987) is correct in saying that the nonlinguistic creature (human infant or nonhuman animal) lives in an eternal present it would seem that the distinction between present, past, and future must be acquired in human childhood.

Time perspective is marked in terms of events: It is events that are past, present, or future. Two other basic temporal concepts derive from events in time: *sequence* (temporal order) and *length* (duration of or interval between events). Events can be sequenced in relation to one another (e.g., getting dressed before breakfast), and the actions that comprise the events themselves are ordered through time (e.g., put on socks before shoes). In a similar way, *length* (distance along the time line) may refer to the duration of an event (e.g., how long breakfast takes) or to the interval between events (e.g., the time between coming home from school and dinner). *Location in time* is also often referenced in terms of events (e.g., bedtime, lunchtime, snacktime). Event *boundaries* are also temporally marked (e.g., time to get up, when we finish dinner). *Speed* is related to the duration of an event (e.g., if you eat quickly, breakfast will be over faster). The *frequency* with which an event has been experienced relates similar experiences to one another along the time axis. All of these concepts can be seen to have a fairly direct relation to the everyday experience of and memory for events. Thus, given the well-established event knowledge of young children (Nelson, 1986), they might be expected to be achieved relatively easily in early childhood.

In contrast, referencing time in terms of units and measuring time in units are, to a greater or lesser degree, arbitrary, socially defined practices. Units of time range from those based on events (e.g., lunchtime), to those based on natural cycles (e.g., morning, day, night; spring, summer, fall, winter), to arbitrary divisions (e.g., minutes, hours, weeks, months). There is an element of conventionality even in the most "natural" units. Lunchtime and bedtime vary across households and cultures, as does the division of day and night and of the seasons; and although the lunar cycle provides a basis for division into months, our 12-month year does not coincide with the 13 months of the lunar year. The fact that the earth circles the sun at a fraction less than $365\frac{1}{4}$ days poses a problem for all calendar constructors.

Additional complexities face children when units of time are measured numerically (e.g., 6 weeks hence; 100 years ago) or are counted as in days of the month (e.g., January 6) and year (e.g., 1950). Units of time are not like apples and oranges, nor like sticks and stones that can be laid out in a line to be counted. Clocks and calendars mark out spaces that visually represent temporal units; these can be counted, but their ambiguous relation to the passage of time may be expected to pose a problem for the child who is learning to use them.

There is an even greater complexity in that conventional systems represent time in series of cycles: 24 hours (two cycles of 12) to the day, 7 days to the week, 4+ weeks to the month, 12 months to the year. Friedman (1982) has explored the extraordinary difficulties children have in dealing with the cyclicity of time.

A factor that enters into and crosscuts all of these conceptual representations is the matter of distance: how close or how far in time from the present an event or a period is. As Fraser (1987) notes, the ability to conceptualize far-off time (past or future) is distinctly human. Piaget (1962) proposed that in the preschool years children need to reconstruct notions related to distant time and space that they have already constructed on the sensorimotor level for near time. And it is commonly claimed that when children begin to express temporal relations in speech, it is in terms of near time, time related closely to the "here and now" (Weist, 1986). A grasp of historical time is achieved relatively late in development, and recent reports of educational achievement assessment suggest that some young adults may retain a very vague conception of historical time. Gould (1987) has traced the development of the concept of geological time, a time scale that for most adults is probably an abstraction that is difficult to grasp. At the other end, the measurement of time in microseconds and even smaller units also lies beyond the conceptual grasp of most adults, much less young children.

The concepts that children are expected to master in this domain can be summarized along the dimensions of relative and absolute time, natural and arbitrary bases of temporal concepts, and the unitization of time. Temporal perspective (past, present, future), temporal sequence, duration, and speed of events are all relative concepts with a natural base in children's experience. Temporal units impose an absolute quality, whether referenced in terms of events or arbitrary conventional units. Both *bedtime* and *yesterday* are definite temporal locations, even though today's bedtime and yesterday's are different from tomorrow's. *Nine o'clock* is absolute in contrast to the relative *after breakfast*.

On the view (offered here) that temporal concepts are understood initially in terms of events and discourse relating to events, it would be expected that relative, nonarbitrary concepts would be acquired more easily than absolute arbitrary units. It should be noted that both, however, require interpretation through language. Although the child's experientially derived event knowledge may provide intuitive support for understanding some temporal concepts, event knowledge does not itself contain such concepts. As for temporal measurement and temporal series and cycles, these concepts require direct teaching by the language community, supported by artifacts such as clocks and calendars.

Thus far, the discussion has assumed the dominant Western time perspective, based primarily on classical physical conceptions of time as atomistic and divisible but homogeneous (all units are equal), its units flowing in linear succession, abstract and objective, unidirectional (not reversible). It is important to keep in mind that this is not the only possible conception of time, a fact that underscores the conventional nature of our time concepts, dependent as they are on construction through language. As McGrath and Kelly (1986) emphasize, there are numerous other possible conceptions of time, including those of Eastern philosophy and Einsteinian physics. A perspective that is of particular importance to the study of the development of temporal concepts is what they refer to as "transactional" time, incorporating a biological perspective. In this perspective

> time is divisible but differentiated, with certain points in time serving as "critical values" (e.g., birth, metamorphosis, cell division, etc.). Therefore, time is experienced as epochal . . . time is regarded as concrete, in that it is a necessary ingredient of many biological processes . . . as relational . . . an experiential time that is in part observer determined . . . time is considered as phasic in passage, and irreversible. Therefore it is developmental in its flow, spiral in form rather than strictly recurrent. (p. 33)

This perspective permeates an alternative "time frame" that is prominent in Western thinking but is at odds along many dimensions with the mathematical conception represented in "clock time." Transactional or biological time is the view that is most frequently presented to young children by Early Childhood educators, in terms of the concepts of birth, growth, aging, and death, as for example through the study of plants and the celebration of birthdays.

That this perspective on time differs from the physical science perspective represented in clock time is not generally recognized, but both children and adults in our society come to understand, at least implicitly, both time frames.[3] As McGrath and Kelly (1986) put it: "In the lay culture, time is thought of as both linear and cyclical; clocks and calendars imply both. We tend to *think about time* as if it were abstract, unidirectional, uniform in passage, divisible, and homogeneous; but we tend to *use time* as if it were concrete, phasic, and epochal" (p. 36). The coexistence of these two competing frames of reference may pose problems for the child who is coming to reorganize an experientially based conceptual system to accord with the culturally defined concepts exhibited through language and other symbolic forms. In a sense, the notion of time as uniform and homogeneous must be laid on top of the experiential sense of time as phasic and epochal. Language provides a way of thinking about and talking about both frames.

Time language

Between the ages of 2 and 3 years most children begin to acquire linguistic terms that mark temporal relations. Languages encode temporal relations in two ways: grammatically, in terms of tense and aspect, and lexically. The former has been much more intensively studied than the latter in the developmental psycholinguistic literature.

Obligatory grammaticization: Tense and aspect. Almost all languages have some system of tense (Comrie, 1985; Traugott, 1978), the grammaticized expression of location in time. (Those that do not have tense as such have lexical forms for marking temporal perspective [Lyons, 1977].) English distinguishes past, present, and future,[4] which can be conceptualized as existing as relative points along a time line. Tense is thus a *deictic* notion, one that depends on the establishment of a "deictic center" in relation to which other points can be located. Tense is distinguished from aspect, which expresses the internal temporal contour of a situation. For example, the distinction between *John is singing* and *John was singing* is one of tense (present vs. past), whereas the distinction between *John was singing* and *John sang* is one of aspect (continuative vs. completive).

Children typically begin to acquire the system of past, present, and future forms and of progressive aspect (-ing) around 2 years of age. Much of the recent discussion of children's acquisition of the system of tense morphology in European languages has been concerned with whether children first use tense to express aspectual notions (e.g., the completion of an action) rather than deictic ones (action in the past), suggesting that they are not sensitive to the present–past distinction per se (Antinucci & Miller, 1976; Bloom, Lifter, & Hafitz, 1980; Weist, 1986). Some studies (Gerhardt, 1988; Weist, Wysocka, Witkowska-Stadnik, Buczowska, & Konieczna, 1984; Weist, 1986) have indicated that children are sensitive to the deictic meaning of tense forms from very early in grammatical development (but see Bloom & Harner, 1989).

There is also some evidence that children first use the past tense to refer to the immediate rather than the remote past (Weist, 1986). However, an analysis of the crib talk of a single child, Emily, between the age of 21 and 36 months suggests that this may be a methodological artifact (Nelson, 1989a) and that when utterances are sampled in a context that supports reference to events from the non-immediate situation children may use past tense to refer to the more remote past (and similarly for the future).

It is noteworthy that children learn to use the grammatical systems of tense and aspect very early, beginning usually before 2 years. Although this does not imply that the relevant concepts are available independent of the language system (and different languages grammaticize different aspects of temporal perspective; see Berman & Slobin, 1987; Slobin, 1987), it suggests that obligatory coding in the language at least makes these dimensions salient. Unlike other aspects of language learning, where the evidence seems to indicate that the child begins with conceptual (semantic) relations that are subsequently grammaticized (see discussions in Levy, Schlesinger, & Braine, 1988), in this case it appears that grammatical coding precedes and leads to semantic conceptualizations (Nelson, 1989a).

Both the "aspect before tense" hypothesis (Bloom et al., 1980) and the evidence from Emily's narratives suggest that the specific past – now contrast represented in tense forms may be constructed in response to linguistic coding rather than being itself a basis from which that coding is learned. Bloom et al. argue that children are first sensitive to the form of action (aspect) rather than to its timing in relation to speech time, the deictic notion of tense. Thus, they tend to restrict past forms to uses in reference to completed actions first, before generalizing to any activity or state prior to the present time.

Emily's narratives indicated that during the time that she was acquiring the tense system (which did distinguish past vs. present) she focused specifically on the now–not now construct. Her monologues were sprinkled with expressions such as "not right now; now sleeping time." Gerhardt (1989) argues that she distinguished only between what was happening now and usual events that take place in the not now (that, as we would say, have taken place or will take place). That is, her first temporal perspective was not a distinction between past and present, but between present and not present. (According to Lyons, 1977, this is the only grammatical contrast that is made in some languages.) Indeed, this fits the notion that I have developed elsewhere (Nelson, 1989b, 1990) that the basic memory system is functional in establishing representations of expected events that form the basis for action in the present and future. Thus, the specific past is not important; what is important is an understanding of usual expected events. Representations of such events are not coded for a specific time in the past or future, but only as general: This is what happens. If this is indeed the case, children must acquire an understanding of the specific past and specific future in contrast to the present as they acquire the grammatical tense system.

Note that the acquisition of the past–present–future reference system proceeds differently for those children described as following an aspect before tense course and for Emily, who seemed first to develop a now–not now contrast. But both proceed from what are assumed to be salient and functional nonlinguistic dimensions of events and event knowledge toward an understanding of events within a culturally conventional, linguistically coded system.

Optional lexicalization: Relations, pseudo-objects. Numerous terms in the language may be used to establish relative or absolute time, generally adverbs, prepositions, and conjunctions, but also nouns that refer to pseudo-objects (*yesterday*, for example, may be used as either an adverb or a noun). Such terms may express location in time (*now, tomorrow, at nine o'clock*), sequence (*first, then, after, before*), or duration or interval (*a long time, five hours*). It is generally noted that lexical terms for temporal concepts and relations are not acquired until after tense and aspect – at least the basic forms of tense and aspect. Temporal adverbs such as *today* and *yesterday* and adverbial clauses beginning with *when* are among the first to be used, enabling children to express relations such as "Yesterday we went to the store" and "When Daddy comes home I can watch TV."

In studies of children's comprehension of *yesterday* and *tomorrow*, Harner (1975) concluded that at first children understood the terms as meaning "not today"; they understood *yesterday* as referring to the past before *tomorrow* referred to the future. The acquisition of the temporal prepositions *before* and *after* and the use of these terms to introduce subordinate clauses is typically delayed for a year or more after the use of temporal adverbs (Weist, 1986). When these uses are mastered, the child is able to express relations such as "Before we had our pizza, we ate the salad."[5] There are, of course, many other lexical items that encode relative temporal concepts (e.g., *while, during, already, since*), but these have been studied in developmental psycholinguistic research much less comprehensively.

Languages also encode the absolute and arbitrary concepts tied to conventional temporal systems, such as those for months, days, years, and hours. Of these, concepts of seasons, holidays, and birthdays are typically expected of young children and are discussed with them explicitly. The other lexical terms tend to be used in discourse but not directly taught until the early school years. Thus, their forms may become familiar to young children, although their reference remains obscure.

French and Nelson (1985) analyzed the use of temporal terms by preschool children who described scripts for familiar events and found that in that context 3- and 4-year-olds used temporal language to express more complex relations than is usually reported at this age. In particular, the expression of relative time (*and then*), as well as the sequencing of events using *before, first,* and *after,* appeared in the scripts of the youngest children. However, language referring to arbitrary conventional measures of time were rarely observed and, when they were, were used inaccurately (e.g., "The cookies have to bake for five hours").

Cognition and the acquisition of time language

Several proposals have been put forward to explain the development of time language in terms of general cognitive development. The two best known are Cromer's (1968) de-centering model and Weist's (1986) four-stage model (see also Slobin, 1982, for some general considerations of the relation of cognition and language using cross-linguistic evidence of the acquisition of verb morphology).

De-centering model. On the basis of his analysis of the use of temporal language – tense, aspect, and temporal terms – by two of Brown's (1973) subjects, Cromer (1968) proposed a developmental scheme derived from Piaget's theory, in particular the notion that young children are centered on the here and now and need to develop the capacity to "de-center." Before de-centering, children are unable to take a perspective other than that of the present, thus delaying the achievement of complex temporal expressions. In particular, Cromer considered the use of the "timeless" verb form (the simple present to express the normative or general case) to be a late achievement for this reason. In reconsidering the "cognition hypothesis," Cromer (1988) has backed away from his earlier conclusion, however. He now takes an interactionist view in which language is composed of a number of subsystems, some of which may be dependent on cognitive achievements and some of which are independent of general cognition. He also reviews evidence consistent with the present argument that some concepts may be derived from language use.

Weist's four-stage model. Miller (1978), Smith (1980), and Weist (1986) describe the development of tense in terms introduced by Reichenbach (1947) of the establishment of relations between speech time (ST), reference time (RT), and event time (ET). Briefly, Weist's claim is that children progress "through a sequence of four temporal systems during the development of the capacity to express increasingly complex configurations of temporal concepts" (1986, p. 357). At first there is a "here and now" system in which ET and RT are frozen at ST. That is, children are not able to talk about events that occur outside the present context. Next, children differentiate ET from ST through the use of contrasting tense forms (e.g., past in contrast to present), but RT is stuck at ST. Thus, a past event may be referred to but not located with respect to a time or an event other than the present. In the third system, RT may be differentiated from ST (e.g., by the use of adverbials such as *yesterday*), but ET is restricted to the RT context. Finally, RT may be established separately from ST, and ET may be separated from both RT and ST. (An example of this might be "Before my brother was born [RT], I used to sleep in my brother's room [ET].") Weist (1986) puts the initial development of the ET system (Stage 2) at about 1,6 to 2,0 and the development of the RT systems, restricted (RTr, Stage 3) and free (RTf, Stage 4), at about 3,0 and 4,0, respectively. Weist sees the progressive establishment of these increasingly complex systems as reflecting stages in cognitive development. Specifically, he ties the initial "here and now" system to children's lack of capacity for "displacement," the capacity to think about events as having occurred in the past or to conceptualize events as occurring in the future. Temporal "de-centration" is held to be required for the establishment of RT(r) relations. And seriation and reversibility are proposed as requirements for RT(f). Although Weist cites findings from the literature to support these suggestions, the evidence for the close coincidence (much less a cause–effect relation) of the cognitive achievements and the linguistic expressions is slight. Moreover, there is some reason to doubt that the developmental course of the expression of ST–ET–RT relations is always as constrained as Weist's description implies.

Evidence from discourse. Evidence from the use of terms in discourse contexts suggests that the development of some aspects of temporal language may not be as delayed as Cromer and Weist found, and thus that the alleged cognitive achievements may not be necessary for their development (or these achievements may come earlier in development). For example, French and Nelson (1985) found that in reporting scripts for familiar events all children from the age of 3 (the youngest observed) used the simple present tense to indicate the normative or general "timeless" case, which Cromer put as a late development that depended on de-centering.

The crib monologues collected from Emily between 21 months and 3 years have provided additional data relevant to this question. Gerhardt's (1988, 1989) analysis of Emily's development of a contrastive system of verb morphology indicates that her initial contrast between simple present and progressive forms was based on discourse contexts – talk about stable, usual, and expected events versus unstable events, respectively. The development of her simple present–past contrast did not reflect an aspectual difference, nor was it restricted to immediate past actions (indeed, past-tense forms were not used for immediate past at first). Rather, the contrast was between those events that were usual or normative (simple present) and those that were recounted as a specific happening in the past – hours, days, or weeks earlier (past tense).

Further analysis (Nelson, 1989a) showed that even at the very beginning of the development of the tense and aspect system (at 22 to 23 months) Emily was capable of expressing RT, ET, and ST independently. An excerpt from a monologue at 23 months is instructive:

My sleep.	ET1 = RT1
Mommy came.	ET2 = RT1
And Mommy "get up, get up time go	
home."	ET3
When my slep and.	RT1 = ET1
And mormor came.	RT1?
Then mommy coming.	ET2 = RT1
Then "get up, time to go hoome."	ET3
Time to go home.	ET3
Drink p-water [Perrier].	ET4
Yesterday did that.	RT1 = ET{1, 2, 3, 4}
Now Emmy sleeping in regular bed.	ST = RT2 = ET5 > RT1

Here ET1 is the first event in the activity sequence, ET2 the second, and so on, and RT1 is the reference time of the first event.

My gloss on this narrative is straightforward, although not without its ambiguities: Yesterday (actually earlier the same day) Emily was sleeping at Tanta's (or perhaps Mormor's) when Mommy (or Mormor) came and told her to get up because it was time to go home. They went home and she drank p-water (Perrier).

Emily displays several characteristics of Weist's Stage 3 (restricted RT): She uses both temporal adverbs (*yesterday, now*) and adverbial clauses (*when my slep*) to establish RT separately from ST. This puts her considerably in advance of the age norms Weist projected. Even more interesting, this indicates that she can manipulate these relations with minimal mastery of the tense system itself. Note the inconsistent use of tenses in this segment: Mommy *came,* mommy *coming;* my *sleep,* my *slept* (and in another version, *my sleeping*). Yet from another perspective, Emily appears to be attempting to contrast tenses to set up temporal relations.[6] For example, in the first two lines: my *sleep* (RT) followed by Mommy *came* (ET); lines 5 and 7: my *slep* (RT), then mommy *coming* (ET). The last three lines also contrast in an interesting way: *drink* (ET3), *did* that (RT = ET{1, 2, 3, 4}, *sleeping* (ST = ET5). Present is used for the event in the narrative, past to indicate RT for the narrative, and progressive to indicate now, ST.

From the point of view of sentence structure, then, this segment represents an imperfect attempt at restricted RT. But when viewed in terms of extended discourse, namely, as an attempt to construct a narrative, the effort is much more impressive. In the narrative, the speaker must go beyond sentential relations to relate events to one another over time. In this simple segment, what Emily has accomplished has been to set up an RT, not for one event, but for a sequence of actions that are ordered in relation to each other. We can envision this in terms of positions along a time line, as follows:

$$RT = ET1 \rightarrow ET2 \rightarrow ET3 \rightarrow ET4 \longrightarrow ST$$

Given these relations, the narrator must first refer back in time to establish the beginning point (my sleeping) and then move forward toward the present in the order of the actions (Events 1, 2, 3, and 4), finally moving to the present to reestablish ST in relation to the totality of the events recounted (yesterday did *that*). When the segment is viewed in this way, it is clear that Emily is not restricted to an RT = ET system, but rather is able to use different events as references for subsequent ones. That is, "mommy coming" serves as the RT for the ET of mommy saying "get up," which serves in turn as the RT for the ET of "drink p-water." The RT system may not yet be entirely free, but at not yet 2 years it is already quite complex.

Emily was a very bright and verbal child, and she might be an exception to Weist's cognitive scheme. However, a major point here is that the ability to manipulate time relations appears in connected discourse before its appearance in single sentences. Thus, conclusions about cognitive constraints drawn from sentence grammars or the use of lexical terms can be misleading. Moreover, the evident ability of this child to set up stable representations and then to manipulate order relations within them is consistent with evidence from other, albeit somewhat older, children. The complexity of thought implied by this ability is impressive. I suggest that we have no firm basis at the present time for expecting general cognitive constraints on the expression of temporal relations. Rather, we should examine the expression of temporal concepts and relations in extended discourse contexts to determine the general course and conditions of their development.

Time concepts and event knowledge

That children's implicit and explicit understanding of time concepts and temporal relations derives from their understanding of events has been emphasized throughout this chapter. Of course, children's understanding of events also depends on their implicit understanding of temporal relations, that is, that one event component precedes and succeeds others, forming an inviolable sequence. That very young children represent knowledge of both familiar and novel event sequences is now well established (Bauer & Mandler, 1989; Nelson, 1986; O'Connell & Gerard, 1985). Causally related events and highly routine events are more successfully sequenced than unfamiliar, arbitrarily related events (Bauer & Shore, 1987; Slackman, 1985), but temporal sequence is apparently a basic dimension of event representations. There is good evidence that both duration and frequency are also basic dimensions for parsing and representing experience (Friedman, 1988; Hasher & Zacks, 1979; Pouthas, 1985).

But dimensions of represented experience are not necessarily easily transformed into concepts codable in language. The case of color is analogous: Bornstein (1975, 1985) showed that infants perceive the color spectrum in divisible categories similar to those that are focal for adults, but it is many years before most children can reliably code these divisions in language. Yet color, unlike time, is visible and can be pointed to, named, and contrasted, and indeed adults frequently spend much time trying to teach color words (Rice, 1980). If time words are acquired early, it would seem that events are salient to children in a way that colors are not. It is true that colors are perceptually salient: Children enjoy brightly colored objects. But color is not usually a functional characteristic; things of the same kind may be different colors, and young children do not generalize words along the dimension of color (E. V. Clark, 1973; Nelson, 1973). In contrast, events are functional in the life of the child (as in that of the adult); it is important to know how routines proceed: when to expect lunch, what the sequence of actions is in the bath routine, what comes first in getting dressed, and so on. Thus, a functional representation system must represent sequence, duration, and frequency. Because they are represented in the child's developing experientially based knowledge system (and not just perceived), they may form a basis for learning linguistic forms that express them.

If it is true that children do not enter the language system with a predefined notion of locating events at specific points along a time line, it is understandable that they might not grasp the meaning of linguistic terms that refer to specific temporal locations (e.g., *yesterday*, *last night*). As we saw earlier, however, young children do have a good sense of *relative* location in time, that is, sequence and simultaneity, indicated by *when . . . then* constructions and exemplified in the excerpt from Emily's monologue presented earlier. Indeed, temporal locations tend to be formulated in terms of events when adults converse with young children (Lucariello & Nelson, 1987). Children are familiar with and use terms such as *lunchtime, bedtime, naptime, time for bath.* These are no doubt the first temporal locative expressions that enable children to mark out the partitions of the day. Note that although these are based in a child's own experience, they are to a degree conventional. Among English-speaking children, British children might understand *dinnertime* and *teatime* but not *lunchtime.* Implicit in this kind of language is the idea that there are specific times during the day when certain events take place and not others.

Learning arbitrary divisions of time that serve to locate events is obviously much more difficult for children. Errors in the use of *yesterday* and *tomorrow* have been widely noted. An example is provided in Emily's narrative quoted earlier when she states, "Yesterday did that." Her mother noted that the episode recounted had taken place that morning, not yesterday. For many children *yesterday* seems to mean any time in the past, or even in the future, whereas *tomorrow* means any time in the future (Harner, 1982).

Another example from Emily's monologues is instructive here, this one when she was just 24 months:

> I can't go down the basement with jamas on.
> I sleep with jamas.
> Okay sleep with jamas.
> In the night time my only put big girl pants on.
> But in the morning we put jamas on.
> But, and the morning gets up . . . of the room.
> But afternoon my wake up and play.
> Play with mommy, daddy.

It is not surprising that Emily tries to locate the activities of her life (and the appropriate clothing) with respect to temporal divisions (nighttime, morning, afternoon) because her parents use such language in their conversations about what will happen "tomorrow morning" or "after your nap." There is something odd about Emily's account, however, in that she has the nighttime and morning clothes reversed. She notes correctly that she sleeps with jamas; is she then confused about *morning, afternoon,* and *night*? We, of course, cannot be sure, but it seems likely that these terms are for her as arbitrary and difficult to place correctly as are *yesterday* and *tomorrow*. (Anecdotal evidence from other parents suggests that children as old as 3 years may have a poor understanding of *morning* and *night*.)

The following conversation with a child who was a bit older than Emily also suggests how terms like *yesterday* are understood in relation to the child's organization of event knowledge. In this case, mother and 3-year-old child (Steven) are driving to nursery school:

S :   This . . . remember the water was here . . . the old puddle was here when it rained tonight?
M: When it rained . . . the other day.
S :   No, it rained yesterday.
M: No, it rained the day before yesterday.
S :   No, it was the day before . . . yest . . . yesterday. It was now yesterday!
M: It was now yesterday?
S :   No, when we were . . . when it was night then . . . nighttime then it was yesterday. When we waked up . . . when we had some supper . . . then we went to bed, then it was nighttime, then the sun was out, then it was nighttime, then it rained, then we waked up, then we . . . then we goed, then we went in that puddle. (Nelson, 1977, pp. 226–227)

In this example it appears that Steven is trying to go backward in time to when it rained (the day before yesterday), even while constrained to ordering events in a forward sequence (i.e., supper, bed, sun, nighttime). Coordinating the forward sequence, necessary to ordering activities in real time, with the backward sequence, necessary when representing events in the past, is obviously a formidable task. It appears to be solved by Steven in terms of a hierarchy of temporal units, with the day sequence retaining its forward order and the sequence of days being reversed. But all of this takes place on a mental representation level with no concrete props to aid in the construction. This very commonplace and seemingly very simple reconstruction turns out to be an extraordinary achievement for the 3-year-old mind!

How are temporal terms learned?

Given that expressions for many temporal relations and concepts are not directly taught to children and cannot be inferred from concrete reference, how are they learned? Several clues from the study of Emily's crib monologues suggest a probable course of development. Emily used her monologues to reconstruct events from the past, to forecast events in the future (based on what her parents told her and her own past experience), and to construct a general account of how things go (Nelson, 1989a). Event narratives were the major component of her monologues, as illustrated in the preceding section. Within these narratives she produced many temporal terms, although as the earlier examples showed, there was often a lack of fit between the actual event parameters and Emily's linguistic expressions relating to them. Still, divorced from the context of the real-world constraints, her use of the terms "sounds right." That is, they were appropriately used in terms of both syntax and narrative discourse. Thus, it appears that she had acquired notions of what syntactic and discourse contexts the terms were useful in (e.g., *yesterday* indicates that talk is about the past; *so* connects two related clauses), without yet attaching any specific meaning to the terms. We can conclude from this that she was following a strategy for acquiring words in discourse contexts that we can call *use before meaning*. (As Gelman and Byrnes note in Chapter 1, this volume, this proposal is consistent with Vygotsky's discussion of the acquisition of word use before meaning. See also Wertsch & Stone, 1985, for a discussion of the implications of this position. The notion of deriving meaning from use is also explicit in Wittgenstein's 1958 analysis of language and language learning.) Use before meaning contrasts with other possible formulations to describe the course of learning, including attributing incorrect meaning or incomplete meaning to the child. Use before meaning implies that the use of a term will at first be tightly constrained to particular discourse and syntactic contexts in which it has been observed in use by others.

Presumably the terms Emily used in this "meaningless" way had been used by her parents or other adults in conversations about events that Emily found interpretable on other grounds, on the basis of her general event knowledge and specific past experience. Then, in talking about the same or similar events herself, she could insert the appropriate words into more or less appropriate slots in her narratives. In the absence of negative feedback, the form might be used again in similar contexts. In the course of using and hearing it used, Emily could attend more and more to the conditions of use implied by adult uses and eventually emerge with a meaning constructed from use that matched that of the adult language.

As an example, in pre-bed dialogues when Emily was 26 months, her father used the phrase *just a minute* only in response to her request to be rocked in her crib ("I will rock you for just a minute"). In a related monologue Emily states that "Daddy came in just a minute and rocked me." This expression had not been previously recorded in use by Emily, and it was used at that time only in the specific context in which it was used by the parent. The assumption here is that Emily's representation of the event of Daddy rocking her had come to include the specification *just a minute*. There is no implication that Emily attached any particular meaning to the phrase, however. That is, *just a minute* did not for her specify a particular duration of time over which the rocking took place.

How would other word-learning theories address this evidence? The claim that she had developed a nonlinguistic concept that fit the expression *just a minute* (or that such an innately specified concept had matured) that could therefore be triggered or acquired seems totally unwarranted. Might there be linguistic constraints that could be invoked to ensure that *just a minute* referred to a parcel of time and nothing else? What kind of constraints could these be? There are many other possible phrases that might complete the father's statement "I will rock you," such as "because you're sick," "until you're sleepy," or "if you stop crying." There is nothing in this discourse situation to support the idea that Emily's hypotheses about the meaning of the phrase must be constrained to the domain of time.

In the present view, the child gradually develops knowledge about the expression as it is used by others and as she uses it herself. For example, the next time Emily wants to be rocked, she is likely to include the phrase and ask Daddy to rock her for just a minute. If she asks him to continue rocking, he might say, "No, that's enough for now; it's more than just a minute." This feedback (which might in other cases be less explicit and require more inferencing by the child) can lead Emily to adjust her understanding of the appropriate use of the phrase. As further observations of its use in other contexts are accumulated, the phrase may become decontexted and generalized to novel situations. Emily may notice that *in a minute* is a closely related phrase and the two may be used interchangeably. Indeed, in the use quoted, the two are conflated. Of course, in everyday speech, these terms do not actually reference minutes as measured in clock time. Eventually, Emily has to adjust her understanding of *minute* to accord with the clock and to know that *five minutes* is a definite period of time, whereas *just a minute* and *in a minute* are used to indicate "not very long at all." Thus, constant adjustment of both her representation of reality and her representation of the possible meanings of words and phrases is necessary as she proceeds through the preschool and into the school years.

This kind of learning must be typical of much word learning in early childhood, forming the basis for the extraordinary rate of vocabulary growth that has been frequently noted. What has been referred to as "fast mapping" (Carey & Bartlett, 1978) may frequently reflect only the acquisition of a word form and some notion of its appropriate context of use. Indeed, this is what the Carey and Bartlett (1978) study of the acquisition of a novel color term indicated; the children in that study did not in fact acquire an accurate understanding of the meaning of the new term, but only its general context of use. In fact, Carey and Bartlett made a distinction between fast mapping and extended mapping; extended mapping seems to apply to the temporal terms discussed here.

The construction of a meaning from use may take a long time. For example, as noted previously, many children do not understand the specific reference of *yesterday* and *tomorrow* before the age of 4 or 5 years. And as Carni and French (1985) showed, 3-year-olds tend not to understand the terms *before* and *after* outside of familiar well-structured events, although they produce them in appropriate familiar contexts. In some cases a child may check his explicit understanding of a term after having used it implicitly for some time. For example, Steven's attempt to reconstruct *yesterday* (quoted earlier) seems to involve a kind of explicit checking of his understanding of this relation.

The hypothesis that children use knowledge of event structure as a framework for acquiring and eventually interpreting words coding temporal relations can be viewed in terms of the coordination of two relational structures, speech and event representations. Consider the representation of Event A *while* Event B (e.g., Mother cooked [A] while child watched television [B]), each represented along a time line, where the vertical arrow represents *now*, or ST:

$$
\begin{array}{lll}
 & A \dashrightarrow & \\
ER & B \dashrightarrow & \underline{\qquad\text{now}} \\
 & & \uparrow \\
 & & \\
SR & \underline{\text{A while B}\quad} & \text{ST} \\
 & & \uparrow \\
\end{array}
$$

(Here ER denotes event representation; SR, speech representation. The horizontal arrows indicate indefinite continuation of activity in the past.) The SR presents the events sequentially, the ER simultaneously. Coordination of the two requires that *while* be recognized as an indicator of simultaneous action. Other representations of this kind for some of the temporal terms that children come to understand are illustrated in Figure 8.1. The importance of learning terms within familiar structured events is brought out by this analysis: Without a prior understanding of the event structure the terminology of the SR could not be interpreted.

In summary, the present proposal is that children rely on event knowledge based on prior experience first to acquire and eventually to interpret the meaning of words that refer to temporal concepts and relations. Those relations that directly reflect the relations represented in event knowledge (relations of sequence, frequency, and some notions of duration) would be expected to take on meaning for children relatively early and to be extended to novel contexts of use relatively easily. Those concepts and relations that are not implicit in children's representations of events (e.g., definite, conventionally determined locations in time, temporal measuring units) would be expected to be understood later and with more difficulty and to be used incorrectly rather frequently. These expectations appear to fit the data from studies of child language, insofar as data are available, rather well. Further study is needed, however, to flesh out the evidence and test detailed hypotheses.

Children's construction of meanings on the basis of event knowledge is only a part of the story, however. The other essential part is experience with language concerned with time, and it becomes important to determine what kind of time language children hear and in what kinds of contexts. How do parents use time language? We are beginning to learn something about this through studies of the way parents talk with their children about the past and the future (Eisenberg, 1985; Hudson, 1990; Sachs, 1983). Lucariello and Nelson (1987) found that mothers tended to talk with their children about past and future events at times when the ongoing activity did not absorb their attention, that is, when there was extra "processing space" that could be given to matters beyond the here and now. These situations involved caretaking activities such as having lunch, when mothers might talk about what had happened that morning or what would happen that afternoon. Mothers used terms with

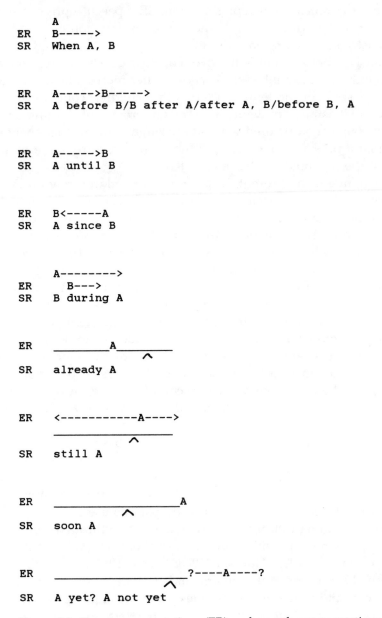

Figure 8.1. Event representations (ER) and speech representations (SR) of some temporal relational terms.

their 2-year-old children locating events in the past such as *today* and *last night,* as well as relative time markers such as *later, after,* and *when,* especially in reference to anticipated future events.

A number of researchers have observed that parents (in our middle-class culture) tend to induct their 2- to 4-year-old children into talk about the past, "memory talk" (Eisenberg, 1985; Engel, 1986; Fivush & Fromhoff, 1988; Hudson, 1986; Sachs, 1983). Many mothers lead their young children through long narratives about what has happened on a particular occasion. In this way, children may come to understand that remembering and talking about particular happenings at a particular point in the past or future have social value. They may then be led to formulate accounts of such events on their own. Learning how to narrate past events and to make plans for future events necessarily involves learning the time language that will clarify sequence, location, and so on. But parents do not teach these terms directly; rather, they are embedded in remembering narratives.

We also observed that Emily's parents' bedtime talk was very largely concerned with talk about anticipated future events and contained references to *tomorrow morning, Saturday, after your nap,* and so on. Table 8.1 illustrates the varieties of uses of temporal language by Emily's parents during the course of pre-bed conversations with her at 26 months (of which *just a minute,* discussed earlier, was an example) and her own uses to express similar concepts in her monologues. This table is revealing of the many complex expressions to which Emily was exposed as well as the several but still limited ways in which her language (if not her concepts) matched those of her parents. Further analyses of these data are currently under way to determine more precisely the restrictions on Emily's uses of the terms in question and their possible generalizations over time.

General implications for the relation between language and thought in development

To recapitulate, children alone could not *discover* time, because (unlike concrete objects) it is not an entity that exists to be discovered. Rather, conceptions of process and change have led different societies to conceptualize time in different ways, and these are conveyed to children through language forms.[7] Children's knowledge of time concepts, even those that are not directly taught, is knowl-

Table 8.1. *Temporal terms used by Emily and her parents*

Parent	Emily
Location	
afternoon	in the morning
earlier	in the night
good night's (sleep)	in the nighttime
morning	now
nighttime	right now
now	when
right now	yesterday
Saturday	
sometime	
Sunday	
time to go to bed	
today	
tomorrow	
tonight	
weekend	
when	
Sequence	
after	and then
afterwards	if
because	cause
so	so
then	when
while (sim)	
Duration	
a little bit	just a minute
a little early	
in the meantime	
in another month	
just a minute	
not quite yet	
not yet	
pretty soon	
until	
yet	
Frequency	
again	again
already	already
betcha	maybe
maybe	
probably	
sometimes	
Other	
any more	any more
birthday	day (fun)
day (fun, nice, busy, mommy and daddy, Tanta)	go night
Good night	long time (as topic)
grow	tomorrow (as topic)
just starting	
new	
till	
times (fun)	
tomorrow (as topic)	

Note: Includes all temporal references in the dialogues and monologues when Emily was 26 months (7 sessions, 231 parent utterances and 101 child utterances).

edge mediated in different ways through language. As such, it exemplifies much of what children must come to know about the world in which they live. The individual child mind is never free to construct a model of the world independent of others who share it, and the individual mind would not get far if it had to construct a model of the complex human world without the linguistically mediated guidance of others. A very large part of what we as adults know we know because we learned it through language. And much of that consists of knowledge that is constituted *in* language; that is, it is not simply a reflection of reality, but a construction of reality.

Putting the matter this way, it seems painfully obvious, and yet, as noted at the outset, most discussions of cognitive development proceed as though language were irrelevant to the issues. In contrast, the analysis here leads to the conclusion that language is central to the discussion; we cannot consider issues of cognitive development without taking the many roles of language into account.

Further, the problem of language acquisition and development is not just determining what influence (if any) general cognition has on the process. Rather, we need to know how general cognition, knowledge representations, and the developing grasp of language terms and structures mutually affect one another in the developing child, and what and how the child adds to knowledge about the world and about the language through transactions with others within the social and cultural milieu. The child develops within a complex system of relationships; we cannot expect to untangle the web all at once.

Thus far, in considering the case of time concepts and time language we have observed three quite different relations between language and cognition, and the roles of language as a mediator of knowledge. First, language may make salient a type of relation that was not previously apparent in a child's nonlinguistic conceptual representations. Present evidence suggests that this may be the case for the tense system, distinguishing past, present, and future. Before acquiring this system children may distinguish only now and not now, or attend only to action relations in the here and now. In this case, the relation that must be expressed grammatically tunes them to a relation to which they had previously been indifferent (see Bowerman, 1982, for related analyses).

Second, nonlinguistic, experientially derived conceptual representations may provide support for acquiring language forms that appropriately express the relations inherent in those representations. This is the relation that is hypothesized to hold between children's event representations and expressions of relative sequence, duration, and frequency (as represented in Figure 8.1). Here cognition, in the form of knowledge representations, supports and influences what language forms are acquired. Terms for relations implicit in events and expressed in parental talk about sequence, duration, and frequency can be learned implicitly, as outlined in the preceding section, through contexted use followed by generalization to other contexts, updating semantic knowledge to accord with speech use. This type of implicit mediated knowledge has only minor effects on the underlying conceptual representations.

Third, language makes possible the construction of abstract concepts and complex representations that cannot be acquired solely from unmediated direct experience because they are culturally constituted through language. Concepts of specific location (*last night*, *Saturday*), measurement (*hours, days, years*), and complex temporal systems such as calendars, and the meaning of terms referencing these, depend on explicit knowledge mediated through language. In this case, concepts constructed in language by members of the culture are conveyed to the young explicitly through talk about the concepts.

Children cannot take advantage of such talk until the ability to use the representational function of language to acquire new knowledge is achieved. They must be able to understand a representation presented by someone else in language as a vehicle for internalizing a new or modified mental representation of reality in order to attain concepts without a basis in direct experience. This ability to amend one's representations of reality or to construct new representations in response to others' talk about states, objects, and events in the world is a crucial achievement of early human childhood that is not shared with other species. This achievement makes it possible for children to compare others' perspectives with their own, as well as to acquire knowledge mediated solely through linguistic means. To arrive at this point children must have acquired sufficient linguistic ability to engage fully in conversations with others about common experiences, the kind of conversations that have been the object of the studies of "memory talk" referred to earlier. Emily seemed to have reached that point by 2 years, but for the majority of children who are less verbal the point seems to come at about 3 or even 4 years (Fivush & Fromhoff, 1988; Sachs, 1983). This is a critical turning point in human development and one that deserves much more attention than it has thus far received.

The distinction being made here between implicit learning of terms that readily map into a child's own conceptual structures and the explicit learning of concepts and terms from adult talk about them is similar in some respects to the distinction that Vygotsky (1986) made between spontaneous and scientific concepts. In Vygotsky's view children do not achieve the level of scientific concepts until adolescence, when concepts become systematized and hierarchized. In the present view the critical shift in the capacity to acquire explicitly mediated knowledge takes place in the preschool years, when children are first able to use language as a vehicle for learning what others know. Certainly much conceptual and semantic development takes place after this point, and these types of linguistic mediation of knowledge continue to characterize learning and knowing throughout life.

The implication here is that there are clear and dramatic shifts in human cognitive development that are a function of language and its development. The first is the shift from being a nonlanguage user (an infant) to becoming a language user that takes place in the second and third years. The second is the shift from being limited to implicit linguistic mediation to the point where explicit linguistic mediation is possible as well. At that point children are opened, for better or worse, to all the possibilities inherent in the rich knowledge systems developed by human cultures. There may be a further shift, in later childhood or early adolescence, as proposed by Vygotsky, when a child's conceptual system may be reorganized in response to the possibilities presented by complexly structured knowledge systems and scientific theories.

It cannot be claimed that all of cognitive development is a function of the developing representational system mediated through language. Nonetheless, it is time to acknowledge the enormously important functions of language in human cognitive development and to study those functions directly. We will find that to do so is to abandon the model of the human child attempting to make sense of the world on her own and to take fully into account the roles that parents and teachers play in these developments. In taking this route we will be following the path of major theorists of the 1920s and 1930s such as Vygotsky, Whorf, Werner, and G. H. Mead. Their theories cannot be adopted without modification in the face of the genuine advances in knowledge of cognitive and linguistic development that have been made over the intervening years; still, the general perspective adopted by these theorists of the child developing within a social, cultural, and linguistic world has implications that we have not yet fully explored. It is time for us to do so.

Notes

1. The first proposition is obviously related to E. V. Clark's (1983, 1987) principle of contrast: Every word contrasts with other words in the lexicon. But because each individual's lexical system is different from every other's, the particular contrasts involved will not match those of a presumed standard or ideal lexicon. Thus, the statement that there are no true synonyms (E. V. Clark, 1987, 1988) may be true for the language considered as an ideal system, but it is unlikely to be true for any given individual. The fact that words exist within a system does not entail that two words cannot occupy the same place within the system. For example, although the dictionary makes subtle distinctions between *couch* and *sofa*, in my idiolect they are interchangeable. Moreover, as pointed out subsequently, the applicability of words shifts with context; thus, contrasts within the system are not stable.
2. Thorndike–Lorge (1944), although dated, was chosen because it reflects children's as well as adult literature, unlike more recent word counts (e.g., Francis and Kucera, 1982; the most frequent time words in these two counts are virtually identical). It seems likely that the most frequently used 500 words have not changed greatly since the Thorndike–Lorge count was undertaken. Only nouns were counted, because they provided the best test case: It is often asserted that children place constraints on the possible reference of nouns, considering them to apply only to objects and object taxonomies. The dichotomization is rough, because a word often has two meanings, one concrete and the other abstract. In most such cases, the word was classified as concrete. For example, *change* was counted as concrete because of its monetary use. The meaning of some of the words counted as abstract could be illustrated by pointing to an exemplar, a symbol, or a representation, but the meaning could not be conveyed in this way. For example, a parent might point to a picture of a crowned figure and say, "That's a king," but the child could not infer the meaning of the word *king* from this example. *King* is clearly a concept that is culturally and linguistically constituted.
3. Working with dual conceptions and representations of time is not unusual. For example, religious calendars, both Christian and Jewish, calculate annual observances according to schemes that differ from the secular calendar. To take a more extreme example, the Balinese observe celebrations dictated by 10 different "weeks" running simultaneously and ranging from 1 to 10 days, the whole forming a year of 210 days. At the same time they follow a Hindu calendar with a standard 12-month year similar to the Western calendar.

4. Not all linguists accept that English codes future independent of modality. Lyons (1977) argues that English (like Indo-European languages in general) makes a fundamental distinction only between past and not past.
5. It is not feasible to review here the extensive literature on the complexities of the acquisitional course of the comprehension of the terms *before* and *after* and their use to express relations between events (see E. V. Clark, 1983; French & Nelson, 1985).
6. Or from another perspective, to set up foreground and background relations in the narrative (see Hopper, 1979).
7. The claim here can be seen to accord to no small degree with Whorfian ideas (Whorf, 1956; see also Lakoff, 1987; Lucy, 1985; Silverstein, 1985; for related ideas see Bowerman, 1985; Slobin, 1987).

References

Adams, A. K., & Bullock, D. (1986). Apprenticeship in word use: Social convergence processes in learning categorically related nouns. In S. A. Kuczaj II & M. D. Barrett (Eds.), *The development of word meaning: Progress in cognitive development research* (pp. 155–197). New York: Springer.

Anderson, R. C., & Ortony, A. (1975). On putting apples into bottles: A problem of polysemy. *Cognitive Psychology, 7*, 167–180.

Antinucci, F., & Miller, R. (1976). How children talk about what happened. *Journal of Child Language, 3*, 169–189.

Au, T. K., & Markman, E. M. (1987). Acquiring word meanings via linguistic contrast. *Cognitive Development, 2*, 217–236.

Augustine, Saint (1950). *The confesions of St. Augustine* (E. B. Pusey, Trans.). New York: Dutton. (Original work written 397.)

Bauer, P. J., & Mandler, J. M. (1989). One thing follows another: Effects of temporal structure on one- to two-year-olds' recall of events. *Developmental Psychology, 25*, 197–206.

Bauer, P. J., & Shore, C. M. (1987). Making a memorable event: Effects of familiarity and organization on young children's recall of action sequences. *Cognitive Development, 2*, 327–339.

Berman, R. A., & Slobin, D. I. (1987). *Five ways of learning how to talk about events: A cross-linguistic study of narrative development* (Working Paper No. 46). University of California, Berkeley, Center for Cognitive Studies.

Bierwisch, N. (1970). Semantics. In J. Lyons (Ed.), *New horizons in linguistics* (pp. 166–184). Harmondsworth: Penguin.

Bloom, L., & Harner, L. (1989). On the developmental contour of child language: A reply to Smith and Weist. *Journal of Child Language, 16*, 207–216.

Bloom, L., Lifter, K., & Hafitz, J. (1980). The semantics of verbs and the development of verb inflection in child language. *Language, 56*, 386–412.

Bornstein, M. H. (1975). Qualities of color vision in infancy. *Journal of Experimental Child Psychology, 19*, 401–419.

Bornstein, M. H. (1985). Colour-name versus shape-name learning in young children. *Journal of Child Language, 12*, 387–393.

Bowerman, M. (1982). Reorganization processes in lexical and syntactic development. In E. Wanner & L. R. Gleitman (Eds.), *Language acquisition: The state of the art* (pp. 319–346). Cambridge University Press.

Bowerman, M. (1985). What shapes children's grammars? In D. I. Slobin (Ed.), *The cross-linguistic study of language acquisition: Vol. 2. Theoretical issues* (pp. 1257–1319). Hillsdale, NJ: Erlbaum.

Brown, R. (1958). *Words and things.* New York: Free Press.

Brown, R. (1973). *A first language: The early stages.* Cambridge, MA: Harvard University Press.

Carey, S. (1978). The child as word learner. In M. Halle, J. Bresnan, & G. A. Miller (Eds.), *Linguistic theory and psychological reality* (pp. 265–293). Cambridge University Press.

Carey, S., & Bartlett, E. (1978). Acquiring a single new word. *Papers and Reports on Child Language Development* (No. 15, pp. 17–29). Stanford, CA: Stanford University, Department of Linguistics.

Carni, E., & French, L. A. (1984). The acquisition of *before* and *after* reconsidered: What develops? *Journal of Experimental Child Psychology, 37,* 394–403.

Clark, E. V. (1973). What's in a word? On the child's acquisition of semantics in his first language. In T. E. Moore (Ed.), *Cognitive development and the acquisition of language* (pp. 65–110). New York: Academic Press.

Clark, E. V. (1982). The young word maker: A case study of innovation in the child's lexicon. In E. Wanner & L. R. Gleitman (Eds.), *Language acquisition: The state of the art* (pp. 390–425). Cambridge University Press.

Clark, E. V. (1983). Meanings and concepts. In P. H. Mussen (Ed.), *Carmichael's manual of child psychology* (4th ed., Vol. 3, pp. 787–840). New York: Wiley.

Clark, E. V. (1987). The principle of contrast: A constraint on language acquisition. In B. MacWhinney (Ed.), *Mechanisms of language acquisition* (pp. 1–34). Hillsdale, NJ: Erlbaum.

Clark, E. V. (1988). On the logic of contrast. *Journal of Child Language, 15,* 317–336.

Clark, H. (1973). Space, time, semantics, and the child. In T. E. Moore (Ed.), *Cognitive development and the acquisition of language* (pp. 27–63). New York: Academic Press.

Comrie, B. (1985). *Tense.* Cambridge University Press.

Cromer, R. F. (1968). *The development of temporal reference during the acquisition of language.* Unpublished doctoral dissertation, Harvard University, Cambridge, MA.

Cromer, R. F. (1988). The cognition hypothesis revisited. In F. S. Kessel (Ed.), *The development of language and language researchers: Essays in honor of Roger Brown* (pp. 223–248). Hillsdale, NJ: Erlbaum.

Dickinson, D. K. (1988). Learning names for materials: Factors constraining and limiting hypotheses about word meaning. *Cognitive Development, 3,* 15–36.

Eisenberg, A. R. (1985). Learning to describe past experiences in conversation. *Discourse Processes, 8,* 177–204.

Engel, S. (1986). *Learning to reminisce: A developmental study of how young children talk about the past.* Unpublished doctoral dissertation, City University of New York.

Fivush, R., & Fromhoff, F. A. (1988). Style and structure in mother–child conversations about the past. *Discourse Processes, 11,* 337–356.

Fodor, J. A. (1975). *The language of thought.* New York: Crowell.

Fodor, J. A. (1981). *Re-presentations.* Cambridge, MA: MIT Press.

Francis, W. N., & Kucera, H. (1982). *Frequency analysis of English usage: Lexicon and grammar.* Boston: Houghton Mifflin.

Fraser, J. T. (1987). *Time the familiar stranger.* Amherst: University of Massachusetts Press.

French, L. A., & Nelson, K. (1985). *Young chldren's knowledge of relational terms: Some ifs, ors, and buts.* New York: Springer.

Friedman, W. J. (Ed.). (1982). *The developmental psychology of time.* New York: Academic Press.

Friedman, W. J. (1988). *Children's knowledge of the duration of familiar events.* Unpublished manuscript, Oberlin College, Oberlin, OH.

Gerhardt, J. (1988). From discourse to semantics: The development of verb morphology and forms of self-reference in the speech of a 2-year-old. *Journal of Child Language, 15,* 337–394.

Gerhardt, J. (1989). Monologue as speech genre. In K. Nelson (Ed.), *Narratives from the crib* (pp. 171–230). Cambridge, MA: Harvard University Press.

Gould, S. J. (1987). *Time's arrow, time's cycle: Myth and metaphor in the discovery of geological time.* Cambridge, MA: Harvard University Press.

Harner, L. (1975). *Yesterday* and *tomorrow*: Development of early understanding of the terms. *Developmental Psychology, 11,* 864–865.

Harner, L. (1982). Talking about the past and future. In W. J. Friedman (Ed.), *The developmental psychology of time* (pp. 141–169). New York: Academic Press.

Hasher, L., & Zacks, R. T. (1979). Automatic and effortful processes in memory. *Journal of Experimental Psychology: General, 108,* 356–388.

Heibeck, T. H., & Markman, E. M. (1987). Word learning in children: An examination of fast mapping. *Child Development, 58,* 1021–1034.

Hopper, P. (1979). Aspect and foregrounding in discourse. In T. Givon (Ed.), *Syntax and semantics: Vol. 12. Discourse and syntax* (pp. 213–241). New York: Academic Press.

Hudson, J. A. (1986, April). *A longitudinal study of memory talk in mother–child conversation.* Paper presented at the International Conference on Infant Studies, Los Angeles.

Hudson, J. A. (1990). The emergence of autobiographic memory in mother–child conversation. In R. Fivush & J. A. Hudson (Eds.), *Knowing and remembering in young children* (pp. 166–196). Cambridge University Press.

James, W. (1950). *The principles of psychology.* New York: Dover. (Original work published 1890.)

Johnston, J. R. (1985). Cognitive prerequisites: The evidence from children learning English. In D. I. Slobin (Ed.), *The cross-linguistic study of language acquisition: Vol. 2. Theoretical issues* (pp. 961–1004). Hillsdale, NJ: Erlbaum.

Labov, W. (1973). The boundaries of words and their meanings. In C.-J. N. Bailey & R. W. Shay (Eds.), *New ways of analyzing variation in English* (pp. 340–373). Washington, DC: Georgetown University Press.

Lakoff, G. (1987). *Women, fire, and dangerous things.* Chicago: University of Chicago Press.

Lakoff, G., & Johnson, M. (1980). *Metaphors we live by.* Chicago: Chicago University Press.

Landau, B., Smith, L. B., & Jones, S. S. (1988). The importance of shape in early lexical learning. *Cognitive Development, 3,* 299–321.

Levy, Y., Schlesinger, I. M., & Braine, M. D. S. (Eds.) (1988). *Categories and processes in language acquisition.* Hillsdale, NJ: Erlbaum.

Lucariello, J., & Nelson, K. (1987). Remembering and planning talk. *Discourse Processes, 10,* 219–235.

Lucy, J. A. (1985). Whorf's view of the linguistic mediation of thought. In E. Mertz & R. J. Parmentier (Eds.), *Semiotic mediation: Sociocultural and psychological perspectives* (pp. 73–97). New York: Academic Press.

Lyons, J. (1977). *Semantics.* Cambridge University Press.

Macnamara, J. (1982). *Names for things.* Cambridge, MA: MIT Press.

Markman, E. M. (1987). How children constrain the possible meanings of words. In U. Neisser (Ed.), *Concepts and conceptual development: Ecological and intellectual factors in categorization* (pp. 255–287). Cambridge University Press.

Markman, E. M., & Hutchinson, J. (1984). Children's sensitivity to constraints on word meaning: Taxonomic vs. thematic relations. *Cognitive Psychology, 16,* 1–27.

McGrath, J. E., & Kelly, J. R. (1986). *Time and human interaction: Toward a social psychology of time.* New York: Guilford Press.

Miller, G. A. (1978). Pastness. In G. A. Miller & E. Lenneberg (Eds.), *Psychology and biology of language and thought* (pp. 167–186). New York: Academic Press.

Nelson, K. (1973). Structure and strategy in learning to talk. *Society for Research in Child Development Monographs, 38* (1–2, Serial No. 149).

Nelson, K. (1974). Concept, word, and sentence: Interrelations in acquisition and development. *Psychological Review, 81,* 267–285.

Nelson, K. (1977). Cognitive development and the acquisition of concepts. In R. C. Anderson, R. J. Spiro, & W. E. Montague (Eds.), *Schooling and the acquisition of knowledge* (pp. 215–253). Hillsdale, NJ: Erlbaum.

Nelson, K. (1985). *Making sense: The acquisition of shared meaning.* New York: Academic Press.

Nelson, K. (1986). *Event knowledge: Structure and function in development.* Hillsdale, NJ: Erlbaum.

Nelson, K. (1988a). Constraints on word learning? *Cognitive Development, 3,* 221–246.

Nelson, K. (1988b). The ontogeny of memory for real events. In U. Neisser & E. Winograd (Eds.), *Remembering reconsidered: Ecological and traditional approaches to the study of memory* (pp. 244–276). Cambridge University Press.

Nelson, K. (1989a). Monologues as construction of self in time. In K. Nelson (Ed.), *Narratives from the crib* (pp. 284–308). Cambridge, MA: Harvard University Press.

Nelson, K. (1989b). Remembering: A functional developmental perspective. In P. R. Solomon, G. R. Goethals, C. M. Kelley, & B. R. Stephens (Eds.), *Memory: An interdisciplinary approach* (pp. 127–150). New York: Springer.

Nelson, K. (1990). Remembering, forgetting, and childhood amnesia. In R. Fivush & J. Hudson (Eds.), *Knowing and remembering in young children* (pp. 317–330). Cambridge University Press.

O'Connell, B. G., & Gerard, A. B. (1985). Scripts and scraps: The development of sequential understanding. *Child Development, 56,* 671–681.

Piaget, J. (1962). *Play, dreams, and imitations.* New York: Norton.

Pouthas, V. (1985). Timing behavior in young children: A developmental approach to conditioned spaced responding. In J. A. Michon & J. L. Jackson (Eds.), *Time, mind, and behavior* (pp. 100–109). New York: Springer.

Putnam, H. (1975). The meaning of meaning. In *Philosophical papers: Vol. 2. Mind, language, and reality* (pp. 215–271). Cambridge University Press.

Putnam, H. (1988). *Representation and reality.* Cambridge, MA: MIT Press.

Quine, W. V. O. (1960). *Word and object.* Cambridge, MA: MIT Press.

Quine, W. V. O. (1977). Natural kinds. In S. P. Schwartz (Ed.), *Naming, necessity, and natural kinds* (pp. 155–175). Ithaca, NY: Cornell University Press.

Reichenbach, H. (1947). *Elements of symbolic logic.* New York: Free Press.

Rice, M. (1980). *Cognition to language: Categories, word meanings, and training.* Baltimore: University Park Press.

Sachs, J. (1983). Talking about the there and then: The emergence of displaced reference in parent–child discourse. In K. E. Nelson (Ed.), *Children's language* (Vol. 4, pp. 1–28). New York: Gardner Press.

Sampson, G. (1980). *Making sense.* Oxford: Oxford University Press.

Shore, C., O'Connell, B., & Bates, E. (1984). First sentences in language and symbolic play. *Developmental Psychology, 20,* 872–880.

Silverstein, M. (1985). The functional stratification of language and ontogenesis. In J. Wertsch (Ed.), *Culture, communication, and cognition: Vygotskian perspectives* (pp. 205–235). Cambridge University Press.

Slackman, E. (1985). *The effect of event structure on children's ability to learn an unfamiliar event.* Unpublished doctoral dissertation, City University of New York.

Slobin, D. I. (1982). Universal and particular in the acquisition of language. In E. Wanner & L. R. Gleitman (Eds.), *Language acquisition: The state of the art* (pp. 128–170). Cambridge University Press.

Slobin, D. I. (1987). Thinking for speaking. In J. Askew, N. Beery, L. Michaelis, & H. Filip (Eds.), *Proceedings of the Thirteenth Annual Meeting of the Berkeley Linguistics Society* (pp. 435–445). Berkeley: University of California.

Smith, C. (1980). The acquisition of time talk: Relations between child and adult grammars. *Journal of Child Language, 7,* 263–278.

Soja, N., & Carey, S. (1986, April). *Constraints on learning: The role of the concept of object.* Paper presented at the International Conference on Infant Studies, Los Angeles.

Thorndike, E. L., & Lorge, I. (1944). *The teacher's word book of 30,000 words.* New York: Columbia University, Teachers College, Bureau of Publications.

Traugott, E. C. (1978). On the expression of spatio-temporal relations in language. In J. H. Greenberg (Ed.), *Universals of human language: Vol. 3. Word structure* (pp. 369–400). Stanford, CA: Stanford University Press.

Vygotsky, L. S. (1986). *Thought and language* (rev. ed.). Cambridge, MA: MIT Press.

Weist, R. M. (1986). Tense and aspect. In P. Fletcher & M. Garman (Eds.), *Language acquisition* (2nd ed., pp. 356–374). Cambridge University Press.

Weist, R. M., Wysocka, H., Witkowska-Stadnik, K., Buczowska, E., & Konieczna, E. (1984). The defective tense hypothesis: On the emergence of tense and aspect in child Polish. *Journal of Child Language, 11,* 347–374.

Wertsch, J. V., & Stone, C. A. (1985). The concept of internalization in

318 K. Nelson

Vygotsky's account of the genesis of higher mental functions. In J. V. Wertsch (Ed.), *Culture, communication, and cognition: Vygotskian perspectives* (pp. 162–179). Cambridge University Press.

Whorf, B. L. (1956). *Language, thought, and reality: Selected writings of Benjamin Lee Whorf* (J. B. Carroll, Ed.). Cambridge, MA: MIT Press.

Wittgenstein, L. (1958). *Philosophical investigations* (3rd ed.; G. E. M. Anscombe, Trans.). New York: Macmillan.

9. Constraints on the acquisition of English modals

MARILYN SHATZ AND SHARON A. WILCOX

Introduction: Modals and language–thought issues

The ability to communicate through language is a benchmark of human competence. Speakers use language to communicate their knowledge and beliefs and to share their community's rules of social order and cultural norms. Modal expressions, because they encode the stances speakers take on propositions, are essential to these two language functions. Consider, for example, a proposition like *John come.* With the addition of a modal, such as *can, may, must,* or *will,* speakers can make a variety of statements about that proposition, from expressing their degree of certainty about the likelihood of the event it encodes to giving permission for the event to occur. If children are to become competent members of their language community, it is crucial that they master their language's modal system.

Because modal expressions encode notions of necessity, possibility, obligation, and permission, they are an important and revealing aspect of language to study with regard to language–thought issues. The use of modals in the epistemic sense (having to do with beliefs, attitudes, and knowledge states) seems to entail the ability to assess one's own knowledge state, to evaluate evidence, and to communicate those assessments to another whose state may be different from one's own. Such abilities, central though they are to a host of cognitive activities, have not regularly been accorded to children younger than 4. Yet children younger than 4 certainly produce modals in their spontaneous speech. Possibly children use these words solely for purposes of social regulation and description, that is, with deontic and dynamic meanings rather than epistemic ones (Palmer, 1979). If children's uses are constrained in these ways, that may be because they are limited cognitively from doing otherwise, or it may be that the input to them is limited. That is, mothers themselves may confine their use of modals to the social sphere. The spontaneous use of modals by parents and children informs us, then, about the important question of children's understanding of knowledge states and the bases of knowledge.

A related issue is the question of how concepts of knowledge state and evidence arise. If children have to develop the capacity to assess knowledge states, where do they get the idea that doing so is important? One possibility is that the language of social regulation, based as it is on notions of warrants for action, provides an entree into the idea of bases for knowledge as well (see Lyons, 1977, for a related suggestion that children acquire understanding of necessity and possibility by analogy to notions of permission and obligation). Indeed, it may be no accident that many of the world's languages use a single set of devices to express both deontic and epistemic notions. Every society, after all, must set definitional standards for both knowledge and authority, and language is the primary source of information about those standards. We suggest that acquiring a language of modality in part involves a process of socialization of cognition in which the cognitive developments underlying epistemic understandings are themselves influenced by the very language being learned. If this is so, it may be inappropriate to speak of cognitive prerequisites to the acquisition of the modal system. A more appropriate model may be a dynamic, interactive one of mutual influence between language and thought.

In what follows, we examine in more detail the characteristics of English modals and consider previously proposed acquisition mechanisms. We go on to review the literature on modal acquisition. We then propose a set of constraints on the acquisition of English modals and conclude with some general comments about the acquisition of a complex grammatical system.

The characteristics of English modals

There are several ways to express modality in English, including the use of modal adverbs such as *maybe* and *certainly* and complement-taking verbs such as *think* and *suppose*. Among the most important devices, and certainly among the earliest that children acquire, however, are the modal verbal constructions, including modal auxiliaries and semiauxiliaries. These constructions are the focus of this chapter, although we make occasional references to the other devices when relevant.

In English the set of modal auxiliaries includes *can, could, may, must, might, should, ought, will,* and *would.* These words are defined as a set not only because they express related meanings but because they share a set of grammatical properties such as contraction, absence of marking on third-person singular, and sentence fronting (Palmer, 1979). In addition, a set of semimodals, *hafta, wanna, gonna, gotta,* and *needta,* which express similar meanings and which share some but not all of the grammatical properties of "true" modals, are often considered along with them in discussions of English modal expressions (Garcia, 1967). In this section, we consider the semantic and syntactic characteristics of these modal expressions, particularly with regard to those that may bear on the nature of the acquisition process.

Semantics: The plurifunctionality of modals

Traditional analyses of modal semantics have focused on the logical relations between necessity and possibility: If a proposition, P, is necessarily true, then its negation, $-P$, cannot possibly be true, and if P is necessarily not true, then its negation, $-P$, cannot possibly be not true. Lyons (1977) notes that expressions of logical necessity are rare in everyday discourse, but he suggests that an intuitive understanding of logical necessity is the basis for everyday language that expresses speaker notions of certainty and obligation. For example, if one is certain that P is true, then one must also be certain that $-P$ is not true, and if one is obligated to do an act, then not doing the act is not permitted. Thus, in logic-based analyses, necessity and possibility are central to the meaning of modals, and the related notions expressed by modals in everyday language, such as desire, prediction, intention, volition, and ability, are peripheral, with little attention given to them. Thus, such analyses do not readily capture the richness of the meanings modals can express.

More recent alternative analyses seek to explicate more fully the richness of the modal system. Coates (1983) analyzes modal meanings according to fuzzy set theory, noting that most modals are plurifunctional.[1] That is, they can express different (albeit related) meanings. The most prototypical meanings lie at the core of the set of meanings, with the least prototypical ones falling in the periphery. For some modals, such as *can*, more than one fuzzy set is required to represent all the meanings expressed. For example, the notions of permission and ability form the cores of two fuzzy sets for *can*, with the notion of possibility defined as the intersection of the two sets.

Talmy (1988) uses the notion of force dynamics to characterize what lies at the heart of modality as "force opposition." In particular, he argues that subjects of modals are seen as agonists constrained or opposed in some way by a force, usually a social one. The various modals express the degree of force exerted on the agonist. Thus, a sentence such as "John must be home by 11" implies that there is an external authority requiring John to be home at a certain hour, even against his will; "John should be home by 11" also implies an external authority opposed to John's staying out past 11, but that authority has less power to enforce its will on John. As for epistemic meanings, by metaphoric extension, these imply an agonist who is forced or compelled to make certain inferences (e.g., "The pear must be ripe now"), presumably on the basis of the knowledge she has.

One advantage of these recent analyses is that they recognize more explictly the plurifunctionality of the modals. Moreover, they attempt to capture the psychological underpinnings of the modal system. Whether fuzzy sets or forces are the appropriate representations of the underlying cognitive structures is not an issue for the present discussion. The importance of these recent characterizations is that they highlight the plurifunctionality of a linguistic system that young children must acquire. Yet plurifunctionality is a characteristic that young language learners try to avoid (Karmiloff-Smith, 1979). Two questions to be asked, then, about the acquisition of the modal system is whether modal input is simplified by the avoidance of plurifunctionality, and whether children, in their early use of modals, demonstrate an avoidance of plurifunctionality. If so, the avoidance of plurifunctionality could be seen as a constraint on the course of acquisition of the modal system.

Syntax: Modals and defective paradigms

English modals have regularly been classified as members of an auxiliary class; indeed, they share grammatical characteristics with the other English auxiliaries, *be*, *have*, and *do*. Yet as Table 9.1 illustrates, auxiliary paradigms are irregular, or defective, ones, with no two auxiliary types having exactly the same set of grammatical characteristics. Thus, it would be perilous for the language-learning child to generalize from one auxiliary class member to another (cf. Baker, 1981; Pinker, 1984).[2]

Acquisition researchers have sometimes ignored the defectiveness of the auxiliary paradigm and have studied the acquisiton of the auxiliary system – particularly the influence of maternal speech on the rate of acquisition – as though it were a unified whole (e.g., Furrow, Nelson, & Benedict, 1979; Gleitman, Newport, & Gleitman, 1984; Newport, Gleitman, & Gleitman, 1977). Although many studies have shown some effect of maternal auxiliary use on child acquisition, the specification of the precise mechanism whereby maternal input affects child output has been hampered by variations in the specifics of the findings from different studies (see Shatz, Hoff-Ginsberg, & MacIver, 1989, for a review). This may not be surprising, because, given the grammatical differences among auxiliaries that must be learned, an approach that glosses over those differences is not likely to result in a satisfactory account of the mechanisms of acquisition.

Pinker (1984) has taken the alternative approach of arguing that the defectiveness of the auxiliary paradigms is the very characteristic governing the kinds of mechanisms that must be postulated to account for acquisition. He proposes that children are constrained from generalizing from one auxiliary type to another inappropriately by a universal principle forbidding the creation and application of general auxiliary paradigms. Instead, children fill in the grammatical paradigms for auxiliaries (as opposed to those for other verbs, where the constraint against generalizing does not apply) on a word-by-word basis as they get specific positive evidence. What makes children able to observe the constraint in the appropriate instances is that words can be identified early as members of the grammatical class AUX on the basis of semantics. The crucial semantic elements involve some combination of tense, modality, aspect, deontic notions, and sentence and discourse notions representing speaker intent (whether what is said involves questioning, negating, or emphasizing). Thus, although he claims that auxiliaries are acquired on a case-by-case basis, Pinker contends that children have a class of AUX to which these words accrue, not *despite* their grammatical dissimilarities, but *because* of them.

Table 9.1. *Constructions diagnostic for category definition*

Type of AUX	Type of construction							
	to complement	Negative contraction	Third-person-*s*	*-ing* on MV	Past on AUX	Past on MV	Infinitive	Nonemphatic declarative
Do	–	×	×	–	×	–	–	–
Be	×	×	×	×	×	×	×	×
Have	×	×	×	–	×	×	×	×
Modal	–	×	–	–	–	–	–	×
Semi-AUX	×	–	0	–	–	–	0	×

Key: ×, Applicable; –, not applicable; 0, variable according to item; MV, main verb.

Several aspects of Pinker's theory are problematic. For one, it assumes that AUX and the constraints attendant on it are universal; but whether auxiliaries are a separate and universal grammatical category is a controversial question among linguists (Gazdar, Pullum, & Sag, 1982; McCawley, 1975; Reuland, 1983). For another, the semantic elements on which the syntactic category bootstraps are varied and nonobvious. It seems unlikely that young children would be able to recognize enough of these consistently on primarily nonlinguistic grounds to assign the AUX label on the basis of semantics alone. Also, a category that is defined by the diversity of its syntactic elements rather than their similarities seems intuitively harder to recognize, and it would be surprising to find it an early acquisition.

Pinker is correct in arguing that relatively few errors in auxiliary use appear in the literature. However, with his argument for word-by-word acquisition based entirely on positive evidence, it is difficult to account for any errors at all, although some certainly do occur. Reliance on the claim that errors are performance-based rather than competence-based seems ad hoc.

Moreover, the postulation of an early category of AUX may not be parsimonious. There is some evidence that if early categorization exists at all, it is based on similarities among elements rather than on an abstract notion of diverse defects among those elements. Children exposed to additional input with the modal *could* at the beginnings of utterances showed faster modal development over time than did children who received the additional instances of *could* in the middle of sentences. Although the facilitation from fronted *could* generalized to other modals, no differences between groups were found for nonmodals, suggesting that the children saw the input as relevant to other modals but not to the nonmodal cases (Shatz, Hoff-Ginsberg, & MacIver, 1989). In a word-by-word acquisition process that depends on the identification of new words as elements in an AUX class, one would have expected either no facilitation at all from the presented *could* instances to other auxiliaries or equal (but minimal) facilitation to all other auxiliaries. Pinker argues that even modals differ among themselves in some grammatical characteristics. However, modals share more major grammatical characteristics with one another than they do with other auxiliaries (see Table 9.1). Given that facilitation of other modals but not nonmodals did occur, it appears that children early on in the acquisition process may indeed create a grammatical class, but one that is narrower (and more consistent grammatically) than that of AUX. We shall return later to the topic of the nature of early grammatical categories and the factors that influence their establishment.

Modals as a complex system

Our brief discussion of some of the semantic and syntactic characteristics of modals should suffice to make it obvious that modals are a complex aspect of language. They cannot be characterized simply or completely consistently on any dimension. Moreover, virtually anyone who has written about modals notes how difficult it is even to define the class, because there are other words in the language, such as *dare, need,* and *let,* that share either grammatical or semantic properties (or both) with the "core" modals (see Palmer, 1979; Talmy, 1988). Children begin to use modals relatively early, when they have a mean length of utterance (MLU) of a little more than 2.0 (Brown, 1973). How do they manage so complex a system? We suggest that there are both internal, child-based, and external, environment-based, constraints on the acquisition path that the modal system takes. These constraints help to make the system more analyzable for a limited-capacity language user. We shall return to the question of the nature of these constraints in the third major section of the chapter. For now, we turn to a review of what is known about modal usage by young children.

The course of modal acquisition: A literature review

In this section, we first consider studies that have described children's modal productions in naturally occurring conversations, usually at home, over a period of time. Most of these studies concentrate on children aged 1,10 to 3,0. We then examine the data on children's performance in a variety of experimental studies, some of which include children up to middle childhood. Finally, we consider the studies that have investigated either the syntactic or the semantic characteristics of the modal input children receive.

Naturalistic longitudindal studies

The onset of modal use. In the work of Brown and his colleagues on acquisition stages I through III (up to age 3,0 and MLU 3.5) of Adam,

Eve, and Sarah, the earliest occurrences (in Stage II) of modal expressions they observed were negative contractions (*can't*) or con-catenatives (*wanna, gonna, hafta*). *Can* and *will* occurred at Stage III, although less frequently than negative contractions or concatena-tives (Brown, 1973; Brown, Cazden, & Bellugi, 1969). As for the se-mantic functions of these early modals, the children used them for general negation and to express notions of desire and intention, as well as what Brown (1973) called "imminence," commentary on an action about to occur. Bloom, Lightbown, and Hood (1975) char-acterized a similar set of verbs, *want to, wanna, going to, gonna, have to, hafta, let's,* and *can't,* as having the meaning of *desire to act.* For two of the children they studied, these verbs were productive at 2,1, for one, they were productive at 1,10, and for the fourth, there were no examples of such verbs by 2,1. Fletcher (1979) reported on two children, one of whom first used *can't* and *won't* at 2,2, with the affirmative forms of these modals following a month later. The sec-ond child was observed between 2,0 and 2,2 using both positive and negative forms of *can* and *will* ("willn't"), as well as *shall.* Another child (Fletcher, 1985) used only *can't* by 2,4, as a general negative marker rather than a modal verb.

Two research groups have examined larger samples of children for the early uses of modals. As part of the Bristol Language De-velopment Study, Wells (1979) time-sampled 60 children along with their mothers every three months from 1,3 to 3,6. He reported the data in terms of (a) the percentage of children who used a modal to express a particular meaning at least once during the period of the study and (b) the age at which at least 50% of the sample used a particular modal to express a particular meaning. By 2,6 only two meanings of *can,* ability and permission, and one meaning of *will,* intention, were being used by half of the sample (Wells, 1985).

As part of a study of auxiliary acquisition, Shatz, Billman, and Yaniv (1986) examined the modal productions of 30 children bi-monthly for a six-month period, beginning when the mean age of the children was 2,2. These children had been selected for an earlier study (Shatz, Hoff-Ginsberg, & MacIver, 1989) because they seemed ready to acquire auxiliaries: When first seen, they were regularly producing subject–verb–object utterances but very few auxiliaries. (Some of them later participated in six weeks of modal enrichment with *could,* as described earlier.) They are an excellent sample to consider for our purposes because the selection procedure identified a large group of children at the very onset of modal production. Examination of more than 3,500 utterances produced by the children at pre-enrichment sessions revealed that only eight children used even one modal form, and only three used two. *Can* and *will* accounted for all but one occurrence of modals, and many of these were in the form of negative contractions. Two of the children used *can* affirmatively while producing no negative modals, suggesting that negative modal constructions, although common, are not necessarily the first forms children use (cf. Klima & Bellugi, 1966). In addition, half of these eight children used one concatenative (either *gonna* or *wanna*), as did seven other children, only one of whom used both.[3]

All the children, including the ones who received no *could* enrichment or no benefit from the enrichment (see Shatz, Hoff-Ginsberg, & MacIver, 1989, for details) developed a modal vocabulary rapidly over the ensuing months. By mean age 2,6, 21 of the 24 children who were still being observed every two months had used at least one modal and one concatenative; of the other three, two had used only modals and one only concatenatives.

Still, the children did not give much evidence of syntactic productivity with modals. Shatz et al. (1986) analyzed the kinds of constructions in which modal words and concatenatives appeared. For this analysis, full forms and contractions were considered as separate types. For example, 'll and *will* were separate word types, as were *can* and *can't*. Word types were then scored for whether they appeared in yes–no questions, yes–no inverted questions, wh-questions, tag questions, declaratives, or imperatives. Although the children produced an average of five different word types, only 18% of these on average appeared in more than one type of construction. Just one child used more than half his words (three of five) in more than one type of construction. Thus, the children had a range of modal words but limited privileges of occurrence for them. Of course, this analysis is limited by the bimonthly sampling procedure and may underestimate the productivity of these forms. However, the data are consonant with those of Fletcher (1979), who argued that the early acquisition of verb forms including auxiliaries is best characterized as piecemeal lexical learning in limited syntactic contexts.

Kuczaj and Maratsos (1983) advanced a related argument that there is no evidence for a general syntactic category of AUX in early auxiliary usage. Nonetheless, they proposed granting something other than item-by-item knowledge to young children. They suggested that children form a separate grammatical category defined by a single syntactic position for those lexical items that appear in initial position in yes–no questions. Their suggestion is based on two kinds of longitudinal data from 16 children who were observed during various periods of development, which covered ages 2,6 to 3,0 for all of them. First, a common pattern was that new modal words occurred earliest in declaratives, appearing in yes–no questions some months later (also see Bellugi, 1967); moreover, both words of related word pairs (*can, could; will, would*) often appeared in declarative contexts whereas only one was used in interrogative contexts. Second, for two of the children studied intensively, the acquisition course of modals in declaratives (as measured by the criterion of 90% correct use in obligatory contexts) was slow and sporadic, whereas several lexical items tended to achieve stability in yes–no questions closer together in time, giving credence to the claim that the children grouped the latter items into a grammatical category having the single common syntactic property of first position in yes–no questions.

The Shatz et al. (1986) data agree on the early predominance of modals in declarative forms. More than 83% of the modal word types observed in their sample by age 2,6 appeared only in declaratives. However, their data on first observed occurrences are equivocal with regard to the claim that initial verbs of yes–no questions emerge together as a class somewhat later. By 2,6, half of the 24 children had already produced one or more of the same word types in yes–no questions, either earlier or in the same observation session, as in declaratives. Also, only three of these children could be said to have had anything like a grammatical cateogry for initial verbs of yes–no questions: Only these three used as many as two different word types in initial position in yes–no questions. Thus, the data suggest that some children use a word in initial position in yes–no questions before declarative use and long before they acquire a group of words with privileges to initial position. Shatz et al. used a first-occurrence measure rather than the 90% criterion, and their subjects were younger than those of Kuczaj and Maratsos. Thus, methodological differences may account to some extent for the differences in findings.

Indeed, the possibility that children start to create some sorts of grammatical categories involving auxiliaries (albeit not adultlike ones) during the second half of the third year receives support from the analyses done by Shatz, Hoff-Ginsberg, and MacIver (1989), although their findings go counter to the specific Kuczaj and Maratsos proposal about the nature of the children's category. In the Shatz, Hoff-Ginsberg, and MacIver (1989) study, a subset of children who received enriched input with the modal *could* in front position exhibited faster growth in the use of modals (both frequency and types of modals), but not other auxiliaries, than did children who received other kinds of input. However, the acceleration was not limited either to the modal *could* or to uses of modals in front position, suggesting that the children had learned something general about the class of modals. If the children had not been able to relate the fronted input to modals in other positions, it is difficult to see how the more general facilitation could have occurred. Thus, Shatz, Hoff-Ginsberg, and MacIver (1989) argue that the early category distinction children make is a modal–nonmodal one, rather than one defined by position.

What kind of mechanism might account for the early categorization of modals together as a class? Gleitman et al. (1984) have suggested that fronted auxiliary input is effective for children because first position is salient to them and because that position tends to be stressed. However, if first position were the facilitative factor, then all auxiliaries that could appear in first position should have been equally facilitated. Moreover, both Shatz, Hoff-Ginsberg, and MacIver (1989) and Fletcher (1985) found relatively little stressing of fronted auxiliaries. One characteristic that distinguishes modals from all other auxiliaries is the absence of third-person singular *s*. On the Shatz, Hoff-Ginsberg, and MacIver tapes, the final consonants of fronted auxiliaries often stood out. Possibly, the phonological difference between *'s* and *c'd* in words like *does* and *could* is especially salient and leads children to differentiate fronted words on the basis of the presence or absence of *s*.

The two proposals for early categorization may not be antithetical to one another. Possibly the differentiation of modals and nonmodals first occurs among the words in an "initial verbs of yes–no questions" category, and then, as further distributional analyses are done (Maratsos, 1982), children recognize other similarities and differences among words across the possible positions in which modals and the other auxiliaries occur. They may then reorganize their categories into modals and nonmodals. Another possibility is that there are several patterns of early category development that can occur in the acquisition of auxiliaries depending on individual differences in children or on the input they receive. Clearly, more research is needed on early grammatical category formation.

In general, however, all the studies taken together produce a fairly consistent picture of early modal development. For English-speaking children, modal use begins gradually, between 1,10 and 2,6, often with a single concatenative or negative modal form appearing in limited syntactic contexts and with a constrained set of meanings. Modal vocabulary growth proceeds fairly rapidly during this early period, while the range of syntactic contexts in which the modals appear changes somewhat more slowly. First modal meanings center on intention, volition, "imminence," and ability or, more often, inability. Relatively few comparable data are available for languages other than English, but Stephany (1986) reports for modern Greek some early modal expressions by children about the same age that again focus on intention and future events.

Development in the preschool years. Beyond 2,6, children develop a broader range of meanings for modal expressions. By 3,3, at least half of Wells's subjects used modals to make predictions and to talk about possibility, obligation, and necessity (Wells, 1985; also see Garvey, 1989). In addition, words other than *can* became multifunctional; for example, *will* expressed both intention and prediction for at least half the sample. In addition, the children increased the number of lexical items they used to express intentions; that is, the plurilexicality of that meaning increased (Wells, 1979). In a study examining the modal development in German-speaking and English-speaking children with a mean age of 2,5, Shatz, Grimm, Wilcox, and Niemeier-Wind (1990) found a similar increase in plurilexicality. Both groups of children showed an increase in the number of different modals used to express particular meanings over the four months they were followed.

Some researchers have argued that increasingly differentiated meanings for particular modals develop at about this time. Shepherd (1981, 1982) reports that the one child she studied originally used both *will* and *gonna* to express volition and intention, but then began to use the former for either distant events or ones that she herself did not control. Gee and Savasir (1985) report that for two 3-year-old girls observed in play together *will* seemed to be reserved for immediate undertakings in which willingness to cooperate was being expressed, whereas *gonna* was used during interactions in which future activities were being planned or organized. The generality of these claims is difficult to evaluate because of the small number of subjects and limited interactional contexts studied. However, the findings of Harner (1982) provide some corroboration of the Gee and Savasir claim. Children aged 3 to 5 were more likely to select toys to which they would have access in the immediate as opposed to the more remote future when asked to "show me the toy you will play with." Harner interprets this preference to mean that children take the immediacy of an action or event and the relative certainty that it will occur to be important components of the early meaning of *will*.

Wells (1985) reports on a second sample of 65 children followed from age 3,3 to 5,0. Most of these children (91%) expressed notions of necessity and possibility by age 5,0, but the development of these meanings largely followed the ones more directly related to the modulation of action (e.g., ability, willingness, permission). Interestingly, less than half the children at 5,0 produced modals with epistemic meanings involving inference or certainty (e.g., "The [toy] train isn't running. It must be off the track"). Several researchers (e.g., Shepherd, 1981, 1982; Stephany, 1986; Wells, 1985) have suggested that meanings involving action and social relations appear earlier than epistemic meanings. Only Choi, who examined the speech of several Korean children, found a different order of development of modal meanings, with a sentence-final suffix for certainty antedating the appearance of desire and intention suffixes. If Choi's findings (reported in Heeschen, Perdue, & Vonk, 1988) are replicated, they would be strong evidence that there is no universal cognitive constraint against the early development of epistemic modal uses.

As for the development of syntactic uses of modals during this period, that, unfortunately, has not been as well documented as the semantic uses. Pinker (1984) reviewed the literature on error data during preschool auxiliary development, including modals. He found virtually no errors on modals in declarative word order or overmarking for tense or person (e.g., *canned, cans, canning*). The lack of overgeneralization errors from such auxiliary forms as *had, does*, and *be + ing* provides some support for the notion of conservative item-by-item acquisition. Bellugi (1971) found that many of the syntactic errors involving auxiliaries in Adam's speech between 3,0 and 4,6 occurred when multiple grammatical operations were required in a single utterance. For example, inversion occurred later with wh-questions than yes–no questions, and inversion was less likely to occur in the wh-questions when a negative was included as well. This error pattern suggests that the grammatical rules may be known but that their application is subject to cognitive processing constraints (see Shatz, 1978a, for a discussion of such constraints).

In summary, the years between 3,0 and 5,0 include a consolidation of the nonepistemic meanings of modals, with an increasing ability to express various meanings with multiple words and to use particular words for more than one meaning. In addition, the epistemic meanings of modals appear with increasing frequency, although their use is still far less prevalent than nonepistemic uses. As with other auxiliaries, there are remarkably few systematic grammatical errors involving modals, suggesting that children do not create a large undifferentiated class of verb forms, or even auxiliaries. Instead, it appears that the acquisition of modals is piecemeal, with early modal categorizations defined more narrowly than the adult grammatical category.

Experimental studies

Experimental studies on modal development have focused either on semantics or on syntax. We consider the latter first and then go on to the semantically focused studies. We conclude this section by considering a set of studies that are not strictly concerned with modals but that examine mental verbs in paradigms related to those used to study modals. Taken together, the studies on mental verbs and modals shed light on the question of whether the early meanings of modals are limited primarily to nonepistemic senses on the basis of a cognitive constraint.

Syntactic data. To examine the syntactic flexibility of modal use in kindergartners through third-graders, Major (1974) used a variety of tasks such as imitating sentences with modals, transforming affirmative sentences into negatives and declaratives into questions, and adding tag questions to affirmatives. She found no clear evidence even in third grade for a set of general syntactic rules governing all modals. For example, second- and third-graders, when asked to turn a declarative, "You may go," into a question, often responded, "Can you go?" substituting a semantically related but more common modal. Younger children were still more inept, sometimes producing either semantically unrelated substitutions ("Will you go?") or ungrammatical, redundant auxiliaries ("Do you may go?").

Consonant with the results of naturalistic studies, Major's work suggests that an adultlike category of modals based on abstract rules is late to develop. However, it is difficult to assess from Major's data just what the nature of the children's categorical knowledge was. There is at least some evidence that they did have some category knowledge. When the children made substitutions, they did so with other modals, rarely replacing a modal with a nonmodal auxiliary (e.g., "Have you fixed it?" for "You ought to fix it"). Incorrect insertions of other auxiliaries resulted in redundancies rather than substitutions, suggesting that the children recognized that nonmodal auxiliaries were inappropriate replacements for modals. Thus, the pattern of substituting one modal for another, especially when they were semantically related, supports the idea of a modal category.

Nevertheless, one cannot determine the basis of the tendency to substitute more common and familiar forms for less common ones. Possibly the children still had a rule limiting the type of modal word that could appear in initial position in yes–no questions, or their behavior could possibly be an artifact of the task; that is, at least the older children might have thought that part of their task was to produce sentences that sounded natural, not just grammatical.[4]

Evidence for the latter alternative comes from the data on transforming affirmatives into negatives. Third-graders made more errors than first-graders on this task because of their preference for contractions. When asked to transform sentences with *shall, may, might,* or *ought to,* they often substituted other modals in contracted form rather than produce a full negative with these forms or an awkward contraction such as *shalln't.* Such behavior suggests a sensitivity to both the naturalness of the language they produced and the syntactic characteristic of contraction that is unique to auxiliaries.

Semantic data. In a study examining the way children organize modal meanings, adult, 12-year-old, and 8-year-old subjects were asked to sort cards, each containing a modal sentence, into piles by similarity of meaning (Coates, 1988). Cluster analyses revealed that the two older groups developed four distinct clusters, although there were some differences in detail between the groups in what was included in each cluster. The youngest group had fewer distinct clusters and showed no evidence of a cluster for epistemic possibility, as did the two older groups. The absence of this cluster in the younger group may have been a consequence of the particular sentence frames in which the modals appeared. For example, a sentence such as "I can visit my grandmother tomorrow" is ambiguous with regard to deontic or epistemic possibility, but young children, more regularly concerned with permission warrants, may be more biased to interpret such sentences deontically than are older subjects. Nonetheless, the relative indistinctness of the younger children's clusters suggests that 8-year-olds do not yet share a wholly conventional system of modal meanings.

Two studies used a different method to examine children's ability to comprehend differences among modal meanings. Hirst and Weil (1982) and Byrnes and Duff (1989) asked children to distinguish between sentences containing modals in two tasks, one an object-search paradigm focusing on epistemic meanings and the other a directive-action paradigm focusing on deontic meanings. In their study, Hirst and Weil asked 54 children aged 3 to 6,6 to distinguish between modals of different strengths. For example, children were asked in the epistemic task to find a peanut hidden in one of two locations after they heard two puppets give them the following hints: "The peanut should be under the box"; "The peanut may be under the cup." In the deontic task, they were asked to say what room a doll would go into after hearing two teachers say, "You must go to the green room" and "You may go to the red room." Hirst and Weil found an ordering of ability to distinguish the strength of the terms such that the greater the distinction in strength between the two modal words, the younger the age at which a distinction was reliably made. They found that by 5,11, all the pairs in the epistemic task were distinguishable, and even the 3-year-olds made some reliable distinctions. On the deontic task, however, only the 6-year-olds made reliable distinctions.

Byrnes and Duff (1989) used similar epistemic and deontic tasks to assess 3- to 5-year-old children's ability to comprehend statements differing in the strength of speaker conviction conveyed by the modal. For example, in one epistemic task, children heard either a statement of strong conviction describing the location of an object ("It has to be under the red cup") or a statement of weak conviction

("It might be under the red cup"). Children of all ages could use the modals to guide their object search, but on the tasks that pitted statements of strong conviction against those of weaker conviction, the two older groups were better at following the hint using the stronger modal than were the 3-year-olds. In general, the children did somewhat better on words that were highly familiar to them (*has to, can't*) than words with which they were less familiar (*might, might not*), although when they received trials with two hints, each of which contained a negative, they found such trials most difficult.

Five-year-olds performed better on both the epistemic and the deontic tasks than did the younger groups. Moreover, the younger groups performed significantly better on the epistemic than on the deontic task. However, as Hirst and Weil point out in interpreting their similar findings, the epistemic task is much more straightforward with regard to the kind of response the child must make. In that task, the subjects must select the location at which they believe (on the basis of hints) a hidden object will be found. In the deontic task, the children must interpret how an actor other than themselves will respond to demands made on them by authority figures. Hence, the tasks, suffering from a disparity in the degree of interpretation they require of the subjects, are bad comparative cases to use to assess children's relative facility with epistemic and deontic meanings. For this reason, the experimental data cannot be taken as evidence against the claims made by natural-language researchers that deontic meanings are primary, forming the early basis of modal meanings.

Nonetheless, 4-year-olds do demonstrate beginning competence with epistemic modals in both the experimental comprehension studies and the studies of natural-language use. An interesting and important question concerns what these early epistemic modals tell us about children's understanding of epistemic meanings. Epistemic modals can express notions ranging from judgments of one's own certainty or uncertainty about a proposition to the marking of an inference or understanding of the inherent undecidability of a problem or the hypothetical nature of a situation. These various notions are likely to develop over an extended period (see Stephany, 1986, for a review). One way to clarify the meaning of the early epistemic modals might be to consider how other terms with a modal character are being used at about the same time. Thus, we turn to studies that have used the forced-choice search paradigm discussed earlier to investigate children's understandings of mental verbs.

Mental verb data. Moore and his colleagues have investigated whether children distinguish among the differences in certainty designated by *know, think, be sure,* and *guess.* In one study, children aged 3,6 to 8,5 were asked to listen to two puppets, each of which gave a clue about where a piece of candy was hidden, and then to search for the candy. The clues pitted *know, think,* and *guess* against one another. Three-year-olds did not distinguish between any of the pairs; all of the other age groups distinguished *know* from the other two terms, but did not distinguish between *think* and *guess* (Moore, Bryant, & Furrow, 1989). In another study, children 3,7 to 6,6 were asked to distinguish between *know, think,* and *be sure.* Again, 3-year-olds did not regularly choose the expression of more certainty over the one of less certainty, whereas the older children did. However, none of the children distinguished between *know* and *be sure* (Moore & Davidge, 1989). The authors argue that the children's ability to distinguish on the basis of certainty (e.g., *know, be sure* vs. *think*) but not factivity (*know* vs. *be sure*) indicates that their knowledge is pragmatically not semantically based.

The work of other researchers for the most part confirms these findings, and at the same time goes beyond them. Using a similar paradigm but a larger set of word pairs in the clues (*see, know, remember, tell, think, guess, want, hope, dream*), Wilcox and Woolley (1989) partially ordered children's preferences for one verb over another with regard to the degree of certainty the verbs convey. Both 4- and 5-year-olds chose *know* over *think* over *hope,* and *remember* over *guess* and *dream.* Thus, children are able not only to distinguish terms dichotomously as indicating certainty or uncertainty, but to place terms on a continuum according to degree of certainty. In a second study, Wilcox and Woolley, unlike Moore et al., found that children as young as 4 were able to distinguish *think* from *guess.*

In general, the forced-choice search task seems to be more suitable than others (e.g., Johnson & Wellman, 1980) for revealing competence with the notion of certainty in children over 4 years of age. Further interesting work with the paradigm could be done comparing the semantic and pragmatic components of modals and mental verbs. For example, if children could distinguish readily between clues like "I know that the cookie is in the box" and "The cookie must be in the cup," it would be evidence that they can distinguish between items of high certainty on the basis of factivity versus inference.

Why are 3-year-olds unable to perform in these tasks? The paucity of epistemic modal uses in their naturalistic data suggests that children simply do not have much knowledge of epistemic meanings before the age of 4 and that their failure in the experimental tasks is a cognitive one, and not merely a problem of task difficulty. However, the possibility that children learning languages other than English acquire epistemic markers early (Choi, 1988) casts doubt on the cognitive constraint explanation. Also, children under 3 have been observed expressing uncertainty, but with *think* in complementizer constructions rather than modals (Bloom, Rispoli, Gartner, & Hafitz, 1989; Shatz, Wellman, & Silber, 1983). It is possible, then, that the absence of epistemic modals in early speech is due not to a cognitive constraint but to input: Parents whose language does not mark epistemic modality as a matter of course may choose to mark epistemic meanings for their young children with complementizer constructions instead of modal auxiliaries. Possibly, modals are reserved in parental speech primarily for deontic uses.

Input studies

Although a number of studies have examined the auxiliary input that children receive from their mothers, few have either broken the auxiliary class down into modal–nonmodal categories or examined the meanings that maternal modals carry. One study of modal meanings in maternal speech compared the frequency and function of modal verbs in the speech of eight German-speaking mothers with those of modal auxiliaries in the speech of eight U.S. mothers as they talked to their children of mean age 2,5, and again four months later (Shatz et al., 1990). Especially relevant here is the categorization of maternal modals as either epistemic or nonepistemic. Fewer than 10% of the mothers' modals carried an epistemic sense. Thus, in the third year of life, children apparently receive little input about the epistemic functions of modals. Shatz et al. are currently examining the maternal speech to see whether epistemic meanings are more frequently carried by other constructions such as *think* in complementizer sentences.

Shatz, Grimm, Wilcox, and Niemeier-Wind (1989) coded modal meanings into eight categories of semantic function, including agreement, intention, permission, obligation, necessity, possibility, conditional, and enablement. For both groups of mothers, intention and possibility were the most frequent meanings conveyed to the children. Almost all the other meanings were at least half as frequent as these two. The children's early modal uses were coded as well, and intention and possibility were found to account for more than two-thirds of the instances of modal use. There were significant correlations between groups of mothers and children on the frequency of modal word types for both languages and a significant correlation on the frequency of semantic categories for German. Thus, it appears that the familiarity of particular lexical items and meanings, as exemplified by the frequencies in maternal speech, has an important bearing on the words and meanings children learn and use frequently.

Nevertheless, children did pick up words and meanings that were relatively rarely used. For example, although only 2% of their utterances expressed necessity, all eight German mothers used the meaning at least once, and as a group they were more likely to do so than were the U.S. mothers. Their children expressed necessity 10 times as often as did U.S. children, using it in 3% of their utterances. Thus, a semantic category need not be particularly frequent for children to pick it up.

Another study confirmed the likelihood that the lexical characteristics of input affect the order of acquisition of modals. Wells (1979) reported that *will* and *can* were the two modals used by 100% of the mothers of his sample of younger children, and they were also the most frequently occurring.

In related work on the auxiliary *have*, Gathercole (1986) compared the use of the present perfect in Scottish and U.S. adults and children to explore Cromer's (1976) claim, based on U.S. children, that the present perfect is a late construction due to cognitive constraints. She found that Scottish adults used the present perfect much more frequently than did U.S. adults and that the construction appeared in the speech of Scottish children much earlier than in the speech of U.S. children. Cross-cultural studies of this sort can be especially helpful in determining whether the order of acquisition of modal meanings is a consequence of universal cognitive constraints or (at least partially) a function of the input children receive.

Research on syntax, focusing not on modals, but on the whole auxiliary system, has also regularly found effects of maternal auxiliary use on child acquisition. Correlating some aspects of maternal speech at one time of measurement with auxiliary growth in children at a later time, researchers have found some positive relations between maternal speech and the frequency of auxiliary use in children. However, this line of research has not produced unequivocal answers to the questions of which specific aspects of the input are efficacious and what the mechanism of facilitation is (for reviews see Hoff-Ginsberg & Shatz, 1982; Shatz, Hoff-Ginsberg, & MacIver, 1989). On the basis of their experimental enrichment study, Shatz, Hoff-Ginsberg, and MacIver (1989) propose that children whose mothers produce a high frequency of fronted auxiliaries have a chance to observe in a highly salient sentence position a grammatical difference among the words that can occur in that position: Modals do not take third-person-singular s, but other auxiliaries do. Having observed this difference, children might then examine the input for other syntactic characteristics that would distinguish verbal elements as modals, nonmodals, or main verbs. Thus, certain characteristics of the input, in combination with two characteristics of the child – the ability to carry out distributional analysis (Maratsos, 1982) and the tendency to be somewhat cautious about making grammatical classifications (Pinker, 1984) – would account for the observed relation between input and acquisition.

In summary, studies on both the syntactic and semantic aspects of modal development strongly suggest that the frequency with which children hear particular forms and meanings affects the course of their acquisition. However, it is also clear that the nature of the input itself cannot fully determine the child's course of acquisition. At the very least, the influence of the input is mediated by the processing characteristics and limitations of the child. We turn now to further discussion of the kinds of constraints that operate on the acquisition of the modal system in English.

Constraints on the acquisition of English modals

We have suggested that the acquisition of modals may be constrained in various ways. We take constraints to be factors that channel or direct the process of acquisition. In the sense that they help to define the course of acquisition, they are mechanisms of development. In this section, we consider a range of constraints that have been proposed to help account for language acquisition, in particular those most relevant to the acquisition of modals. In discussing each constraint, we ask whether the data just reviewed provide evidence for it. We also suggest additional studies that would help clarify the nature and role of various constraints. Finally, we propose that different constraints may apply at different times in development and that theorists arguing for constraints in the past have largely ignored this possibility (but see Behrend, 1990).

The applicability of constraints to modals

The general notion of constraints operating on the language acquisition process is a familiar one. It has been recruited by theorists of various persuasions to address several well-known problems connected with language acquisition. One major problem concerns the fact that children are able to achieve the language of their community, without direct tuition, on the basis of input that underdetermines the output (Chomsky, 1975). The kinds of constraints that attempt to address this problem are ones that limit the set of possible grammars from which a child can select; that is, universal grammatical properties of language are postulated that narrow the possibilities among which a child must choose. Thus, the data that are available to children need only be rich enough to allow them to choose among possibilities available to them by virtue of their being human (Baker, 1979; Hornstein & Lightfoot, 1981). The difficulty with this approach is that the effort to identify universal grammatical properties upon which linguists can agree has been a slow and painstaking process, and thus far it has not produced a formal analysis of either modals or auxiliaries that results in an accepted explanation of the ways acquisition is constrained (for some attempts in this vein see Baker, 1981; Hyams, 1986).

Moreover, as Grimshaw (1981) noted, even if there were an accepted set of formal principles of universal grammar, they would not likely address the question of how children accomplish the language-learning task over time; to explain the course of acquisition requires attention to substantive relations between form and function, as well as the cognitive characteristics of the learner. Some of the constraints that address the latter concern focus on the kinds of information young children are likely to notice and understand and the kinds of inductive inferences they make on the basis of incomplete information. Examples relevant to auxiliaries and modals can be found in Gleitman et al. (1984) and Shatz, Hoff-Ginsberg, and MacIver (1989) and have already been discussed. Although further research on the way children's attentional and perceptual capacities constrain acquisition would be most welcome, there can be little doubt that these cognitive processing capacities are a constraining factor (see Shatz, 1978a, 1987, for further discussion of this point).

Others have proposed constraints that focus on the form–function relation. The notion that children have a universal grammatical category of AUX to which they can assign elements of their language on the basis of semantic information is an example of a substantive form–function relation that constrains the nature of auxiliary acquisition (Pinker, 1984; Wasow, 1981). However, we have already questioned the viability of accounts like Pinker's, which require that young children have a sophisticated semantic and categorical understanding, on the grounds of both plausibility and empirical evidence that does not support the early establishment of an AUX category.

Another, more general constraint on the relation between form and function that has been proposed is the principle of contrast (Clark, 1987). This principle states that any two linguistic forms differ in meaning in some way. It is appealing from a developmentalist's point of view because of its simplicity. Even a young child, able to recognize only phonological differences in form, would be inclined to search for differences in meaning, without having to know what those meanings were when form differences were first noticed. Applying the contrast principle to modals does little to explain the acquisition of syntactic knowledge, but it has some interesting implications for meaning acquisition.

One implication for the acquisition of modal meaning is that children should be disinclined to assign the very same meaning to two modal forms, for example, to assign the meaning of permission to both *can* and *may* or the meaning of prediction to both *will* and *gonna*. Another is that if mental verbs such as *think* are used to express relative certainty, there should be a reluctance to use modals such as *must* and *might* to express the same meaning, especially when they already serve other functions such as expressing obligation. Thus, the principle of contrast helps to explain why children have been observed making systematic distinctions between closely related modals such as *will* and *gonna* (cf. Gee & Savasir, 1985; Harner,

1982) and why epistemic uses of modals do not occur at the same time as other epistemic constructions in children's speech. At the same time, one can ask why, if the principle of contrast is as pervasive as Clark (1988) argues, one finds an early stage in which words like *will* and *gonna* are not differentiated (Shepherd, 1981, 1982). Possibly this principle operates only at certain times in development. We shall return later to the question of why constraints might not be exercised continually.

Is the principle of contrast necessary to explain the course of development of modal meanings, or can the influence of input account as well for the data? Certainly, early maternal uses of modals are overwhelmingly nonepistemic. As we suggested earlier, the encoding of epistemic functions first with mental verbs and not modals may be a consequence of the input children receive. Whether the input also favors monolexicality within the modal system requires further investigation. The data from the Shatz et al. (1990) study of German and U.S. mothers suggest that, at least for their broadly defined semantic categories such as intention, possibility, and necessity, mothers do not restrict the expression of one meaning to one form; on average, mothers used two forms to express each meaning. Further research is needed, however, before one can conclude that a tendency to use only one form for each meaning is generated by the child's following of the contrast principle. For example, it would be useful to know whether children make finer (or different) distinctions between *will* and *gonna* than do the adults who regularly speak to them.

At present, then, we cannot, with the data at hand, decide between the principle of contrast and the influence of input as explanations for the course of modal meaning acquisition. However, a substantive cognitive constraint against epistemic understanding can be eliminated as an appropriate explanation for the lateness of modal epistemic uses. If there were such a substantive cognitive constraint, one would not expect to find epistemic instances with mental verbs in the second half of the third year of life (Bloom et al., 1989; Shatz et al., 1983).

Yet a substantive cognitive constraint of that sort may well operate before age 2,6 and may even have consequences after it ceases to operate. Such an early cognitive constraint, along with selective input, apparently facilitates a primary tie between modals and nonepistemic meanings. Very young children frequently hear modal forms with nonepistemic meanings, and their first modal uses suggest that they have assigned modals to a nonepistemic meaning domain. Later, when the constraint is no longer operating, children might notice both *think* and modals in contexts that express relative certainty, but they might initially prefer to choose the previously unassigned mental verb form rather than the previously assigned modal forms to express the new meaning. Although Clark argues that the principle of contrast blocks only synonymy and not homonymy, there may nonetheless be some avoidance of homonymous forms, especially when both forms fall into the same grammatical class. It would be useful to know whether homonymy is indeed avoided in such cases. Certainly some of Karmiloff-Smith's work suggests that it would be (Karmiloff-Smith, 1979). It would also be useful to modify the search tasks that have been so successful in discovering 4-year-olds' knowledge of certainty to enhance the performance of children under 4 and to determine whether children can assess the degree of certainty expressed in such protocols as well with modals as they can with mental verbs.

If the principle of contrast is at work, why would children ever start to use modals to express notions of relative certainty once they have assigned such notions to mental verbs? One possibility is that these are complex notions, with shades of meaning depending on the contexts of their use becoming more apparent to the child as time goes on. There is some suggestion in the literature that this is the case. On the basis of experimental data testing children's modal reasoning under a variety of conditions, Pieraut-Le Bonniec (1980) argued that children do not have complete understanding of the complex notion of certainty until adolescence; for example, her subjects did not demonstrate an understanding that some things are undecidable until about age 10. It would be useful to know whether, when children reach the point of using both mental verbs and modals to express relative certainty, they mark subtle distinctions of meaning by the differential choice of forms.[5]

Changes in constraints as a function of development

What, then, can be said about the nature of the constraints that operate on children's acquisition of modals? First, there seems to be a variety of constraints that operate on modal acquisition. For one, input, although not usually considered a constraint by theorists, potentially falls under our definition of constraints as factors that channel or direct the process of acquisition. We have seen that modal input to young children is limited in meaning, focusing on nonepistemic uses, and may indeed be a constraint on the course of modal meaning acquisition. For another, there may be a substantive cognitive constraint, before 2,6, channeling children's attention to conditions on actions. Children younger than 2,6 seem to pick up most easily those meanings related to intentions and the ability to carry out actions. At the same time, they are sensitive to deontic meanings: German children pick up notions of obligation from their mothers despite their relative rarity in input. Corroborating the notion of a substantive cognitive constraint is the fact that Shatz et al. (1983) found no epistemic uses of mental verbs in children's speech before 2,6.[6] An additional useful test of the cognitive constraint hypothesis would be to examine the acquisition of languages that require inflections encoding epistemic meanings such as the evidentiary basis of assertions and that therefore must appear in children's input. If epistemic meanings are acquired earlier in such languages, that would be evidence against the hypothesis.

As for constraints on syntactic knowledge, the empirical findings suggest that children first create narrow grammatical categories for modal words, based on selected morphological and phonological characteristics or, possibly, on positional privileges of occurrence. The lack of evidence for an initial abstract category of AUX argues against a universal grammatical constraint operating early in acquisition. Rather, children seem to use surface syntactic properties to bootstrap their early classificatory knowledge (see Gleitman, 1990). Children's early categorical behavior provides evidence for the view that there may be a general principle of categorization that leads children to look for various sorts of similarities, even among symbolic objects like words, on which inductive inferences can be based (see Gelman & Coley, Chapter 5, this volume).

Whether a more abstract universal constraint has an influence on later reorganization of children's grammatical categories remains an open research question. There are two sources of support for the possibility that a universal grammatical constraint functions at a later time in development. For one, others have argued that universal grammatical constraints are triggered on a maturational schedule, rather than functioning throughout the period of early language development (Gleitman, 1981; Roeper, 1978). For another, both of the two very different constraints on meaning already discussed, those of input and cognition, appear to operate in a time-bound fashion. Children are eventually exposed to epistemic modals: In the German–U.S. study, some mothers had begun to produce modal epistemics by the second observation period, when the children's average age was 2,9. Also, we have already noted that any substantive cognitive constraint against epistemics appears to have been outgrown by the second half of the third year. Thus, there is considerable support for the idea that constraints do not operate continually during the course of acquisition.

The notion that constraints operate in a time-bound fashion suggests that the constraints themselves have limits. A full developmental theory of how constraints govern the course of development would have to explain just what these limits are and how they control the time-bound activation of various constraints. A complete theory is beyond the scope of this chapter, but we provide two examples of the factors that might limit the operation of various constraints. The first example depends on the notion that one constraint might block the operation of another. Suppose that a child, in assigning meaning to the words *will* and *gonna*, hears them in similar contexts on separate occasions but fails because of cognitive processing limitations to check whether the meaning assigned to the word heard second has already been assigned elsewhere in the lexicon. Then, the two words could exist simultaneously with the same meaning until such time as the child noticed the synonymy. At that point, the principle of contrast, blocked from operating earlier by a cognitive processing constraint, would come into play.

The second example illustrates why a child might be led at a later time to notice something (like synonymy) that he had failed to notice earlier. Suppose that the child then notices grammatical similarities between *will* and *gonna* (such as the fact that both words take nonfinite verb forms and neither is marked for third-person singular). The grouping of these words together on syntactic grounds (guided by the principle of categorization) may facilitate attention to and comparison of their meanings relative to one another. Such a comparison should lead to the differentiation of meaning between the two words (on the basis of the principle of contrast), but it might facilitate as well the recognition that there is a semantic "field" of related meanings that are encoded by a special grammatical class whose elements selectively share a set of properties. That is, children might then come to recognize the AUX class as one whose members are related on both semantic and syntactic grounds. Thus, the level of knowledge a child has in one domain may facilitate the operation of some constraint in another domain. Indeed, it is reasonable to assume that the operation of some constraints will trigger the operation of others, just as on other occasions constraints can have blocking effects.

A reasonable model of constraints on the acquisition of modals, then, would be one in which the constraints change with the developmental status of the child. Not only do the input data to the child change, but what the child perceives the input data to be changes (White, 1981). As the child develops both cognitively and grammatically, what she has already learned determines in part what she will notice next. In some sense, then, a major constraint on acquisition is the acquisition process itself (Shatz, 1987). Because each child's input and cognitive history is somewhat different, we should not be surprised to find some individual differences in the language acquisition process as well, although the common findings discussed previously suggest that the general outlines of beginning modal acquisition are shared by most children, probably because the very early cognitive constraints (both substantive and processing ones) are universal. Any universal grammatical constraints, whenever they operated, would also mitigate individual differences.

Conclusions

The acquisition of a complex and irregular system

Linguists and psychologists agree that English modals are a complex and irregular part of the English language. At best, universal principles of grammar are likely to constrain their acquisition only minimally, because much of their character is both language-specific and "defective." Thus, one would expect that they would be difficult to acquire. But what does "difficult to acquire" mean? Apparently, as Pinker's review of error data tells us, it does not mean that many errors will be committed. Indeed, the pattern is quite the opposite: Relatively few errors occur. What "difficult to acquire" seems to mean is that the adultlike generalizations pertaining to the modal system, with regard to both semantics and syntax, are relatively late in coming. Instead, children make narrower classificatory generalizations and use heuristics such as the avoidance of plurifunction-ality and plurilexicality initially to assign meaning to form conser-vatively.

Progress toward the adult system could be achieved as old con-straints no longer operate and new ones are called into play. For example, as a child develops cognitively and as input broadens, the child has the opportunity to notice new meanings for modals that may not have occurred or may have gone unnoticed previously. The system must accommodate these while still adhering to basic prin-ciples of language organization such as the principle of contrast, and this constraint itself may encourage still further analysis of subtle differences in meaning or use. Similarly, increased attention to syn-tactic and semantic similarities among modals and other auxiliaries may force reorganization of earlier, narrower categories into a more general, abstract one. Over the course of acquisition, then, the var-ious constraints operating on the system produce a convergence on the adult model.

The generality of a converging constraints model

The kind of acquisition pattern we have proposed should hold more generally for the acquisition of other complex and irregular com-ponents of languages. That is, one would expect that the interplay of constraints would produce a course of acquisition characterized by early narrow generalizations, limited understanding of mean-ings, and reorganizations over time, as the system converged onto the adult model. We would expect the acquisition of such systems to recruit many, if not all, of the kinds of constraints we have enu-merated: input, cognitive processing, substantive cognitive, form–function relational, and universal grammatical. However, we would expect that the particular roles of the constraints would vary with the specific component of the language being acquired. Obviously, this means that the details of any analysis of the acquisition of a particular language-specific component have limited application to other components.

Nonetheless, a converging constraints model has some major ad-vantages as a model of language acquisition. For one, it provides a broad theoretical framework that is accountable to the data of ac-quisition. For another, it clarifies what kind of data can be appro-priately considered evidence for or against a particular constraint.

For example, that children do not always appear to be observing the principle of contrast is not necessarily, in the converging constraints model, evidence against the principle.

The model also acknowledges the influence on development of both nature and nurture and allows for their relative power to be assessed by empirical evidence. Finally, it allows for the simultaneous consideration of two questioins: How does a child learn any language at all, and how does a child learn a particular language? When these questions are not juxtaposed, the magnitude of a child's accomplishment is diminished, and the subtlety of the language acquisition process is lost.

Investigating language–thought relations with modal expressions

In closing, we return to the question motivating this volume: the relations between language and thought. We have suggested that modal expressions may be constrained by a substantive cognitive limitation in children, but that such a constraint may be very short-lived. Additional constraints on the use and function of modal expressions may come from children's understanding of how a linguistic system functions – for example, that two forms should have different meanings or that grammatical classes are based on a single shared privilege of occurrence. Further constraints may be placed on both language and cognitive development by the input children receive. Cultures use modal expressions to socialize children into culture-specific foundations of belief and social order. It stands to reason that the input to a child will reflect cultural priorities on these important topics, as well as views about what the child is capable of understanding at a given point in time. All these factors combine to make the relations between language and thought neither simple nor unidirectional. Indeed, what makes the study of linguistic and cognitive development intriguing is that it is not.

Notes

1. We use the term *plurifunctionality* rather than *polysemy* to indicate that the range of meanings expressed by particular modals in varied contexts may have pragmatic bases as well as semantic ones (see Garvey, 1989; Gee & Savasir, 1985). Hence, the term refers to the broadest range of meanings a word can express.
2. In Table 9.1 we provide an informal characterization of the kinds of dif-

ferences among auxiliary types in grammatical privileges of occurrence children might notice. See Pinker (1984) for more formal and detailed analyses of the ways in which auxiliaries and even modals differ from one another.
3. We have counted here only the explicit concatenatives and not alternative forms such as *want* + *verb* or *going* + *verb* to make the data analogous to Brown's. However, one can argue, at least on semantic grounds, for including such alternatives in analyses of early modal expressions.
4. It would be interesting to know how adults would fare on Major's (1974) tasks. They might even find some of the "correct" responses sufficiently unnatural that they would be disinclined to follow abstract rules in all cases.
5. Clark's position would be that there must be such subtleties, even if they are differences in register or attitude, which some would argue are pragmatic and not semantic.
6. See Shatz (1978b) for another kind of evidence that children under 2,6 focus on the conditions for action.

References

Baker, C. L. (1979). Syntactic theory and the projection problem. *Linguistic Inquiry, 10,* 533–582.

Baker, C. L. (1981). Learnability and the English auxiliary system. In C. L. Baker & J. J. McCarthy (Eds.), *The logical problem of language acquisition* (pp. 296–329). Cambridge, MA: MIT Press.

Behrend, D. (1990). Constraints and development: a reply to Nelson (1988). *Cognitive Development, 5,* 313–330.

Bellugi, U. (1967). *The acquisition of negation.* Unpublished doctoral dissertation, Harvard University, Cambridge, MA.

Bellugi, U. (1971). Simplification in children's language. In R. Huxley & E. Ingram (Eds.), *Language acquisition: Models and methods* (pp. 95–119). New York: Academic Press.

Bloom, L., Lightbown, P., & Hood, L. (1975). Structure and variation in child language. *Monographs of the Society for Research in Child Development, 40*(2, Serial No. 160).

Bloom, L., Rispoli, M., Gartner, B., & Hafitz, J. (1989). Acquisition of complementation. *Journal of Child Language, 16,* 101–120.

Brown, R. (1973). *A first language: The early stages.* Cambridge, MA: Harvard University Press.

Brown, R., Cazden, C., & Bellugi, U. (1969). The child's grammar from I to III. In J. P. Hill (Ed.), *Minnesota Symposium in Child Psychology* (Vol. 2, pp. 105–117). Minneapolis: University of Minnesota Press.

Byrnes, J., & Duff, M. (1989). Young children's comprehension of modal expressions. *Cognitive Development, 4,* 369–387.

Chomsky, N. (1975). *Reflections on language.* New York: Pantheon.

Clark, E. (1987). The Principle of Contrast: A constraint on acquisition. In B. MacWhinney (Ed.), *Mechanisms of language acquisition: Proceedings of the 20th Annual Carnegie Symposium on Cognition* (pp. 1–33). Hillsdale, NJ: Erlbaum.

Clark, E. (1988). On the logic of contrast. *Journal of Child Language, 15,* 317–335.

Coates, J. (1983). *The semantics of the modal auxiliaries.* London: Croom Helm.
Coates, J. (1988). The acquisition of the meanings of modality in children aged eight and twelve. *Journal of Child Language, 15,* 425–434.
Cromer, R. R. (1976). The cognitive hypothesis of language acquisition and its implications for child language deficiency. In D. M. Morehead & A. E. Morehead (Eds.), *Directions in normal and deficient child language* (pp. 283–333). Baltimore: University Park Press.
Fletcher, P. (1979). The development of the verb phrase. In P. Fletcher & M. Garman (Eds.), *Language acquisition: Studies in first language development* (pp. 261–284). Cambridge University Press.
Fletcher, P. (1985). *A child's learning of English.* Oxford: Blackwell Publisher.
Furrow, D., Nelson, K., & Benedict, H. (1979). Mothers' speech to children and syntactic development: Some simple relationships. *Journal of Child Language, 6,* 423–442.
Garcia, E. (1967). Auxiliaries and the criterion of simplicity. *Language, 43,* 853–870.
Garvey, C. (1989, April). *The modals of necessity and obligation in children's pretend play.* Paper presented at the biennial meeting of the Society for Research in Child Development, Kansas City, MO.
Gathercole, V. C. (1986). The acquisition of the present perfect: Explaining differences in the speech of Scottish and American children. *Journal of Child Language, 13,* 537–560.
Gazadar, G., Pullum, G., & Sag, I. (1982). Auxiliaries and related phenomena in a restrictive theory of grammar. *Language, 58,* 591–638.
Gee, J., & Savasir, I. (1985). On the use of *will* and *gonna*: Toward a description of activity-types for child language. *Discourse Processes, 8,* 143–175.
Gleitman, L. R. (1981). Maturational determinants of language growth. *Cognition, 10,* 103–114.
Gleitman, L. R. (1990). The structural sources of verb meanings. *Language Acquisitiion, 1,* 3–55.
Gleitman, L. R., Newport, E. L., & Gleitman, H. (1984). The current status of the motherese hypothesis. *Journal of Child Language, 11,* 43–79.
Grimshaw, J. (1981). Form, function, and the language acquisition device. In C. L. Baker & J. J. McCarthy (Eds.), *The logical problem of language acquisition* (pp. 165–182). Cambridge, MA: MIT Press.
Harner, L. (1982). Immediacy and certainty: Factors in understanding future reference. *Journal of Child Language, 9,* 115–124.
Heeschen, C., Perdue, C., & Vonk, W. (1988). *Annual Report 1988.* Nijmegen: Max Planck Institute for Psycholinguistics.
Hirst, W., & Weil, J. (1982). Acquisition of epistemic and deontic meaning of modals. *Journal of Child Language, 9,* 659–666.
Hoff-Ginsberg, E., & Shatz, M. (1982). Linguistic input and the child's acquisition of language. *Psychological Bulletin, 92,* 3–26.
Hornstein, N., & Lightfoot, D. (1981). Introduction. In N. Hornstein & D. Lightfoot (Eds.), *Explanation in linguistics* (pp. 9–31). London: Longman Group.
Hyams, N. M. (1986). *Language acquisition and the theory of parameters.* Dordrecht: Reidel.
Johnson, C., & Wellman, H. (1980). Children's developing understanding of mental verbs: Remember, know, and guess. *Child Development, 51,* 1095–1102.

Karmiloff-Smith, A. (1979, June). *Language as a formal problem-space for children*. Paper presented at the MPG/NIAS Conference on Beyond Description in Child Language, Nijmegen.

Klima, E., & Bellugi, U. (1966). Syntactic regularities in the speech of children. In J. Lyons & R. Wales (Eds.), *Psycholinguistic papers* (pp. 333–353). Edinburgh: Edinburgh University Press.

Kuczaj, S., & Maratsos, M. (1983). Initial verbs of yes–no questions: A different kind of general grammatical category. *Developmental Psychology*, *19*, 440–444.

Lyons, J. (1977). *Semantics* (Vol. 2). Cambridge University Press.

Major, D. (1974). *The acquisition of modal auxiliaries in the language of children*. The Hague: Mouton.

Maratsos, M. (1982). The child's construction of grammatical categories. In E. Wanner & L. R. Gleitman (Eds.), *Language acquisition: The state of the art* (pp. 240–266). Cambridge University Press.

McCawley, J. (1975). The category status of English modals. *Foundations of Language*, *12*, 597–601.

Moore, C., Bryant, D., & Furrow, D. (1989). Mental terms and the development of certainty. *Child Development*, *60*, 167–171.

Moore, C., & Davidge, J. (1989). The development of mental terms: Semantics or pragmatics? *Journal of Child Language*, *16*, 633–641.

Newport, E. L., Gleitman, H., & Gleitman, L. R. (1977). Mother, I'd rather do it myself: Some effects and noneffects of maternal speech style. In C. Snow & C. Ferguson (Eds.), *Talking to Children: Language input and acquisition* (pp. 109–150). Cambridge University Press.

Palmer, F. R. (1979). *Modality and the English modals*. London: Longman Group.

Pieraut-Le Bonniec, G. (1980). *The development of modal reasoning: Genesis of necessity and possibility notions*. New York: Academic Press.

Pinker, S. (1984). *Language learnability and language development*. Cambridge, MA: Harvard University Press.

Reuland, E. J. (1983). Government and the search for AUXes: A case study in cross-linguistic category identification. In F. Heny & B. Richards (Eds.), *Linguistic categories: Auxiliaries and related puzzles* (pp. 99–168). Dordrecht: Reidel.

Roeper, T. (1978). Linguistic universals and the acquisition of gerunds. In H. Goodluck & L. Solan (Eds.), *Papers on the structure and development of child language* (University of Massachusetts Occasional Papers in Linguistics No. 4, pp. 1–36). Amherst: University of Massachusetts.

Shatz, M. (1978a). The relationship between cognitive processes and the development of communication skills. In C. B. Keasey (Ed.), *Nebraska Symposium on Motivation, 1977* (Vol. 25, pp. 1–42). Lincoln: University of Nebraska Press.

Shatz, M. (1978b). On the development of communicative understandings: An early strategy for interpreting and responding to messages. *Cognitive Psychology*, *10*, 271–309.

Shatz, M. (1987). Bootstrapping operations in child language. In K. E. Nelson & A. Van Kleeck (Eds.), *Children's language* (Vol. 6, pp. 1–22). Hillsdale, NJ: Erlbaum.

Shatz, M., Billman, D., & Yaniv, I. (1986). *Early occurrences of English auxiliaries in children's speech*. Unpublished manuscript. University of Michigan, Ann Arbor.

Shatz, M., Grimm, H., Wilcox, S., & Niemeier-Wind, K. (1989, April). *The uses of modal expressions in conversations between German and American mothers and their two-year-olds.* Paper presented at the biennial meeting of the Society for Research in Child Development, Kansas City, MO.

Shatz, M., Grimm, H., Wilcox, S., & Niemeier-Wind, K. (1990). *Modal expressions in German and American mother–child conversations: Implications for input theories of language acquisition.* Unpublished manuscript. University of Michigan, Ann Arbor.

Shatz, M., Hoff-Ginsberg, E., & MacIver, D. (1989). Induction and the acquisition of English auxiliaries: The effects of differentially enriched input. *Journal of Child Language, 16,* 121–140.

Shatz, M., Wellman, H., & Silber, S. (1983). The acquisition of mental verbs: A systematic investigation of the first reference to mental state. *Cognition, 14,* 301–321.

Shepherd, S. C. (1981). *Modals in Antiguan Creole, child language acquisition, and history.* Unpublished doctoral dissertation, Stanford University, Stanford, CA.

Shepherd, S. C. (1982). From deontic to epistemic: An analysis of modals in the history of English, creoles, and language acquisition. In A. Ahlqvist (Ed.), *Papers from the 5th International Conference on Historical Linguistics* (pp. 316–323). Amsterdam: Benjamins.

Stephany, U. (1986). Modality. In P. Fletcher & M. Garman (Eds.), *Language acquisition: Studies in first language development* (pp. 375–400). Cambridge University Press.

Talmy, L. (1988). Force dynamics in language and cognition. *Cognitive Science, 12,* 49–100.

Wasow, T. (1981). Comments. In C. L. Baker & J. J. McCarthy (Eds.), *The logical problem of language acquisition* (pp. 324–329). Cambridge, MA: MIT Press.

Wells, G. (1979). Learning and using the auxiliary verb in English. In V. Lee (Ed.), *Cognitive development: Language and thinking from birth to adolescence* (pp. 250–270). London: Croom Helm.

Wells, G. (1985). *Language development in the preschool years.* Cambridge University Press.

White, L. (1981). The responsibility of grammatical theory to acquisitional data. In N. Hornstein & D. Lightfoot (Eds.), *Explanation in linguistics* (pp. 241–283). London: Longman Group.

Wilcox, S. A., & Woolley, J. D. (1989, April). *Children's evaluation of statements of belief as sources of information.* Paper presented at the biennial meeting of the Society for Research in Child Development, Kansas City, MO.

10. Acquisition and development of *if* and *because:* Conceptual and linguistic aspects

JAMES P. BYRNES

Introduction

It has long been held in psychological and philosophical circles that important insights into the nature of cognitive processes can be gained through an analysis of the connectives *if* and *because* (Traugott, ter Meulen, Reilly, & Ferguson, 1986). In particular, *if . . . then* statements serve the important linguistic function of expressing fundamental cognitive processes such as inference and prediction, and *because* statements figure prominently in the cognitive processes of argumentation and explanation. Moreover, while the structure and function of these connectives make them particularly useful for describing causal relations, they are also ideally suited for characterizing a variety of other relations among objects or events.

Linguistically, these connectives are important to study because *if* and *because* constructions fall within the category of "complex" sentences (as opposed to "simple" or "compound" sentences). Specifically, such constructions often consist of the embedding of one sentence into another. For example, in "If today is Tuesday, the bill is overdue," each of "Today is Tuesday" and "the bill is overdue" could stand alone. Developmental psycholinguists have found it important to study how children progress from the connectiveless juxtaposition of sentences to the integration of sentences within a single connective construction (e.g., Hood & Bloom, 1979). In addition, an adequate semantic analysis of *if* constructions has proved to be quite a complex and vexing issue and one that has generated a great deal of interest (Fillenbaum, 1986). The elusiveness of the meaning of *if* for adults makes one wonder how children ever come to acquire *if* constructions. The semantic complexities are further com-

I wish to thank Susan Gelman for very helpful comments on a draft of this chapter.

plicated by (and of course not independent of) complexities of the pragmatics of subordinating conjunctions (Bates, 1976). These issues are described more fully in subsequent sections.

In the present chapter I proceed by separately describing the conceptual and linguistic aspects of *if* and *because* to give a sense of what is acquired. After describing each aspect, I introduce research bearing on the acquisition and development of this aspect. Following this exposition and literature review, I explore the theme of the book with respect to the case of connectives. In particular, I consider the nature of the interrelations between the conceptual and linguistic aspects in detail.

What is acquired: Conceptual and linguistic components

This section is concerned with the conceptual and linguistic components of *if* and *because* expressions. For organizational and expository purposes only, I describe what is acquired using the traditional distinction between syntactic, semantic, and pragmatic aspects of expressions, being mindful that these categories are in reality nonorthogonal. In addition, I adopt Slobin's (1979) notion shared by Clark (1983) and others that concepts and meanings are distinct. More specifically, I assume that language selectivity evokes or "picks out" aspects of the conceptual domain for expression. Within this assumption, I first describe conceptual components prerequisite to the use of *if* and *because*, then describe the linguistic components of *if* and *because* expressions. Relevant developmental research is introduced following the description of each component.

Conceptual components

Some of the primary concepts expressible by *if* expressions, *because* expressions, or both include the following: causality, noncausal conceptual relations, social rules, and procedural knowledge. Of course, this list is not exhaustive but is merely representative. I discuss each of these forms of knowledge in turn.

Causality. Both *if* and *because* can be used to express causality. However, *if* and *because* express distinct aspects of specific causal relations. In particular, whereas *if* expressions convey the *covariance relation* between cause and effect, *because* expressions describe the causal *mechanism* between cause and effect (Byrnes & Gelman, 1990). That is, in expressions of the form "If *X* happens, *Y* happens," event *X* is the cause and event *Y* is the effect. What is explicitly described is the co-occurence of events *X* and *Y*, not the mechanism by which event *X* brings about event *Y*. An example would be "If you turn that knob, the light will go on."

In contrast, *because* statements explain *why* a cause brings about an effect. In addition to knowing that causes and effects consistently covary (*principle of covariance*), that causes precede effects (*principle of temporal priority*), and that causes and effects frequently occur in close temporal succession (*principle of temporal contiguity*), one's knowledge of causal relations also includes mental models of the way that each cause brings about its effect (Bullock, Baillargeon, & Gelman, 1982). Moreover, each mental model represents an inferred mechanism (Piaget, 1974). It is precisely this mechanism, detailed or not, that is referred to by a *because* expression. An example would be "It's colder in the winter because of the angle of the sun's rays."

A reasonable assumption is that once children's knowledge of causal relations has developed to the point where they can encode co-variance relations and are capable of constructing mechanisms within causal explanations, they are capable of expressing this knowledge using *if* and *because* (provided that the appropriate linguistic apparatus is available). Bullock et al. (1982) and Shultz and Kestenbaum (1985) reviewed the research regarding children's knowledge of causal principles such as covariance and temporal priority and found that even 3-year-olds possess knowledge of these principles. Moreover, Bullock et al. (1982) provide data showing that a number of 3-year-olds recognized that a cause would no longer produce its effect when a causal mechanism was inactivated. Keil (1979) provides suggestive evidence that this form of insight into mechanisms is present in even younger children. Although the causal knowledge required in these experiments is far from sophisticated, it can at least be said that by age 3 children's knowledge of covariance relations and mechanisms is developed sufficiently for expression of this knowledge using *if* and *because*.

Noncausal conceptual relations. *If* and *because* expressions can also be used to describe a variety of conceptual relations other than causality. In particular, *if* can be used to describe categorical relations such as that between an object and one of its properties (e.g., "If it is a diamond, then it is very hard") or between a superordinate class and one of its subclasses (e.g., "If it's a dog, then it's a mammal"). Indeed, Quine (1950) argues that class inclusion forms the conceptual foundation for conditional implication. *If* can also serve an indexical or symbolic function wherein some stimulus or event is described to indicate or refer to some outcome meaningfully. For example, "If it's red, that means you should stop" or "If the light goes on, that means it has finished its cycle."

Other conceptual relations do not appear to be as directly expressible using *if* as causality, categorical knowledge, and indexical relations. In particular, each of causality, categorical, and indexical relations are essentially two-term relations where one term in the relation is stated in the antecedent clause (e.g., the cause) and the other term is stated in the consequent clause (e.g., the effect). The relation between the terms (e.g., causality), however, is not explicitly stated and there appears to be no need to do so. Other two-term relations such as spatial relations (e.g., *on top of*) or temporal relations (e.g., *before*) are not expressible in the same way as the aforementioned relations.

With respect to the relation between *because* and noncausal conceptual relations, it can again be emphasized that *because* appears to function exclusively within explanations. In discussing the role of explanations in children's cognition, it is useful to invoke the "child as theorist" metaphor employed in several contemporary accounts of conceptual development (e.g., Carey, 1985; Gelman & Coley, Chapter 5, this volume; Keil, Chapter 6, this volume; Wellman, 1985). Specifically, it can be said that children possess naïve "theories" regarding taxonomic hierarchies that might be called naïve biologies and have theories regarding the causes of human behavior that might be called naïve psychologies, and so on. Each theory consists of an organized body of knowledge wherein important ontological distinctions among relevant subject-matter entities are made. Moreover, a primary function of any theory is to provide explanations (Nagel, 1961). Therefore, it can be said that *because* expressions serve as a linguistic means of conveying explanations derived from one's theories. Regarding physical causality, *because* statements derive from a naïve physics (e.g., "It broke because the rock is hard"). But of course there exists the need for explanatory *because* expressions outside the realm of physical causality that derive from various naïve theories such as psychology (e.g., "He is sad because he was punished'') or zoology (e.g., "It's an animal because a dog is a kind of animal'').

In sum, once children have acquired knowledge of subclass– superclass relations, object–property relations, and indexical relations, they can express this knowledge using *if*. Regarding the evidence for knowledge of hierarchical relations in young children, the reader is referred to Markman, Chapter 3, this volume; Waxman, Chapter 4; Gelman and Coley, Chapter 5; and Callanan, Chapter 12. Regarding object–property relations, Younger (1985) demonstrated the ability of 10-month-olds to distinguish perceptual categories by clusters of attributes, and Gelman and Markman (1985) showed that 4-year-olds were quite adept at discriminating among novel nouns and adjectives. Regarding indexical relations, Piaget (1952) describes the important role that indexical relations play in the symbolic function available (at least) by age 2. As is the case for causality, therefore, categorical and indexical relations seem to be available for expression by *if* in the early preschool period.

With respect to *because*, once children have acquired conceptual knowledge in the form of naïve theories, they are capable of expressing this knowledge in the form of *if* and *because* expressions. Wellman (1985) provides evidence that 3-year-olds possess a reasonably sophisticated theory of "mind." Similarly, whereas Carey (1985) reports substantial change in children's knowledge of taxonomic relations (i.e., a naïve zoology) between ages 4 and 10, 4-year-olds nevertheless possess what is necessarily a theory (see Gelman & Coley, Chapter 5, this volume, for a fuller discussion of theories).

Social rules. At this point it is useful to make a distinction between knowledge in the *epistemic* domain and that in the *deontic* domain. Put simply, the epistemic domain of knowledge concerns causal, categorical, spatial, and temporal relations. The deontic domain of knowledge concerns comprehension of social rules, moral obligation, and so on (see Shatz & Wilcox, Chapter 9, this volume). All of the conceptual relations expressible by *if* and *because* described so far concern knowledge in the epistemic domain. Certain relations in the deontic domain are also expressible using *if* and *because* constructions.

With respect to *if*, a variety of social rules can be expressed. In particular, any social rule that consists of a relation between certain behaviors and a certain outcome can be stated in an *if* construction. Generally, the social rules determine which kinds of behaviors are permissible or desirable and which are not. Such social rules are implicit in threats (e.g., "If you don't sit still, you'll be in trouble") and in promises (e.g., "If you eat your vegatables, I'll give you ice cream"). In some respects, *if* statements based on social rules are causal in that the performance of certain acts are said to lead to or cause certain outcomes. The causal mechanism, however, resides in adherence to social rules and conformity to power relations.

With respect to *because,* social rules are referred to in the context of explanations. One can imagine a child who wishes to know why she is not permitted to engage in a desired activity (e.g., playing), or why she must engage in a nondesired activity (e.g., eating vegetables), and a parent who refers to some social rule or power relation within an explanation. In effect, *if* statements describe the relation between the performance of certain behaviors and their consequences, and *because* statements explain this relation in terms of the existence of social rules. Clearly, very young children comprehend the issue of conformity to social rules, as any parent can attest. Both compliance with and defiance of a parental rule imply comprehension of the social rule. It can be said that when social rules can be grasped, children can comprehend *if* and *because* expressions based on these rules.

Procedural knowledge. Procedural knowledge is "how to" knowledge, that is, knowledge of the steps involved in the performance of an activity (e.g., Anderson, 1982). It is typically contrasted with *declarative* or, equivalently, *conceptual* knowledge (Byrnes, 1988), which consists of an organized network of concepts for a given domain. What has been described here as a "theory" defines conceptual knowledge. So we might have conceptual knowledge of a taxonomic hierarchy (i.e., subclass–superclass relations) and also procedural knowledge of how to sort pictures into categories. Similarly, we might have conceptual knowledge of the number system and procedural knowledge regarding how to add multidigit numbers, multiply, count, and so on.

With respect to *if* statements, computer scientists are well aware of how such statements can be used to describe condition–action sequences. The statement "If *X* is greater than 5, go to line 10," for example, is an instance of a condition–action sequence. That *if* statements are useful in the context of programming implies that they would work well in the more general class of cases of which condition–action statements are a specific case, that is, giving instructions. Hence, in any context in which instructions are given, sentences of the form "If condition *X* exists, do action *Y*" are appropriate. What this means is that when children become cognitively mature enought to follow "how to" instructions, they may become capable of comprehending *if* expressions stating the instructions. Rogoff, Malkin, and Gilbride's (1984) review of recent research on the role that parents play in the problem-solving endeavors of their infants suggests that the ability to follow "how to" instructions is present quite early. Moreover, Piaget's (1952) discussion of means–end problem solving in infants illustrates procedural knowledge in infants (Mandler, 1983).

Unlike other conceptual domains described so far in which both *if* and *because* play a role, it would appear that only *if* statements are appropriate for procedural knowledge; that is, one cannot give "how to" instructions with *because*. However, one can explain *why* the steps to follow are those defined by *if* statements.

Summary. It has been shown that causal relations, a variety of noncausal conceptual relations, social rules, and procedural knowledge are appropriate conceptual domains for *if* and *because* expressions. It has also been suggested that by the early preschool period children's knowledge within these domains appears to be at a level of development suitable for the appropriate use of *if* and *because* expressions. In a subsequent section on the semantics of *if* and *because*, I review the early acquisition data and consider which of these knowledge domains appear to form the conceptual foundations of young children's *if* and *because* utterances.

Linguistic components

In addition to the conceptual foundations of *if* and *because* expressions, of course, children also need to acquire the linguistic knowledge necessary for the comprehension and production of well-formed *if* and *because* utterances. The present section considers this issue by discussing the syntactic, semantic, and pragmatic aspects of these expressions separately. Although the distinction between syntax, semantics, and pragmatics is artificial, it serves as a useful organizational device for presenting the components and relevant data.

Considerations of syntax

Both *if* and *because* constructions consist of a main clause and a subordinate clause (Scholnick & Wing, 1982). The subordinate clause is said to be of a different syntactic "rank" than the main clause (Jespersen, 1968) and is introduced by a conjunction. Thus, in "If today is Tuesday, the bill is overdue," the portion "If today is Tuesday" is the subordinate clause and the portion "the bill is overdue" is the main clause. Constructions containing subordinate conjunctions are considered *complex* syntactic devices wherein components that could stand alone without connective words (e.g., "Today is Tuesday," "The bill is overdue") are embedded within a single structure. In this respect they are similar to relative clause constructions.

Andersson (1975) reviews the adequacy of the various syntactic definitions of subordinate clause that have been given in the past, including (a) "a subordinate clause is a clause that cannot be an utterance by itself," (b) "a subordinate clause is an 'S-node' clause which is not a root," (c) "a subordinate clause is a clause introduced by a subordinating conjunction," and (d) "a syntactically subordinate clause is a clause that is introduced by a complementizer." He argues in favor of (d), given that a number of falsifying cases for (a) through (c) can be generated easily and (d) permits desirable corollaries regarding possible transformations.

Traditionally, subordinate clauses are said to be attached to the main clause at the adverbial node of the phrase structure. The structural details of this subordination, of course, depend on which of the available theories of phrase structure one adopts. Within Jackendoff's (1977) "X-bar" theory, for example, it is assumed that subordinating conjunctions are prepositions with sentential complements rather than adverbs. That is, a sentential complement is attached to a prepositional phrase node, which is itself attached to the adverbial node of the main-clause phrase structure. This and similar arrangements make for a phrase structure in which the functional role of the subordinating clause is to modify the assertion of the main clause. In the earlier example, a speaker modifies the assertion "the bill is overdue" using the additional subordinate clause "If today is Tuesday." In this case, the modifier serves to qualify the truth of what is asserted in the main clause.

The linguistic status of connectives also depends on the nature and number of grammatical categories that one's theory of grammar specifies. Within the original generative semantics account (e.g., Lakoff, 1971; McCawley, 1971), the category of *connectives* was subsumed under the category of *predicate* (Newmeyer, 1986) as part of the general structure "predicate (noun phrase 1, noun phrase 2)." As already, mentioned, Jackendoff (1977) subsumes the category *subordinating conjunction* under the universal category *preposition*, and adds the other universal categories of *verb, modal, particle, noun, article, adjective, degree word*, and *adverb*. These categories are distinguished mainly by whether or not these forms can take subjects, objects, and complementizers. Given that subordinating conjunctions are treated as prepositions, they are "[−subj, +obj, +comp]." This distinguishes them from particles such as *up*, which are "[−subj, +obj, −comp]." Pinker (1984) largely adopts the X-bar theory of phrase structure and assumes that children have innate knowledge of these universal categories. The acquisition of subordinating conjunctions would presumably involve children's learning that subordinating conjunctions as input words are instances of the class of *preposition* as well as learning the recursive rules involved in attaching a sentential complement to the adverbial node of the main clause. Of course, the adoption of a different syntactic theory would make for a different description of what is learned.

Unfortunately, the issue of which syntactic theory is "correct" is not resolved, making it difficult to generate specific predictions and explanations regarding the acquisition and developmental course of subordinating conjunctions. However, the acquisition data themselves can perhaps be used to decide among alternative linguistic descriptions. For example, if subordinating conjunctions are treated as a subcategory of prepositions, one would presumably predict that "prototypical" instances of the major category, that is, prepositions, would be acquired before instances of the subcategory, that is, subordinating conjunctions, much like what occurs in the acquisition of nouns (Callanan, Chapter 12, this volume; Rosch, 1978; Waxman, Chapter 4, this volume). If, however, subordinating conjunctions are systematically acquired before prepositions, or there is no systematic order of acquisition, it would appear that subordinating conjunctions form their own category.

Leaving this aside for now, it is necessary to describe two further syntactic issues before turning to semantic and pragmatic issues. In addition to learning which input words instantiate the category of subordinating conjunction as well as the recursive rules involved in subordination, it has been said that children acquire a further piece of syntactic knowledge. Specifically, they come to know the relation between clause order and the temporal order of events described in *if* and *because* expressions. For those expressions that describe a sequence of events (i.e., Event 1 followed by Event 2), a general rule applies: Regardless of whether the connective is found in the first or second clause, the event described in the clause containing the connective (i.e., the subordinate clause) happened first, and the event described in the main clause happened second (Emerson, 1979, 1980). In other words, *if* and *because* signal that the event described immediately after them happened first. It is for this reason that both of the expressions "If stock prices fall, there will be a recession" and "There will be a recession if stock prices fall" signal that stock prices will fall before a recession. The same is true for *because* expressions. "Because Mary came in, John left" and "John left because Mary came in" describe the same temporal sequence of events. The general rule regarding clause order also specifies that a sentence such as "John left because Mary came in" describes a different temporal sequence than "Because John left Mary came in."

However, perhaps a more general rule should be specified in order to account for clause-order effects found in *if* and *because* expressions that do not refer to event sequences. It is also true that "If it is a dog, then it is a mammal" and "If it is a mammal, then it is a dog" describe different relations, but the aspect of temporal order of events does not apply here. Similarly, there is no discernible temporal order in "A dog is a mammal because it bears live young," but it, too, says something different than "A dog bears live young because it's a mammal." It would appear that a more general rule can be derived from the distinction between subordinate and main clauses. The synonymy or lack of synonymy in all of our examples results from the consistency or lack of consistency in the subordination of specific clauses to the main clause. As mentioned earlier, subordinate clauses modify main clauses (and not vice versa) as a specific consequence of structural relations. This asymmetric order relation is analogous to order effects that occur when two adjectives modify a noun. For example, "the large red ones" refers to a different class of objects than "the red large ones." The order effects found for both subordinating conjunctions and adjectives can be said to be determined by which words or clauses occupy which nodes of the phrase structure. Hence, the "temporal-order constraint" (Emerson, 1979, 1980) really is a specific case of the more general grammatical relation between main and subordinate clauses.

A final syntactic consideration concerns the distinction between subordinate and coordinate constructions. Part of children's grammatical knowledge entails the ability to categorize the phrase structure of component clauses in terms of being "identical" versus "nonidentical." This distinction is implicit in, and essential for, knowing when the conjunction reduction (CR) transformation applies (Bresnan, 1979). Given two clauses such as "John writes books" and "Mary writes books," one applies CR when transforming "John writes books and Mary writes books" into the coordinate structure "John and Mary [both] write books." CR can apply only when the phrase structures in the components are identical. In subordinate constructions, the phrase structures are not identical and CR cannot apply without anomaly. For example, one may not reduce "John writes books because Mary writes books" into "(*) John because Mary writes books" using CR.

In sum, with respect to syntax, children essentially need to learn which input words instantiate the category of *subordinating conjunctions*, how to embed the subordinate clause appropriately within the main clause, and how to distinguish between subordinate and coordinate constructions on the basis of the identity or nonidentity of the phrase structures of the component clauses. In the following section, I discuss the acquisition data regarding this grammatical knowledge.

Acquisition data: Syntax. In the following discussion of the research regarding children's knowledge of the syntactic components of *if* and *because* expressions, I consider first the longitudinal spontaneous-production studies of very young children and then describe the experimental studies that involved older children.

Hood and Bloom (1979) reported that in their longitudinal study of 2-year-olds, children in natural discourse contexts began making causal statements without connectives. Hence, they simply juxtaposed independent clauses or used some other form. Over the span of multiple observations as children approached the age of 3, the proportion of statements without connectives declined steadily such that by the last sample less than half of the tokens were connectiveless. The first connective used for causal statements was *and*, but by the last session it was replaced by *because* (M = 38%) and *so* (M = 18%). *If* causal expressions occurred far less frequently than *and*, *because*, and *so*. In a separate study, Bloom, Lahey, Hood, Lifter, and Fiess (1980) reported that for three of four children, connectives were acquired in the order *and, because, if.* Therefore, children seem to master syntactic coordination before mastering subordination (cf. Werner & Kaplan, 1963). Furthermore, the average age of emergence for *because* was 32 months (range, 27–35 months) and that for *if* was 34 months (range, 32–38 months). In her review of other longitudinal studies Bowerman (1986) reported similar ages of onset. In addition, in a cross-sectional study of children's descriptions of familiar event sequences (e.g., birthday parties), Byrnes and Duff (1988) found that the incidence of *if* expressions increased significantly from 1% to 3% of total utterances between the ages of 3 and 4.

As to clause order, Hood and Bloom (1979) reported that whether *if* and *because* occurred in the first or second clause varied among children, as did the children's consistency in this regard. Only 6% of all utterances, however, violated the temporal-order constraint, and 79% of these errors were made by a single child. No 3- or 4-year-old made such an error in Byrnes and Duff's (1988) study. These findings demonstrate that children seem to master structural subordination in an errorless fashion.

An additional finding of Hood and Bloom (1979) worth noting concerned the relation of maternal input to clause order: The clause-order preference and level of consistency in an individual child was very similar to that of his mother. Hence, children who used an effect–cause order had mothers who used this order, children who were inconsistent in their use had mothers who were inconsistent, and so on.

The conclusion one may draw from spontaneous-production studies, then, is that children seem to master the syntactic structures of *if* and *because* in the early preschool period and simply increase their use of these connectives with age. Experimental studies with older children, however, seem to contradict this conclusion. In particular, in these studies, children were presented with a variety of tasks including (a) providing main clauses given subordinate clauses (Piaget, 1928), (b) deciding which of two picture sequences match *because* and *if* sentences (Emerson, 1979, 1980), (c) deciding which of two *because* sentences matches a picture sequence (Kuhn & Phelps, 1976), (d) judging whether sentences describing correct and reversed causal sequences are sensible or anomalous (Corrigan, 1975; Emerson, 1979, 1980; Johnson & Chapman, 1980), (e) modifying sensible sentences into anomalous ones and anomalous ones into sensible ones on the basis of temporal order (Emerson, 1980), (f) judging whether *because* and *if* sentence pairs that describe identical or opposite temporal sequences are synonymous (Emerson & Gekoski, 1980), and (g) recalling (Johnson & Chapman, 1980) or recognizing (Emerson & Gekoski, 1980) sensible-order or anomalous-order sentences. Across all of these studies, a consistent pattern emerges: A substantial number of children do not appear to grasp the temporal-order constraint until around age 8 or 9. Younger children's responses seem to reflect a disregard for temporal order in that they treat sentences such as "Woodstock fell out of his nest because he was jumping up and down" the same as "Because Woodstock fell out of his next, he was jumping up and down."

How do we reconcile the conclusion of the spontaneous-production studies that 3- and 4-year-olds comprehend the temporal-order constraint with the conclusion of the experimental studies that children do not comprehend this constraint until age 8 or 9? First, it can be said that the ability to produce one's own well-formed expressions of a particular kind appears earlier in development than the ability to comment on or judge this kind of expression made by others (Brown, 1973; Karmiloff-Smith, 1986; Slobin, 1979; Vygotsky, 1962). Hence, the metalinguistic judgments required in the experimental studies underestimate children's ability. In support of this argument, Byrnes and Gelman (1990) used a recall method that did not require metalinguistic judgments and found no reversed-clause errors in 6-, 8-, and 10-year-olds.

Second, in most studies, researchers intentionally employ causal content where cause and effect could reasonably interchange so as to remove "semantic supports" and allow for assessments of "abstracted" syntactic knowledge (e.g., Emerson, 1979, 1980). However, this method makes the erroneous assumption that syntax and semantics are independent or separable. Again, the temporal-order constraint really derives from the issue of which clause is subordinated to which clause. This subordination has inseparable semantic consequences. One can also presume that children's familiarity with the causal sequences affects how well they can map linguistic expressions onto their knowledge (Byrnes & Gelman, 1990).

Third, all of the experimental tasks require substantial cognitive processing and are often considered to be confusing even by adults. All one need do is read any of the methods sections of any of the studies (or the present chapter!) to gain a sense of the difficulty of processing multiple *if* and *because* sentences simultaneously. Clearly, there are increases in children's general processing capacity after the preschool period. Moreover, the removal of semantic supports increases the processing difficulty, thereby attenuating developmental differences.

Therefore, it is my contention that the syntactic structures of *if* and *because* are mastered in the preschool period. The primary developmental improvement concerns frequency of use, metalinguistic access to the class of conjunctions, and the ability to process multiple expressions simultaneously. The wider use may also reflect children employing *if* and *because* to express an increasing variety of conceptual relations other than specific forms of causality.

Semantic considerations

In addressing the semantics of connectives, one soon finds that the approaches applied to category terms such as generating lists of necessary and sufficient features or analyzing prototypes cannot be applied to *if* and *because*. That is, they appear at first blush to be semantically "empty" (Bresnan, 1979). Questions such as "What kinds of objects, actions, events, or relations do they refer to?" have been difficult, to say the least, to answer.

Regarding the issue of whether these terms are semantically "empty," it is useful to determine whether meaning is added when one compares juxtaposed, connectiveless pairs of clauses with their corresponding subordinate constructions. For example, it appears that meaning changes when one moves from (1) to (2):

(1)   The bill is overdue. It is Tuesday
(2)   The bill is overdue if it is Tuesday.

What appears to be added is not something new regarding reference relations between the respective clauses and objects or states of affairs in the world. Rather, what is added and conveyed to the listener is the speaker's *certainty* about the truth of the reference relations. This matter, however, falls in the realm of pragmatics, and I discuss it in the next section.

Regarding *because*, we do not find the same kind of change in meaning. Consider the differences in meaning between (3) and (4):

(3) He fell down. The floor is slippery.
(4) He fell down because the floor is slippery.

The speaker's certainty about the truth of the events is not modified here. What *because* seems to do in this case is *make explicit* the causal connection between the first and second sentences in (3). Presumably, the speaker would add the *because* only if there was some possibility that the causal connection would not be inferred from merely juxtaposing the sentences as in (3). One can imagine several scenarios in which it would be necessary to be explicit to avoid misinterpretation.

It is useful to consider dictionary listings for *if* and *because* in order to gain a sense of their full range of meanings. For *if*, one finds the following entries, listed in order of most primary meanings: (a) "in the event that," (b) "allowing that," (c) "on condition that," and (d) "whether." Hence, the expressions "If it rains today, we'll get wet" and "In the event that it rains we'll get wet" are treated as synonymous. In effect, underlying each of these expressions is knowledge of at least two possibilities: It will rain later and it will not rain. Therefore, *if* placed before a clause whose content we can call p changes the meaning from "p is the only possibility" to "p and not-p are both possible, and in the case of p . . ."

Therefore, adjoining a clause to *if* causes the content of the clause to be arrayed within a set of possibilities consisting of at least p and its negation. Since the negation of p (e.g., "It doesn't rain") can be instantiated in a variety of unspecified ways, the number of possibilities can extend beyond two. The use of *if* further functions to *select* from this set the possibility of p and *relate* this possibility to the content of the second clause.

The second entry for *if*, that is, "allowing that," functions in the context of argumentation where the *if* clause introduces a discourse *topic* (as opposed to *comment*) whose validity is perhaps only provisionally agreed upon by all parties in the discourse (Haiman, 1986). An example of such a *concessive if* would be "Even if you major in psychology, you'll get a job." Haiman (1986) argues that the function of *if* is similar to that of diacritics (auxiliary signs or labels) in that they indicate that the semantic relationship between clauses is something more than the relationship one would infer from their linear order. It is for this reason that *if* can take on both causal and concessive readings, whereas coordinate structures and paratactic structures (coordination of elements without conjunctions) can typically take on only the first. The "allowing that" meaning of *if* occurs in contexts in which one party admits of both the possibility of "*p*" and "not-*p*" but the other party is biased toward "not-*p*." In some respects such *if*s function as counterfactual constructions for the listener.

With respect to *because*, there are two primary dictionary entries: (a) "for the reason that" and (b) "for the fact that." It would appear that *because* simply condenses these longer expressions into a single term. Again, however, it is necessary to note that "reasons" need not be only causal explanations, but any kind of explanation based on social rules or naïve theories, and so on.

One may note in passing that the paraphrases for *if* and *because* entail the conjunctive use of *that*, which has been studied in the context of subordinating sentential complements or the role of the complementizer (e.g., Pinker, 1984). This seems to support grammatical theories that treat *if* and *because* in similar ways as *that*.

Historically, the semantics of *if* has been treated under the truth-functional approach of logicians (e.g., Quine, 1950), though this approach is by no means adequate. In this view, the meaning of connectives derives from the truth status of component propositions. In particular, the statement "If today is Tuesday, the bill is overdue" is true if any of the following three component instances is true: (a) "Today is Tuesday and the bill is overdue," (b) "Today is not Tuesday and the bill is not overdue" (e.g., it's Monday), or (c) "Today is not Tuesday and the bill is overdue" (e.g., it's Wednesday). In addition, the meaning of an *if* statement is also said to derive from knowing which instances falsify it. For this example, if the case (d) "Today is Tuesday and the bill is not overdue" were true, the *if* statement would be false. This combination of having cases (a) through (c) true and case (d) false is said to semantically define *conditional implication*, or the "conditional" for short. The truth conditions for the conditional imply that the antecedent (e.g., "Today is Tuesday") is a *sufficient but not necessary condition* for the consequent (e.g., "the bill is overdue") (Byrnes & Overton, 1988). That is, the antecedent can bring about the consequent on its own, but it is not the only way to bring it about. In this example, the truth of "Today

is Tuesday" is a sufficient condition for the truth of "the bill is overdue," but it is not a necessary condition since it would also be true
when "Today is Wednesday." For this reason the converse implication, "If the bill is overdue, then today is Tuesday," is not necessarily true given case (c). Thus, conditionals reflect one-way,
asymmetrical implication relations from antecedent to consequent.
Of note is the fact that truth-functional analysis is a *reference* theory
of meaning and to know the meaning of *if* is to know which cases
it refers to and which cases it excludes.

Within this scheme, specific subsets of the four possible combinations of negated and affirmed phrases are used to define the
meaning of any given connective uniquely. Thus, *if* is distinct from
and in that if the clauses were linked by *and* instead of *if* as in "Today is Tuesday and the bill is overdue," then only case (a) could be
true and all other cases must be false. Similarly, *if* is distinct from
the connective *if and only if*, which defines *biconditional equivalence*
among events. Whereas case (c) can be true for the conditional, it
must be false for the biconditional. In essence, biconditionals describe a perfect correlation between events where the antecedent is
a necessary and sufficient condition for the consequent; that is, the
antecedent is described to be the only way to bring about the consequent. Moreover, unlike the conditional, a biconditional and its
converse both hold (e.g., "Today is the 10th if and only if it is my
birthday").

Logicians endeavored to express these definitions in abstract formulas in the process of trying to describe the universal, language-
independent, and content-independent "laws of thought" (e.g.,
Frege, 1952). For any true *if* statement with antecedent "*p*" and consequent "*q*," then, the following combinations were said to be true:
"*p* and *q*," "not-*p* and *q*," "not-*p* and not-*q*." Moreover, the case "*p*
and not-*q*" was false. The tidiness of this semantic system and the
political sway of logical positivists such as Russell and Quine resulted in the general adoption of this approach.

It did not take long, however, before individual philosophers discovered cases that conformed to the abstract definition but were
nonetheless meaningless or nonsensical. For example, "If vinegar is
acid, then men have red beards" turns out to be a true statement,
because the proper cases turn out to be true and the case "Vinegar
is acid and men do not have red beards" is false. In addition, in the
context of deriving axioms through mathematical manipulation of

the contentless formalisms, an axiom was proved which stated that one may validly prove the truth of any conditional (e.g., "If Bush is president, then Mars is a red planet") from the truth of its negated antecedent (e.g., "Bush is not president") (Pieraut-LeBonniec, 1980).

These "paradoxes of implication" led some to propose various ways of placing constraints on the semantic content of *if* expressions. In the context of developing a modal logic, Lewis and Langford (1932) proposed a "strict implication," or *entailment* constraint: The antecedent must entail the consequent. Anderson and Belnap (1962) further developed this notion, which essentially specifies that in asserting an "if *p* then *q*" statement, one asserts that the case "*p* and not-*q*" is impossible. For example, in saying "If it rains, we'll get wet," the speaker believes and conveys to the listener that the case "It rains and we don't get wet" is impossible. Entailment, however, is really an aspect of a logical system's metalanguage by which one proves formulaically the logical *consistency* of the propositions "*p*" and "*q*," which in turn means that the case "*p* and not-*q*" is logically excluded. Technically, entailment is not proved by specific semantic contents, because proving by content moves one down from the metalanguage to the level of the language (Quine, 1950). Regardless, this formal constraint has the indirect effect of limiting possible contents. Hence, the meaningless examples provided earlier would be excluded.

Bates (1976) employs Puglielli and Ciliberti's (1973) semantic theory for *if*, which is based partly on generative semantics notions and partly on the notion of entailment. Here, both *if* and *because* share the same semantic core "ENTAIL (proposition X, proposition Y)," which is a specific instantiation of "predicate (argument 1, argument 2)." *If* and *because* are distinguished by differing presuppositions about the truth of what is stated. I discuss these differing presuppositions in the next section on pragmatics.

Whereas on the surface the entailment solution appears to have merit, it unfortunately does not describe the semantics of *if* and *because* any more adequately than truth-functional theory. This is because a variety of *if* statements produced by speakers fail the entailment test. Specifically, speakers often assert *if* expressions when they feel the consequent is merely *likely* given the antecedent, not only when it is absolutely certain. This is particularly evident when one adds a modal qualifier as in "If it rains today, we may get wet."

Moreover, it is virtually impossible to come up with an *if* statement whose content truly conforms to entailment since the case "*p* and not-*q*" is always possible for all contents. For example, even so-called analytic statements based on semantic definitions such as "If it is a dog, then it is a mammal" could turn out to be falsified if the linguistic culture changes the definitions of individual terms (e.g., a dog is no longer considered to be a mammal). This has clearly happened in the case of the classification of *whale*.

We are left, then, with the formulation described earlier, that *if* functions semantically to place the content described in the subordinate clause within a set of possibilities consisting at least of the cases "*p*" and "not-*p*." It then functions first to select the case "*p*" and then to relate it to a case "*q*" through a causal or other relation. This account is not unlike the "possible-worlds" approach (Stalnaker, 1984) but is much more parsimonious. For reasons of cognitive economy and efficiency, one need not assume that a child who constructs an *if* expression imagines all the possible worlds and states of affairs in which this statement would be true. Rather, the child imagines the one possible context in which the relation described holds, and groups all other outcomes implicitly under "not-*p*" or, roughly, "all other cases." At a minimum, the relation described is one of "covariance" or "co-occurrence" between the contents described in the antecedent and consequent. This general relation is instantiated in a variety of relations including causal, subclass–superclass, object–property, and indexical. *Because*, in contrast, relates the antecedent and consequent through an explanation relationship, permitting the case "*p*" and excluding the possibility of the case "not-*p*."

Considering one's semantic theory from the standpoint of the speaker as opposed to the standpoint of a formalizing theorist, one never encounters "paradoxes of implication," because the speaker does not wish to combine units of knowledge nonsensically, but rather wishes to relate them causally, and so on. Keeping this perspective obviates the need to place constraints on a formal system imposed on speakers from without. The principal problem with both the truth-functional and entailment approaches is that they do not incorporate content effects, that is, the nature of the relation between antecedent and consequent, into their semantic theories. This is akin to the problem of a theorist who believes that the semantics of categorical terms consists of lists of necessary and sufficient features but who does not incorporate or consider important the specific necessary and sufficient criteria for individual categorical terms.

Acquisition data: Semantics. Again I consider the developmental data from the standpoint of the early acquisition studies and of experiments using school-aged children. Regarding early acquisition studies, the issue of semantics can be approached from the perspective of what children seem to be talking about in their first *if* and *because* expressions.

Bloom and Capatides (1987) analyzed the semantic content of Hood and Bloom's (1979) *if* and *because* expressions. They first divided the age range (i.e., 26 to 38 months) into four developmental periods. In the first period, Period A, children made causal expressions without connectives. The beginning of Period B marked the point where the children first used connectives productively. Basing their semantic interpretation on context, they discovered two broad categories of *causal* meaning: objective and subjective. Objective meaning was evidential and fixed in the physical world. It had to do with physical order in the world that was associated with actions and perceptions (e.g., tripping over a cord). The other category, subjective meaning, concerned causal relations that were not fixed or self-evident and were based on personal, affective, or sociocultural beliefs (e.g., *red* means "stop").

Bloom and Capatides found that causal statements, both with and without connectives, most often expressed subjective meanings in each of the four periods ($M = 62\%$). Moreover, subjective meaning was always more frequent in sentences without connectives. When connectives first occurred in Period B, subjective meaning was less frequent in sentences with connectives than in sentences without connectives, and more than half of the causal statements with connectives expressed objective causality. Therefore, the acquisition of connectives in Period B was associated with the expression of objective meaning. Presumably, children's *if* and *because* statements expressed only these two categories of causality since the authors did not report that children produced noncausal *if* and *because* expressions. However, the category of subjective meaning seems to include what I labeled indexical relations and social rules in the conceptual basis section of this chapter. At least in this early period, then, children do not appear to express *if* or *because* statements that describe the conceptual categories of noncausal conceptual relations (e.g., object–property relations), nor do they express procedural knowledge using *if*.

Regarding semantic development beyond the preschool period, there is a set of studies on comprehension of *if* whose methods were based on the truth-functional approach of logicians. I am not aware of any similar studies of the semantics of *because* involving school-aged children. In these studies, children were presented with sentences constructed with *if* and other connectives (e.g., *and, or, if and only if*) and stimuli such as pictures or objects that proved the sentence either true or false. In particular, the stimuli instantiated one of the four possible combinations of "*p* and *q*," "not-*p* and *q*," and so on. For example, the children were given the sentence "If it is red, then it is a triangle," shown a red circle, and asked whether the *if* sentence was true. In these studies children younger than 8 generally treated *if* as *conjunction* in that for sentences such as "If it is red, then it is a triangle," they responded that the case *red triangle* (i.e., "*p* and *q*") proved it true and the other three possible cases (i.e., "not-*p* and *q*," etc.) proved it false. Children between the ages of 8 and 12 included both "*p* and *q*" and "not-*p* and not-*q*" in the set of instances proving *if* statements true, thereby treating *if* as *if and only if*. For example, both the cases *red triangle* and *blue square* were said to prove the example sentence true. Finally, from approximately age 13 onward children added the case "not-*p* and *q*" to the set of instances proving *if* statements true, thereby treating *if* as a logician would (Byrnes & Overton, 1988; Lawson, 1983; Moshman, 1979; O'Brien & Overton, 1980; Overton, Byrnes, & O'Brien, 1985; Paris, 1973; Staudenmayer & Bourne, 1977; Sternberg, 1979; Taplin, Staudenmayer, & Taddonio, 1974). One can lower the age of onset for these various patterns somewhat by using meaningful causal relations as opposed to abstract or arbitrary content and by pointing out that the antecedent is only one way to bring about the consequent (e.g., Byrnes & Overton, 1988). Nevertheless, even with such measures the earliest that consistent conditional patterns are found is age 10 or 11. At all ages except adulthood, the biconditional pattern predominates. Even adults, however, generate only 50% conditional patterns without hints about other causes and 80% conditional patterns with hints (Byrnes & Overton, 1988). Therefore, the logician's truth table does not appear to be the basis for the semantics of *if* even for adults.

I can add that the conjunctive as opposed to the biconditional pattern in 6- to 8-year-olds is probably an artifact of the truth-testing task. In a recent study using French and Nelson's (1985) "script" method, I found several cases in which children successfully stated an "If *p* then *q*" sentence and then stated its converse, "If not-*p*, then not-*q*" (Byrnes & Duff, 1988). In a context of describing familiar event sequences that contain variation or alternative courses of action (e.g., *lunchtime*), 4-year-old children said things like "If I eat at home, I drink milk. If I eat at school, I drink juice." French and Nelson (1985) reported similar findings. These patterns reflect a biconditional meaning in that the case "*p*" is said to go with case "*q*," and the case "not-*p*" is said to go with "not-*q*."

Pragmatic considerations

In the preceding discussion of semantic considerations, the artificiality of the distinction between semantics and pragmatics was evident. It became clear that pragmatic aspects of the discourse context (e.g., topic vs. comment), the speaker's certainty about the truth of her utterances, possibility, what the speaker is trying to say, and so on, play a significant role in the meaning of *if* and *because*. In addition to acquiring the requisite conceptual, syntactic, and semantic knowledge described so far, then, children must also gain insight into pragmatic functions of *if* and *because*. I consider the pragmatics of these terms from two standpoints: (a) the pragmatic concepts conveyed and (b) speech act theory.

Each term in the class of subordinating conjunctions expresses a specific speaker attitude toward the truth of his expression (Bates, 1976; Kartunnen, 1971; Scholnick & Wing, 1982, 1983). Specifically, *because, when,* and *although* convey to the listener that the speaker believes or is fairly certain about the truth of the semantic content of each of the clauses. Thus, in saying "It broke because it was old," the speaker believes two things: that "it broke" and that "it was old."

In contrast, *if* in combination with verbs in the indicative mood and *unless* convey to the listener that the speaker is uncertain about the truth of what is stated individually in each clause. Thus, in saying "If it is raining, we'll get wet," the speaker conveys uncertainty about two things: that "it is raining" and that "we'll get wet." Recalling an earlier point, it can be seen that the additional meaning that *if* imparts to juxtaposed clauses is the speaker's attitude of uncertainty.

In contrast, *if* in combination with verbs in the subjunctive mood conveys to the listener that the speaker disbelieves, or, equivalently, is certain about the falsity of, what is stated in each clause. Thus, in saying "If John had come to the party, Mary would have been embarrassed," the speaker conveys certainty about the falsity of two things: that "John came to the party" and that "Mary was embarrassed." Such *if* statements are usually referred to as *counterfactuals*.

In addition to the speaker's attitude about the truth of the individual components, there is also the matter of the speaker's attitude about the *relation between* the components or clauses. In particular, in *because* statements, the speaker is certain not only about the truth of the individual clauses, but also that the consequent is true because of the truth of the antecedent. Thus, in saying "It broke because it is old," the speaker conveys certainty about or belief in the causal relation between antecedent and consequent. Thus, for *because* the speaker is certain about the antecedent's truth, the consequent's truth, and the truth of the relation between the antecedent and consequent.

Such consistency in conveyed belief is not the case for *if*, however. Whereas the speaker conveys uncertainty about the truth of the antecedent and the truth of the consequent, she conveys *certainty* about the relation between clauses. For example, in saying "If it is raining, we'll get wet," the speaker in essence is saying "I'm not sure whether or not it will rain, or whether we'll get wet, but if it *does* rain, then we *will* get wet." This interclause certainty is formalized in the logician's definition of entailment described earlier; that is, given the truth of the antecedent, the consequent is necessarily true or, equivalently, the case "*p* and not-*q*" is impossible.

I should note that the issue of whether a given connective conveys certainty or uncertainty is not absolute. It would appear that the boundary between the categories *certain* and *uncertain* is fuzzy. One may conceive of a speaker's belief as arrayed along a continuum ranging from *absolute disbelief* at one extreme and *absolute belief* at the other (Byrnes & Gelman, 1990). When one feels very certain that the antecedent and consequent are true, one uses *because, when,* or *so* (e.g., "Mary became embarrassed because John went to the party"). When one feels very certain that the antecedent and consequent are false, one uses *if* with verbs in the subjunctive mood (e.g., "If John had gone to the party, Mary would have been embarrassed"). When one feels relatively more certain about the truth of some state of affairs but not strongly certain, one uses *if* with verbs in the indicative mood (e.g., "If John is going to the party, Mary will be embarrassed"). Again, however, certainty and uncertainty pertain here to the likelihood that what is stated in the individual clauses will come about. The speaker's belief in the interclause relation is one of certainty for all of the preceding three examples. Regarding the individual clauses, then, a speaker who has experienced John's going to the party and Mary's embarrassment or who received credible secondhand knowledge to that effect would be misleading the listener by using *if* with a verb either in the subjunctive mood or in the indicative mood. An expression more faithful to the speaker's knowledge would be constructed with *because, when,* or *so.*

As a second pragmatic consideration, I use Searle's (1976, 1983) *speech act theory* to describe how speakers use *if* and *because* expressions to have various effects on the listener. Searle argues that most utterances can be categorized as an instance of one of five kinds of speech acts: *representatives, directives, commissives, expressives,* and *declarations.* Each of these utterance types can be distinguished with respect to (a) what the speaker's purpose or intent is in uttering it, (b) whether the speaker utters the expression to get the "words to match the world" or the "world to match the words," and (c) the speaker's psychological state.

The purpose of uttering instances of the representative class is to "commit the speaker (in varying degrees) to something's being the case, to the truth of the expressed proposition" (Searle, 1976, p. 10). The speaker is trying to get the words to match the world and conveys the psychological state of "belief" to the listener. *If* expressions certainly fall within the class of representatives in that they can be used to make *assertions* about the way the speaker believes the world to be (e.g., "If it's a dog, then it's a mammal"), *predictions* about the way the speaker believes the world will be at some later time (e.g., "If inflation rises, interests rates will go down"), and *counterfactuals* about the way the speaker believes the world could be. To conceive of a counterfactual state of affairs, the speaker mentally negates or falsifies his knowledge about the way things are (e.g., "If John had come to the party, Mary would have been embarrassed"). In essence, the speaker has the sole intention of informing the listener of some piece of information that the listener did not know, had forgotten, or was not considering at the moment. Two utterance types related to these major categories are *suggestions* whereby the speaker believes that the listener would want to know that her actions can bring about some desirable outcome (e.g., "It will come out better if you use this paper"), and what I call here *permissives*, whereby the speaker informs the listener that some constraint on her behavior has been lifted (e.g., "You don't have to eat it if you don't want to"). Suggestions appear to be a subclass of predictions that specifically concern the listener's following successful procedures and that are generally stated in the second person. Non-suggestion predictions generally lack these two features. Finally, permissives are like assertions and predictions but unlike counterfactuals in that the main clause standing alone without the *if* clause would still function as the same kind of speech act. The *if* clause makes the truth of the content of the main clause conditional on the truth of the subordinate clause.

Each of assertive, predictive, counterfactual, and instructional *if* expressions has a fairly distinct and prototypical syntax. That is, one may keep the same content and change one kind of representative into another by altering the syntax. This alteration largely entails verb tense, verb mood, and the presence or absence of auxiliaries. Verb aspect does not appear to play a significant role here. The alterations in speech act as a result of changes in linguistic form demonstrate that pragmatics and syntax are by no means independent. However, it is best to conceive of prototypical as opposed to defining syntactic constructions in this regard.

There are also *because* utterances that are instances of the class of representatives. However, *because* expressions typically can only be assertions (e.g., "It broke because it was old"), predictions (e.g., "It will break soon because it is old"), and permissives (e.g., "You may go out because you were a good boy"). In *because* permissives, the subordinate clause explains why the permission given in the main clause was granted. Speaking more generally, all *because* assertions function to explain. In addition, there is usually no syntactic way to form a *because* counterfactual because the addition of auxiliaries to past-tense verbs creates ill-formed expressions (e.g., "(*) It would have broken because it had been old"). Moreover, there does not appear to be an easy way to make suggestions or give instructions with *because*.

In contrast to uttering representatives, the purpose of uttering instances of the directives class is to get the listener to do something. Hence, the speaker tries to get the world to match the words and conveys the psychological state of "desire" to the listener. Three primary kinds of *if* directives are *threats* (e.g., "If you don't eat your dinner, I won't give you dessert"), *orders* (e.g., "You must sit down, if you want to eat"), and *instructions* (e.g., "If line 10 is larger than line 11, place a '0' in line 12"). A fourth category, *requests,* includes questions, because questions also ask the listener to do something, that is, give information. This is the primary way of using *if* to make a request (e.g., "Would you go if Harry went?"). There are also forms such as "Give that to me, if you don't mind," in which the subordinate clause is more a politeness device than a modifier of the main clause. Finally, one cannot generally make *because* threats or give *because* instructions, but one can ask questions containing *because* and explain one's orders using a *because* (e.g., "You must go to bed because you were bad").

If threats are often syntactically identical to suggestions and other predictions of the representative class. They cannot be distinguished by the presence of negation because threats can be stated positively (e.g., "If you keep on drinking, I'll leave you"). Rather, they appear to be distinguished on the basis of whether the speaker has personal control over the outcome, whether the outcome is aversive to the listener, and whether the aversive outcome is contingent on certain future behaviors on the part of the listener. For Searle, they differ primarily as to purpose and psychological state conveyed.

The third kind of speech act category consists of *commissives,* the purpose of which is to commit the speaker to some future course of action. The speaker tries to get the world to match the words and conveys the psychological state of "intention" to the listener. *Promises* are the primary form of an *if* commissive (e.g., "If you eat your dinner, I'll give you dessert"). Unlike unconditional promises in which the speaker describes an intention to engage in some behavior that is presumably desirable to the listener, *if* promises make the speaker's fulfillment of a commitment contingent on some behaviors on the part of the listener. Like suggestions and threats, promises are a subclass of predictions. One may also make *because* promises in which the subordinate clause functions to explain the reason for the speaker's commitment to provide a desirable outcome (e.g., "I'll give you dessert because you ate your dinner").

An interesting phenomenon is that *if* promises become threats through a distributed negation: "If you eat your dinner, I'll give you dessert" becomes "If you don't eat your dinner, I won't give you dessert" (Fillenbaum, 1977, 1986). In this respect, a threat is a kind of promise in which one promises *not* to provide a desirable outcome. In addition, any *if* promise can be made a synonymous *and* promise (e.g., "Eat your dinner and I'll give you dessert"), and any *if* threat can be made a synonymous *or* threat (e.g., "Eat your dinner or I won't give you dessert") (Fillenbaum, 1977, 1986). These facts further demonstrate that syntax and pragmatics are intimately linked.

Fillenbaum (1977, 1986) also describes the close relation between the pragmatics and semantics of *if*. Basing his analysis on Geis and Zwicky (1971), he argues that threats and promises alter the number of possible instances (i.e., "p and q," "not-p and q," etc.) referred to. In particular, when a speaker says, "If you mow the lawn, I'll give you five dollars," he does not intend the listener to infer that payment will occur even if the lawn is not mowed (i.e., "not-p and q"). Similarly, when a parent says, "If you don't stop yelling, you'll be in trouble," she does not intend to convey that the child will be in trouble even if the child stops yelling (i.e., "not-p and q"). However, the instance "not-p and q," as well as "p and q" and "not-p and not-q," are defining instances in a truth-functional analysis. Therefore, the truth-functional definition is not appropriate for threats and promises. Moreover, the nonapplicability of the case "not-p and q" is true for all other speech act categories except for assertives and predictions.

Finally, Searle's (1976) last two speech act categories of expressives and declarations do not appear to pertain to either *if* or *because*. In expressives, the purpose is simply to express the speaker's psychological state without a desire to get the words to match the world or vice versa. Such expressions as "I apologize" or "I want to thank you" are examples. The successful performance of an instance of the class of declarations brings into being some state of affairs. For example, "I hereby appoint you deputy" is a declaration. *If* would apply to these categories only if one could make conditional apologies, congratulatory remarks, declarations, and so on. *Because* would apply only if one were to explain the content of one's expressives and one's declarations. In sum, *if* and *because* expressions seem primarily to instantiate the classes of representatives, directives, and commissives.

Acquisition data: Pragmatics. I consider the issue of children's knowledge of the pragmatics of *if* and *because* in two ways. First, I apply the classification scheme based on Searle (1976) to the spontaneous speech samples of Berko Gleason, Perlmann, and Greif (1984), Byrnes and Duff (1988), and McCabe, Evely, Abramovitch, Corter, and Pepler (1983). Second, I briefly review several experimental studies on this topic.

In applying the speech act categories to the spontaneous-production data, I relied on context as well as an individual utterance's syntax to guide my coding. I excluded secondhand reports of someone else's *if* or *because* statements (e.g., "He said that if I go, I should tell him") as well as *if* statements expressing the nonconditional meanings in the form *see if, know if, tell if,* and *ask if.* The excluded utterances comprised 9% of the total.

The Berko Gleason, Perlmann, and Greif (1984) corpus was made available to me through the Child Language Data Exchange System (see MacWhinney & Snow, 1985). The context for this data set included children and parents conversing over the evening meal. The 13 children ranged in age from 3,0 to 5,3. I divided utterances into parent-to-parent, parent-to-child, and child-to-parent and categorized them using Searle's (1976) scheme. The data are presented in Table 10.1. What becomes apparent when one inspects the table is that when parents speak to each other or to their children using *if* and *because* statements, most of their utterances fall within the representative class. Generally, then, parents use these statements to provide information. In addition, the distribution of kinds of utterances within a given class seem to vary with differing power relations and relative knowledge between speaker and listener. For example, whereas the *if* representatives of parents speaking to one another included predictions and assertions, when parents were speaking to their children the main categories were permissives and suggestions. Similarly, when parents spoke to one another, *if* directives were mostly in the form of requests. However, when they spoke to their children, *if* directives included threats and orders and *because* directives included orders. In contrast, when children addressed their parents, the majority of *if* statements were not representatives, but directives in the form of questions. Hence, chil-

Table 10.1 *Speech act categories of Berko Gleason, Perlmann, and Greif (1984)*

if statements	*because* statements
PARENT-TO-PARENT UTTERANCES	
Representatives (63%)[a] Predictions (47%)[b] Assertions (33%) Counterfactuals (20%)	*Representatives* (95%) Assertions (100%)
Directives (37%) Requests (questions) (67%) Requests (nonquestions) (22%) Instructions (11%)	*Directives* (5%) Requests (questions) (100%)
Commissives (0%)	—
PATENT-TO-CHILD UTTERANCES	
Representatives (60%) Permissives (56%) Assertives (33%) Suggestions (7%) Counterfactuals (4%)	*Representatives* (86%) Assertives (96%) Predictions (4%)
Directives (36%) Threats (38%) Requests (questions) (38%) Orders (18%) Instructions (6%)	*Directives* (14%) Requests (25%) Orders (75%)
Commissives (4%) Promises (100%)	—
CHILD-TO-PARENT UTTERANCES	
Representatives (29%) Assertions (25%) Suggestions (25%) Counterfactuals (25%) Predictions (25%)	*Representatives* (100%) Assertions (100%)
Directives (71%) Requests (questions) (100%)	—
Commissives (0%)	—

Note: I thank Jean Berko Gleason, Brian MacWhinney, and Catherine Snow for making these data available to me.
[a]This figure reflects the percentage of total utterances that were representatives.
[b]This figure reflects the percentage of representatives that were predictions.

dren were generally more likely to seek information than provide it. However, all of the children's *because* statements were explanations and were uttered in order to provide information. Finally, it can be seen that *if* statements comprised a greater variety of speech acts than *because* statements. In particular, the average number of subcategories (e.g., predictions) per category (e.g., representatives) for *if* was 2.63, whereas that for *because* was 1.40. Thus *if* is a more multifunctional connective than *because*. As a result, children actually heard more *if* statements addressed to them (61%) than *because* statements (39%).

For contrastive purposes, I applied the speech act categories to data in Byrnes and Duff (1988) and McCabe, Evely, Abramovitch, Corter, and Pepler (1983). In Byrnes and Duff (1988), 3- to 4-year-old children spoke to an experimenter about five familiar event sequences (birthday parties, getting dressed, etc.). The corpus consisted entirely of child-to-adult utterances. Subjects described these sequences in response to questions of the form "What happens at _____? [e.g., birthday parties]" (see French & Nelson, 1985). After we grouped utterances according to speech act categories, it was found that 94% of children's *if* and 100% of their *because* expressions were representatives. The majority of these were assertives (*if*, 88%; *because*, 100%). For *because*, the majority attempted to explain their own or another's behavior. Furthermore, the 4-year-olds were significantly more likely than the 3-year-olds to utter *if* and *because* expressions and demonstrated substantially more knowledge about the event sequences using these expressions. Therefore, preschoolers are fully capable of producing *if* representatives given background knowledge. Even though the high percentage of *if* representatives in this sample contrasts sharply with the much lower level produced by Berko Gleason et al.'s (1984) children, this higher percentage is not surprising given that children were specifically asked to provide information in Byrnes and Duff (1988).

I further applied speech act theory to McCabe et al. (1983), even though the data I used consisted only of examples the authors provided in a table. The table listed semantic categories the authors believed they discovered in utterances produced within dialogues between pairs of older and younger siblings aged 2,10 to 7,3. Although these examples by no means constitute a corpus, I analyzed them nevertheless given the possibility that power–knowledge relations might figure prominently in the interchanges. In contrast to the studies of Berko Gleason et al. (1984) and Byrnes and Duff (1988), in which few directives were produced by children (other than questions), 23% of the examples listed in McCabe et al. were directives in the form of threats, orders, and nonquestion requests. One can presume that the majority of these were produced when older siblings addressed younger siblings.

To summarize the speech act analysis of spontaneous-production data, it can be said that in a discourse context, parents are most likely to provide information to their children about "the way things are" through *if* and *because* statements, but also are likely to attempt to control their children's behavior using threats and orders. That few *if* statements issued by parents to children were promises reflects the fact that parents primarily provide information to and impose power over their children using *if* and *because*. Children, in contrast, seem largely to "practice" forming grammatical *if* expressions in the context of asking *what if* questions, and forming *because* expressions in explanation attempts. As children grow older, they gain knowledge (about event sequences, causality) and have more opportunities to impose power over younger siblings. These changes may provide more opportunities to use *if* and *because* statements as representatives and *if* statements as directives.

Further developments in pragmatic knowledge beyond the preschool period have been assessed in several experimental studies. Scholnick and Wing conducted three studies on children's knowledge of the pragmatic concepts that *if* and *because* as well as several other subordinating conjunctions convey (Scholnick & Wing, 1982, 1983; Wing & Scholnick, 1981). The subjects in these studies were as young as age 6 and as old as 21. In the original task, children listened to tape-recorded *if* and *because* utterances made by a ficticious astronaut who described objects on a strange planet. After hearing a statement (e.g., "This is a monkey if it has two hands"), children were asked to judge the speaker's belief in the truth of the main clause (e.g., "Does he believe it's a monkey?") and the subordinate clause (e.g., "Does he believe it has two hands?"). They had the choices of "Yes," "No," or "He's not sure." Since *if* statements with indicative verbs convey uncertainty, the correct response to both questions was "He's not sure." Since counterfactual *if* statements with subjunctive verbs convey disbelief (e.g., "If this were a monkey, it would have two hands"), the correct answers were "No" for each question. For *because* statements (e.g., "This is a monkey because it has two hands"), however, the correct response to both questions was "Yes" since *because* conveys certainty. Across three studies, Scholnick and Wing found that it was not until children were age 8 or 9 that they appeared to know that *if*-indicative conveys uncertainty, *if*-subjunctive conveys disbelief, and *because* conveys certainty.

However, as already argued regarding experimental studies of the temporal-order constraint, Scholnick and Wing's method may have underestimated younger children's knowledge because metalinguistic judgments were required. That is, children may know implicitly that *if* conveys uncertainty and *because* conveys certainty but may be unable to reflect upon this knowledge consciously for several years until it becomes explicit. In support of this claim, Byrnes and Gelman (1990) used a recall method that did not require metalinguistic judgments and discovered implicit knowledge of pragmatic concepts in 6-year-old children. Similarly, Bates (1976), Kuczaj (1981), and Byrnes and Duff (1988) found comprehension of counterfactual *if* statements in preschoolers using a questioning, *what if* format.

Across both the spontaneous-production studies and experimental studies, then, it can be said that whereas children demonstrate a nascent understanding of the pragmatics of *if* and *because* in the late preschool period, this knowledge expands and consolidates up to age 6 or 7, when it is available only on an implicit, "use-in-context" level. By age 8 or 9, this broad implicit knowledge becomes explicit and available to conscious reflection.

Conceptual and linguistic interrelations in development

At the beginning of this chapter I made the assumption that concepts and meanings are distinct and that language evokes aspects of conceptual domains for expression (see Clark, 1983; Slobin, 1979). Having described the conceptual domains that seem to underlie *if* expressions (i.e., causality, categorical relations, indexical relations, social rules, and procedural knowledge) and *because* expressions (i.e., "theories"), as well as having described the linguistic aspects of these expressions, I am now in a better position to consider possible interrelations between thought and language. I set forth three proposals that differ from the traditional approaches of Piaget, Vygotsky, Whorf, and Chomsky (see Byrnes & Gelman, Chapter 1, this volume) and consider *if* and *because* in the context of these proposals.

The first proposal derives from Karmiloff-Smith's (1986) three-phase theory. In the context of describing children's learning of the French determiner system, Karmiloff-Smith proposes that three phases are discernible in the acquisitional data. In the first phase, individual instances of a class of terms (e.g., *the* and *a* of the class of determiners) are learned separately as unanalyzed particles. The various instances are not treated as members of a larger class, and children cannot analyze or comment on these terms metalinguistically. In the second phase, the instances cohere into a system in a way that appears to be an unconscious construction by children. That is, a new emergent system is evident but children cannot analyze or comment on it metalinguistically. Further, Karmiloff-Smith notes two striking features of this system: (a) It occurs in the absence of negative feedback about how the individual terms are used in the first phase (because there are few if any errors in the first phase), and (b) the system that children form often specifies erroneous uses of the terms. For example, children unnecessarily created the phrase *un de* as a means of distinguishing between the "some" and "one" meanings of *un*. This finding is similar to the well-known phenomenon of overgeneralization in which children misapply a rule (e.g., add *-ed* to terms such as *go* after they have been correctly using the term *went* for some time). The unconscious flavor of the system changes are reminiscent of Piaget's (1952) notion of equilibration, although equilibration is said to occur as a result of contradictions, not successes. In the third phase, the system changes to reflect the adult usage of terms, and children are able to reflect upon this system metalinguistically.

It would be interesting to see whether the class of subordinating conjunctions goes through an analogous three-phase development. If so, one would expect that in the first phase, *if* and *because* would be learned in an unanalyzed, disjoint fashion. In the second phase, they would cohere into a (possibly defective) system, and in the third phase children would be able to reflect on this system metalinguistically. I am unaware of whether a longitudinal data base such as that of Hood and Bloom (1979) would support this account but it would be an interesting avenue to pursue.

If such a three-phase pattern were found, between-phase changes could well have conceptual consequences. In particular, it is possible to imagine a hypothetical case in which a child uses *if* only to make causal predictions and uses *because* only to make causal assertions. When the conjunction system unconsciously coheres, *if* and *because* are categorized together. As a result of this change, *if* may take on a new function in the making of assertions, and *because* may take on a new function in the explanation of predictions. Such functional changes in turn open new opportunities for expressing relations other than causality. That is, one need not make only causal assertions. When this recognition occurs, structural similarities between causal relations and other conceptual relations (e.g., class inclusion) are discovered as a result of their being expressible by the same connectives. Hence, the linguistic phenomenon of systems cohering leads to new uses of terms, which in turn lead to conceptual integration.

A second proposal derives from a means–goal approach to problem solving. Specifically, concepts and intentions serve as the starting point for the construction of linguistic expressions. The child has conceptual knowledge (e.g., an understanding of causality) and propositional stances (e.g., uncertainty) that he wishes to express but lacks the syntactic device for doing so. This state of having a goal and needing to devise the means for attaining the goal is common to any problem-solving situation. What is lacking in the language example is procedural knowledge regarding how to express one's intentions syntactically. Parents' modeling of the proper expressions as well as of correlative structures in the form of questions about their children's probable intentions provides children with the necessary information. Once expressions are acquired, their use modifies conceptual relations as described in reference to the three-phase theory. This cycle of goal–use–conceptual change continues dynamically. This second proposal differs from the first in terms of an emphasis on intentionality and problem solving.

A third proposal derives from the notion of *bootstrapping*. Bereiter (1985) describes the utility of a linguistic bootstrapping operation in the context of considering the tenability of a constructivist approach to learning. He rightly notes that no one has developed a convincing counterproposal to Fodor's (1975) indictment of constructivism. Specifically, Fodor (1975) argues that the only way a child could conceivably construct or invent a relation between concepts is if she already understood or knew this relation a priori. In essence, this "constructivism paradox" reaffirms Fodor's nativism. Bereiter (1985) suggests that constructivism may yet be a tenable account if one permits a subset of components of cognition to be innate and one from which others are derived by way of a bootstrapping operation. Thus, in searching to create a novel conceptual relation that resolves contradictions that have arisen, the child derives this novel relation by way of an analogy mapping from linguistic structural relations.

I propose that structural relations inherent in coordinate (e.g., *and*) and subordinate constructions (e.g., *if* and *because*) form the basis of the classificatory conceptual relations of *equivalence class* and *class inclusion*. Specifically, I make a controversial claim that whereas preschool children's early categorical concepts are organized primarily on the basis of prototypes (Rosch, 1978), perceptual similarity, and characteristic features, older children's concepts are organized primarily on the basis of defining features (Keil & Batterman, 1984). This is not to say that older children lack prototypes, but that they have two kinds of representation available (see Osherson & Smith, 1981). When categories are based on defining as opposed to characteristic features, children form *equivalence classes* in which any instance of a class is equally representative of the class because it possesses the defining criteria. Thus, categories demonstrate relative flexibility in the substitutability of instances within frames such as "X is a bird."

Without the notion of bootstrapping, explaining the acquisition of categories based on defining features within a constructivist approach leads again to the constructivist paradox. An explanation that avoids this paradox would be one according to which children construct equivalence classes through an analogy mapping with coordinate structures in the language domain. Recall that in order to form coordinate structures and apply conjunction reduction, the components must be identical in grammatical form. Similarly, in order to explain the construction of hierarchical categorical structures based on defining features, I propose that children construct such structures through an analogy mapping with subordinate structures in the language domain. The acquisition data would seem to be at least consistent with this proposal in that children master coordination and subordination before demonstrating equivalence classes and hierarchical organizations of equivalence classes. I might again note that my proposals regarding the course of conceptual development are by no means mainstream.

Although the details and empirical consequences of these three proposals still have to be worked out, it is clear that they are distinct from prior language–thought proposals in several ways. First, unlike Whorf's they admit of a thought representational system that is equally as important as a language system. Unlike Piaget, they assume that language affects thought and is not simply a tool for the expression of ideas. Unlike the Chomsky–Fodor proposal, there is not a one-to-one correspondence between internal-language (i.e., thought) predicates and natural-language predicates. Rather, there is more of a dynamic asynchrony between these systems, which precipitates the conceptual and linguistic (syntactic, semantic, and pragmatic) developments described in this chapter. Whereas each of the proposals has merit, I favor the third because it permits the specification of multiple bootstrapping operations, which can be verified empirically.

Conclusions

From the description of the conceptual and linguistic components of *if* and *because* expressions, I hope it is apparent that children need to acquire substantial knowledge in order to produce and comprehend a full range of *if* and *because* expressions. It is also apparent, however, that children acquire most of this knowledge between the ages of 3 and 8. This is quite an impressive accomplishment, but also one that is necessary given the key role that such expressions play in the context of problem solving, inference making, argumentation, and so on.

Furthermore, whereas a great deal is known about the nature and development of these expressions, there is still much more to learn. In particular, the intricate relations between syntactic, semantic, and pragmatic issues must be more fully worked out than has been done here, and empirical data on children's knowledge of these relations must be collected. Moreover, longitudinal studies of cycles of conceptual change following linguistic change and vice versa should be conducted in order to explore which of the language–thought proposals have the most merit.

References

Anderson, A. R., & Belnap, N. D. (1962). The pure calculus of entailment. *Journal of Symbolic Logic, 21*, 19–53.

Anderson, J. R. (1982). Acquisition of cognitive skill. *Psychological Review, 89*, 369–406.

Andersson, L.-G. (1975). *Form and function of subordinate clauses.* Göteburg: University of Göteburg Press.

Bates, E. (1976). *Language and context: The acquisition of pragmatics.* New York: Academic Press.

Bereiter, C. (1985). Toward a solution of the learning paradox. *Review of Educational Research, 55*, 201–226.

Berko Gleason, J., Perlmann, R. Y., & Greif, E. B. (1984). What's the magic word? Learning language through politeness routines. *Discourse Processes, 7*, 493–502.

Bloom, L., & Capatides, J. B. (1987). Sources of meaning in the acquisition of complex syntax: The sample case of causality. *Journal of Experimental Child Psychology, 43*, 112–128.

Bloom, L., Lahey, M., Hood, L., Lifter, K., & Fiess, K. (1980). Complex sentences: Acquisition of syntactic connectives and the semantic relations they encode. *Journal of Child Language, 7*, 235–261.

Bowerman, M. (1986). First steps in acquiring conditionals. In E. C. Traugott, A. ter Meulen, J. S. Reilly, & C. A. Ferguson (Eds.), *On conditionals* (pp. 285–307). Cambridge University Press.

Bresnan, J. W. (1979). *Theory of complementation in English syntax.* New York: Garland.

Brown, R. (1973). *A first language.* Cambridge, MA: Harvard University Press.

Bullock, M., Baillargeon, R., & Gelman, R. (1982). The development of causal reasoning. In W. Friedman (Ed.), *The developmental psychology of time* (pp. 209–254). New York: Academic Press.

Byrnes, J. P. (1988). Formal operations: A systematic reformulation. *Developmental Review, 8*, 1–22.

Byrnes, J. P., & Duff, M. A. (1988). Young children's comprehension and production of causal expressions. *Child Study Journal, 18*, 101–119.

Byrnes, J. P., & Gelman, S. A. (1990). Conceptual and linguistic factors in children's memory for causal expressions. *International Journal of Behavioral Development, 13*, 95–117.

Byrnes, J. P., & Overton, W. F. (1988). Reasoning about logical connectives: A developmental analysis. *Journal of Experimental Child Psychology, 46*, 194–218.

Carey, S. (1985). *Conceptual change in childhood.* Cambridge, MA: MIT Press.

Clark, E. V. (1983). Meanings and concepts. In P. H. Mussen (Ed.), *Handbook of child psychology* (Vol. 3, pp. 787–840). New York: Wiley.

Corrigan, R. (1975). A scalogram analysis of the development of the use and comprehension of "because" in children. *Child Development, 46*, 195–201.

Emerson, H. F. (1979). Children's comprehension of 'because' in reversible and non-reversible sentences. *Journal of Child Language, 6*, 279–300.

Emerson, H. F. (1980). Children's judgment of correct and reversed sentences with 'if.' *Journal of Child Language, 7*, 137–155.

Emerson, H. F., & Gekoski, W. L. (1980). Development of comprehension of sentences with 'because' and 'if.' *Journal of Experimental Child Psychology, 29*, 202–224.

Fillenbaum, S. (1977). Mind your *p*'s and *q*'s: The role of content and context in some uses of 'and,' 'or,' and 'if.' In G. Bower (Ed.), *The psy-*

chology of learning and motivation (Vol. 11, pp. 41–100). New York: Academic Press.

Fillenbaum, S. (1986). The use of conditionals in inducements and deterrents. In E. C. Traugott, A. ter Meulen, J. S. Reilly, & C. A. Ferguson (Eds.), *On conditionals* (pp. 179–195). Cambridge University Press.

Fodor, J. A. (1975). *The language of thought.* Cambridge, MA: Harvard University Press.

Frege, G. (1952). *Translations from the philosophical writings of Gottlob Frege* (P. Geach & M. Black, Eds.). Oxford: Blackwell Publisher.

French, L. A., & Nelson, K. (1985). *Young children's knowledge of relational terms: Some ifs, ors, and buts.* New York: Springer.

Geis, M., & Zwicky, A. M. (1971). On invited inferences. *Linguistic Inquiry, 2,* 127–132.

Gelman, S. A., & Markman, E. M. (1985). Implicit contrast in adjectives vs. nouns: Implications for word-learning in preschoolers. *Journal of Child Language, 12,* 125–143.

Haiman, J. (1986). Constraints on the form and meaning of the protasis. In E. C. Traugott, A. ter Meulen, J. S. Reilly, & C. A. Ferguson (Eds.), *On conditionals* (pp. 215–225). Cambridge University Press.

Hood, L., & Bloom, L. (1979). What, when, and how about why: A longitudinal study of early expressions of causality. *Monographs of the Society for Research in Child Development, 44*(6, Serial No. 181).

Jackendoff, R. (1977). *X-bar syntax: A study of phrase structure.* Cambridge, MA: MIT Press.

Jespersen, O. (1968). *The philosophy of grammar.* London: Allen & Unwin.

Johnson, H. C., & Chapman, R. S. (1980). Children's judgment and recall of causal connectives: A developmental study of 'because,' 'so,' and 'and.' *Journal of Psycholinguistic Research, 9,* 243–260.

Karmiloff-Smith, A. (1986). From meta-processes to conscious access: Evidence from children's metalinguistic and repair data. *Cognition, 23,* 95–147.

Kartunnen, L. (1971). Counterfactual conditionals. *Linguistic Inquiry, 2,* 556–569.

Keil, F. C. (1979). The development of young children's ability to anticipate the outcomes of simple causal events. *Child Development, 50,* 455–462.

Keil, F. C., & Batterman, N. (1984). A characteristic-to-defining shift in the development of word meaning. *Journal of Verbal Learning and Verbal Behavior, 23,* 221–236.

Kuczaj, S. A. (1981). Factors influencing children's hypothetical reference. *Journal of Child Language, 8,* 131–137.

Kuhn, D., & Phelps, H. (1976). The development of children's comprehension of causal direction. *Child Development, 47,* 248–251.

Lakoff, G. (1971). On generative semantics. In D. D. Steinberg & L. A. Jakobovits (Eds.), *Semantics: An interdisciplinary reader in philosophy, linguistics, and psychology* (pp. 232–296). Cambridge University Press.

Lawson, A. E. (1983). The acquisition of formal operational schemata during adolescence: The role of the biconditional. *Journal of Research in Science Teaching, 20,* 347–356.

Lewis, C. I., & Langford, C. H. (1932). *Symbolic logic.* New York: Century.

Mandler, J. M. (1983). Representation. In P. H. Mussen (Ed.), *Handbook of child psychology* (Vol. 3, pp. 420–494). New York: Wiley.

MacWhinney, B., & Snow, C. (1985). The child language data exchange system. *Journal of Child Language, 12,* 271–296.

McCabe, A. E., Evely, S., Abramovitch, R., Corter, C. M., & Pepler, D. J. (1983). Conditional statements in young children's spontaneous speech. *Journal of Child Language, 10,* 253–258.

McCawley, J. D. (1971). Where do noun phrases come from? In D. D. Steinberg & L. A. Jakobovits (Eds.), *Semantics: An interdisciplinary reader in philosophy, linguistics, and psychology* (pp. 218–231). Cambridge University Press.

Moshman, D. (1979). Development of formal hypothesis-testing ability. *Developmental Psychology, 15,* 104–112.

Nagel, E. (1961). *The structure of science.* New York: Harcourt, Brace, & World.

Newmeyer, F. J. (1986). *Linguistic theory in America.* New York: Academic Press.

O'Brien, D. P., & Overton, W. F. (1980). Conditional reasoning following contradictory evidence: A developmental analysis. *Journal of Experimental Child Psychology, 30,* 44–61.

Osherson, D., & Smith, E. E. (1981). On the adequacy of prototype theory as a theory of concepts. *Cognition, 9,* 35–58.

Overton, W. F., Byrnes, J. P., & O'Brien, D. P. (1985). Developmental and individual differences in conditional reasoning: The role of contradiction training and cognitive style. *Developmental Psychology, 21,* 692–701.

Paris, S. G. (1973). Comprehension of language connectives and propositional logical relationships. *Journal of Experimental Child Psychology, 16,* 278–291.

Piaget, J. (1928). *Judgment and reasoning in the child.* Totowa, NJ: Littlefield, Adams.

Piaget, J. (1952). *The origins of intelligence in children.* New York: International Universities Press.

Piaget, J. (1974). *Understanding causality.* New York: Norton.

Pieraut-LeBonniec, G. (1980). *The development of modal reasoning: Genesis of necessity and possibility notions.* New York: Academic Press.

Pinker, S. (1984). *Language learnability and language development.* Cambridge, MA: Harvard University Press.

Puglielli, A., & Ciliberti, A. (1973). Il condizionale. *Atti del VI Convego Internazionale della Societa Linguistica Italiana.* Rome: Bulzoni.

Quine, W. V. O. (1950). *Methods of logic.* New York: Holt, Rinehart, & Winston.

Rogoff, B., Malkin, C., & Gilbride, K. (1984). Interaction with babies as guidance in development. In B. Rogoff & J. V. Wertsch (Eds.), *Children's learning in the "zone of proximal development"* (pp. 31–44). San Francisco: Jossey-Bass.

Rosch, E. (1978). Principles of categorization. In E. Rosch & B. B. Lloyd (Eds.), *Cognition and categorization* (pp. 27–48). Hillsdale, NJ: Erlbaum.

Scholnick, E. K., & Wing, C. S. (1982). The pragmatics of subordinating conjunctions: A second look. *Journal of Child Language, 9,* 461–479.

Scholnick, E. K., & Wing, C. S. (1983). Evaluating presuppositions and propositions. *Journal of Child Language, 10,* 639–660.

Searle, J. R. (1976). A classification of illocutionary acts. *Language in Society, 5,* 1–23.

Searle, J. R. (1983). *Intentionality.* Cambridge University Press.

Shultz, T. R., & Kestenbaum, N. R. (1985). Causal reasoning in children.

In G. J. Whitehurst (Ed.), *Annals of child development* (Vol. 2, pp. 195–249). Greenwich, CT: JAI Press.

Slobin, D. I. (1979). *Psycholinguistics* (2nd ed.). Glenville, IL: Scott, Foresman.

Stalnaker, R. C. (1984). *Inquiry.* Cambridge, MA: MIT Press.

Staudenmayer, H., & Bourne, L. (1977). Learning to interpret conditional sentences: A developmental study. *Developmental Psychology, 13,* 616–623.

Sternberg, R. J. (1979). Developmental patterns in the encoding and combination of logical connectives. *Journal of Experimental Child Psychology, 28,* 469–498.

Taplin, J. E., Staudenmayer, H., & Taddonio, J. L. (1974). Developmental changes in conditional reasoning: Linguistic or logical? *Journal of Experimental Child Psychology, 17,* 360–373.

Traugott, E. C., ter Meulen, A., Reilly, J. S., & Ferguson, C. A. (1986). *On conditionals.* Cambridge University Press.

Vygotsky, L. S. (1962). *Thought and language.* Cambridge, MA: MIT Press.

Wellman, H. M. (1985). The child's theory of mind. In S. R. Yussen (Ed.), *The growth of reflection* (pp. 169–206). New York: Academic Press.

Werner, H., & Kaplan, B. (1963). *Symbol formation.* New York: Wiley.

Wing, C. S., & Scholnick, E. K. (1981). Children's comprehension of pragmatic concepts expressed in 'because,' 'although,' 'if,' and 'unless.' *Journal of Child Language, 8,* 347–365.

Younger, B. A. (1985). The segregation of items into categories by ten-month-old infants. *Child Development, 56,* 1574–1583.

IV. The role of social interaction

11. The language of thinking: Metacognitive and conditional words

ELLIN KOFSKY SCHOLNICK AND WILLIAM S. HALL

> The consistency of human behavior, such as it is, is due entirely
> to the fact men have formulated their desires, and subsequently
> rationalized them, in terms of words. . . . For evil, then, as well
> as for good, words make us the human beings we actually are.
> Huxley (1962, pp. 4–5)

Slobin (1979) notes that human culture, social behavior, and thinking could not exist as we know them in the absence of language.
Although we are inclined to agree with both Slobin's and Aldous
Huxley's assessments of the importance of language in our lives, it
is not entirely clear how best to define that importance. This di-
lemma has bedeviled thoughtful persons since at least the beginnings of philosophical inquiry. In this chapter we begin with a brief
review of the language–thought controversy and an analysis of the
roots of the problem, and then describe some research that addresses the issue.

A taxonomy of theories

Huxley and Slobin represent a traditional and persistent hypothesis
in psychology, that language and thought are equivalent and that
language is primary. In the behaviorist tradition, thought was considered to be subvocal speech. In contemporary psychology, knowledge is characterized as semantic understanding. A concept is a dictionary definition or an encyclopedia entry. Planning, problem
solving, and reasoning, all examples of thought, require that knowledge used to access them be coded and stored. Although there is
much debate about the form in which coding takes place, words are
among the most obvious candidates. Contemporary cognitive psychology has proposed other alternatives that are also linguistic, such

as propositions (Frederiksen, 1975; Kintsch, 1974), prototypes, and features. Propositional models interrelate concepts in an abstract network. The links between concepts in semantic networks are largely sentential. Feature models break down concepts into semantic components, such as *human* and *female*.

There are two other views of the relation between language and thinking. The converse view accepts equivalence but claims that cognition is primary, and language is simply a verbal description of thought. The third view claims overlap, but not equivalence. There is thought without language. Everyday observations of behavior support this third possibility. People grope to find words or the best way to express an idea. Artists and composers provide other examples.

The third view, that of overlap, raises issues of influence, and here, too, there are opposing ideas: those of unidirectional influence and of bidirectional influence. Unidirectional views claim either that language influences thought or that thought influences language. From the bidirectional perspective language and thought influence one another. An example of the unidirectional view is Piaget's (1969) account of language and thinking before adolescence. He claimed that language and thought have the same roots, in sensorimotor actions. Language is but one by-product of children's growing representational skills. The emergence of the symbolic function produces language and operative thought. However, cognitive development proceeds on its own and actually paces linguistic development. That is, children cannot use language unless they possess the concepts to which words refer. Further, Piaget argued that the child's intellect grows through interaction with things and people in the environment, and to the extent that language is involved in these interactions, it may amplify and facilitate development in some cases, but it does not in itself bring about cognitive growth.

Brown (1973) literally took up the Piagetian view to explain children's early multiword sentences. Investigating corpora of children from a wide variety of cultures, Brown found eight semantic relations prevalent in their speech. He argued that the frequency of these relations in the speech of children from such a wide variety of cultural backgrounds was due to the fact that they "constitute the linguistic expression of sensorimotor intelligence, or the kind of basic understanding . . . that children everywhere form during the first two years of life" (Brown, 1973, p. 174). In contrast, Bowerman (1988) has demonstrated more recently that children's early use of spatial markers is very much dictated by the linguistic distinctions made in their native language.

Piaget's theory does introduce bidirectional or mutual influence into formal operations. In adolescence, alone, language begins to play a more important role in thinking, being a necessary but not sufficient influence on thinking. Teenagers reason about verbal propositions and use language to monitor reasoning. Thus, language provides the capacity for self-reflection and a means of representing thought, while thought continues to refine semantic concepts and relations.

Vygotsky (1962) also argued for mutual influences on development, but he posed a different course for the interaction of speech and thinking. He described the origin of thought as the internalization of communicative speech, a process taking place in the preschool period. At that point language and thought develop in parallel; later they diverge; and eventually, with the acquisition of literacy, metalinguistic and higher-order reasoning skills interact.

Roots of the controversy

Definitions of language and thinking

Why have so many diverse views been offered about the relationship between language and thought? Perhaps differences arise because the theories do not describe the same entities, and they propose different types of influence. They work from different definitions of the nature of language and cognition, two multifaceted domains. For example, in their discussions of the connection between thought and language, Piaget and Chomsky (Piatelli-Palmerini, 1980) did not pose similar models of either area. Chomsky adopted a computational model of thinking processes, and Piaget, a logical model of thought structure. Chomsky emphasized the syntactic structure of language, and Piaget was concerned with the capacity for signification and the content of semantic schemes. The lack of consensus on the nature of language and thinking inevitably produces divergent views on their relation.

Moreover, from some theoretical perspectives neither cognition nor language is homogeneous. Spatial cognition may differ from solving verbal analogies both in the way that information is represented and in the kinds of operations that must be performed on representations during the course of thinking (Kosslyn, 1981). Each domain requires symbol manipulation, but the nature of the symbols and the way they are processed may differ. Language is also multifaceted. Although theories of sentence interpretation may integrate each dimension of language, the nature of phonological, syntactic, semantic, and pragmatic representations may differ, as may the operations and abilities needed to manipulate those representations to appreciate and apply linguistic rules. Even within each facet of language, there may be subtle, but important differences in the way content is acquired, symbolized, and processed depending on the material. This is particularly likely to be the case with the pragmatic and semantic uses of language. For example, different abilities may be recruited to learn the names of objects, internal states, and logical connectives. Because language is multifaceted and thinking is domain-specific, generalizations about the relations between language and thinking are also likely to be multifaceted and domain-specific.

Consequently, it is necessary to analyze any domain to determine what specific role language and cognition could play in its construction. In addition, task analysis is needed. The behaviors chosen as indices of understanding can bias generalizations about the language–thought relation. For example, in studying spatial development, the role of language and thinking in the mastery of spatial vocabulary may differ from their role in the acquisition of the ability to predict the outcome of figure rotation. Therefore, any discussion of the language–thought relation requires careful theoretical analysis of the content area in order to specify the particular role that language and thinking play in the acquisition of knowledge. That analysis is a prerequisite for determining whether generalizations about one domain will apply to others.

Nature of influence

Another source of differences among theories is the diversity of models of influence (Flavell, 1972). Language and thought may influence one another in at least four ways. First, one may be the necessary prerequisite of the other, as when Brown (1973) suggests that object permanence underlies the ability to label events and their recurrence. Second, a weaker view is that knowledge in one area may be sufficient to produce progress, but it is not the only source of development because there are potential alternative influences. For example, we may gain knowledge of spatial locations through direct perception, deduction, or verbal descriptions (Case, 1985). Third, one domain can modulate another, either facilitating or damping acquisition, activation, and utilization of skills (Overton, Byrnes, & O'Brien, 1985). For example, it may be harder to express a concept in one language than another, or in one syntactic frame than another. Finally, one process may provide a context for practicing the other, as when children exercise reasoning skills in conversation. Verbal rehearsal of procedures for problem solving may make their use less effortful.

In summary, we argue that the degree of overlap between language and thought may depend upon the content domain a theory attempts to describe. Similarly, whether language is the producer, by-product, or equal partner of thought in development may depend on the content area studied and the actual role that each process is thought to play.

The view that language–thought relations are diverse and multidirectional has a cost. It may fragment the language–thought question into an infinite series: language and thinking about space, time, objects, actions, and so on. But there is much to be gained from specifying why the study of a particular content area is potentially revealing of the relation between language and reasoning. A specification of the role of language and thought in a given domain can also provide a basis for choosing other domains in which language and thought might play similar roles.

In this chapter we discuss two areas in which the interaction of language and thought is mandatory: metacognitive language and logical connectives. Each involves the acquisition of terms to describe thinking. We take the position that talking about thought is not the same as thinking. If this is the case, the language of thinking and the language by which thinking is expressed must involve interactions between the two realms. Because the focus is on the language of cognitive processing and because the data used in the discussion are drawn from conversational protocols, linguistic influences are heavily emphasized. In each area language is an integral component of thinking because it enables the language learner to transcend the immediate and to take a more reflective view of the self as cognizer and of the reality that concepts and language represent.

We will proceed by examining each area separately, metacognitive language and the use of subordinating conjunctions with a focus on *if*. We begin with a description of the semantic structure of each content area. Next we discuss theories about the role of language and thinking in structuring awareness of cognitive processes and logical relations. We then report data from conversations between children and adults that reveal how conversational partners understand the semantic structure of the domain. We use these data to evaluate the theories about the role of language and thinking in acquiring a metacognitive and logical lexicon. Finally, we evaluate whether there is any commonality between explanations of the role of linguistic and cognitive influences in the acquisition of a lexicon for monitoring awareness of thinking and for expressing the products of reasoning.

Metacognitive language: The internal-state lexicon

An overview

Internal-state language describes beliefs, ideas, thoughts, and intentions. It is language by which we signal to ourselves and others that we are engaged in some form of internal processing of events, and it is the language by which we identify that others are engaged in internal processing. It is important to note, however, that metacognition cannot be equated with internal-state language. The use of *think*, for example, is not synonymous with thought, and thoughts need not be verbal. Rather, we claim that every meaningful use of an internal-state word indicates an act of metacognition by the speaker. Language plays two roles, then, in metacognition. First, it allows us to gain access to our internal states, to monitor and transform them. Language plays an important role in metacognition, because it is a tool for monitoring. Second, discussions of the behavior of others may provide information about the situations and behavioral cues by which to judge that others are engaged in cognitive processing. Consequently, we make two major assumptions about this domain of language. (a) The terminology used to describe internal states can be used by individuals to gain access to those states and monitor them. (b) That terminology can also be a subject of reflection and enable the individual to understand and interrelate aspects of mental functioning to one another. Distinctions among *see, think,* and *know* may lead the individual to ponder the relation of thought and perception, and belief versus hypothesis (Hall & Nagy, 1987).

The syntax of internal-state words

The major task of children in acquiring an internal-state vocabulary is the same as that of researchers – to define states and to make distinctions among them. We begin with a description of the general domain before discussing in detail one part of it, metacognitive language. Internal-state words appear in several syntactic categories. In many cases, they appear as verbs with the human experiencer as subject or object, as in sentences (1) through (4). Sometimes, as in sentences (5) and (6), internal states are expressed as abstract nouns and, in other cases, as in sentences (7) and (8), as adjectives.

(1)   I *think* you should invite him.
(2)   Jack *knows* the answer.
(3)   It *annoys* him.
(4)   It finally *dawned* on me that . . .
(5)   It's the *thought* that counts.
(6)   That would be a hard *choice* to make.
(7)   He was *angry*.
(8)   She was *delighted*.

The semantics of internal-state language

Internal-state words can be classified into four semantic categories describing (a) cognition, (b) affect, (c) perception, and (d) intentions and desires (Hall & Nagy, 1987). *Cognitive* words describe consciousness, knowledge, and understanding (*aware, remember*), directed attention (*notice*), thinking (*concentrate*), and mental states relative to a proposition (*belief, guess*) as well as mental acts relative to a proposition (*pretend, make-believe*). *Affective* words describe feelings and emotions (e.g., *afraid, angry, ashamed, blue, delighted*). The *perceptual* category includes two subcategories – the five senses (e.g., *see* and *hear*), as well as more "internal" senses (e.g., *dizzy, thirsty, ache*). Words belonging to the *intentions and desires* category cover several semantic subclasses, including wants and desires (*like*), intentions, plans, purposes, determination (*resolve*), willingness (*volunteer*), and choice and decision (*pick*).

Problems of definition. The preceding examples are prototypes of internal-state language, but in some instances the boundary is fuzzy so that it is not always clear whether a word refers to an internal state. Fuzziness of boundaries is also intertwined with a different kind of fuzziness. Words and meanings are not synonymous. The lexical units of a language can differ from "words" in that a word can have several distinct and unrelated meanings, not all of which refer to internal states. In the case of idioms, more than one word comprises a lexical unit, as in *feel blue.* We discuss three boundary problems: determining the focus of word meanings; evaluating causatives; and distinguishing the act from the object of perception.

The complexity of word meanings makes the task of classifying words as members of the internal-state lexicon anything but trivial. It is often difficult to determine whether a word focuses primarily on an internal state. We illustrate this with an analysis of the word *lie.*

> To say that someone is lying says something both about their beliefs (they don't believe what they are saying) and their intentions (they intend to deceive the addressee). This deliberate deception involves the internal states of the addressee as well: the liar intends for the addressee to believe both the content of the lie, and that the liar believes what he/she is saying. Notice how complex the internal state component of the meaning of *lie* is: the person lying has intentions about the beliefs of the addressee, including the addressee's beliefs about the intentions and beliefs of the person lying. (Hall & Nagy, 1986, p. 31)

Despite the similarity of the word *lie* to many words in the internal-state domain, it is not an internal-state word because the internal-state component of the meaning of the word *lie* is not its primary and focal component. Rather, the focus is on producing an untruth.

The same issue applies to *causatives.* Some causatives appear to be candidates for the internal-state lexicon because their overall meaning contains internal-state meanings. The claim is readily apparent in the following list of causatives:

persuade	cause to believe
convince	cause to believe
fool	cause to believe something not true
mislead	cause to believe something not true
deceive	cause to believe something not true
teach	cause to learn
distract	cause to cease momentarily to pay attention

However, the suitability of members of this list for classification as internal-state words is not always clear. They belong in this category when their intent is to describe a change in internal state. Words like *anger*, *sadden*, and *deceive* imply or include change of an internal state as a major part of their meaning. In contrast, lying to someone does not guarantee a change in the listener's belief. Words like *persuade, convince, distract, fool,* or *mislead* cannot be evaluated as internal-state words without contextual evidence that there is a change in internal state and that the focus is on the change in the state itself, not on the act that produced it. The *convinced* of "I am *convinced* that he's right" refers to an internal-state meaning. "John *distracted* him" says nothing about John's internal state, but "He was *distracted*" does.

A related issue arises in the perceptual category of internal-state words. A distinction must be made between the act of perception and the content or object of perception. The distinction can be illustrated with the words *red* and *see*. The word *red* is clearly perceptual in some sense, and it relates to internal states in some significant way; yet it seem inappropriate to label it an internal-state word. *Red* describes a percept or concept. The word *see* (or *hear*), in contrast, refers to the process or experience of perceiving; it is clearly an internal-state word and would be so classified.

The semantic–pragmatic distinction. In categorizing a word as referring to an internal state, the listener must also take into account the speaker's communicative intent. Internal-state words are sometimes used to communicate about something else. A distinction must be made between semantic and pragmatic uses. A semantic use occurs when the literal internal-state meaning of a word contributes directly to the intended meaning of the utterance containing it. The use of the word *know* in the following utterance illustrates this point:

(9) Jack *knows* the answer.

Barring unusual contextual constraints, the intended meaning of this utterance refers to Jack, knowledge, and the answer to some question; that is, the literal internal-state meaning of *know* plays a straightforward and obvious role in determining the meaning of the utterance. The same claim cannot be made for sentence (10):

(10) You *know*, Jack could play shortstop.

In this sentence, under normal circumstances, *know* is not used to convey anything about knowledge itself. It is an attention getter.

The literal meaning of the word *know* does not contribute to the propositional content of the sentence. Pragmatic use describes those cases in which the literal internal-state meaning of a word contributes indirectly, if at all, to the intended meaning of an utterance.

Pragmatic uses of internal-state words often appear in *indirect speech acts*, that is, utterances whose intended meaning can be inferred from the literal meaning by principles of conversation (Gordon & Lakoff, 1971). Sentences (11) and (12) illustrate this usage:

(11)   Do you *want* to take out the garbage, please?
(12)   You *know* what I'll do. I'll talk to the boss about it.

Internal-state words have a second pragmatic function, as conversational devices and mannerisms. They appear in highly stereotyped phrases containing internal-state words that have either completely, or almost completely, lost their internal content, as in the following:

(13)   You *know*, I should do something about that leak.

Hedges, which use primarily cognitive internal-state words to convey uncertainty, are a third pragmatic usage of internal-state words. An illustration is

(14)   It's going to rain, I *think*.

Attentional devices are a fourth and final pragmatic use of internal-state words. These words are used primarily to get the addressee's attention. They include the imperative of verbs like *look*, as in "*Look* what I did." Another use occurs in questions and reduced questions with *see*, such as "You *see* that?"

In summary, we have presented some of the problems and issues associated with defining internal-state words as indicators of metacognition and with determining the boundaries of these words. We have examined four major subclasses: cognitive, perceptual, affective, and intentional words. The boundary problems in this area arise from lexical ambiguity and from difficulties in determining whether an internal-state component in a complex word meaning is the central component of that meaning. We have also outlined two basic categories of usage, the semantic and pragmatic. This distinction depends on whether the lexical meaning of an internal-state word contributes directly, indirectly, or not at all to the intended meaning of the utterance in which it occurs.

Implications for linguistic development. Problems in defining the boundaries of internal-state words have implications for understanding lexical acquisition. One boundary problem is that internal-state words differ from other words. Many words have objective referents, allowing children to verify the mapping of a word to an object, attribute, or action. Children can learn by ostensive definition. In contrast, mental states are ephemeral, private, and intangible (Wellman & Estes, 1987). They vary in accessibility. We have feelings of forgetting, or of knowing, but not necessarily of thinking. A second problem is that it is often difficult to separate the act of thinking or perceiving from its content. To become aware of these states, the mental processor must step away from the content to monitor the self.

The history of psychology (Overton, in press) reflects a struggle between those who claim that internal states, such as knowledge, are the product of external influences as opposed to those who attribute their construction to an active mental processor. So it is not surprising that language itself is fuzzy about internal versus external referents and that the language learner would have a similar problem in constructing a mental-state lexicon. We suggest that the language learner will begin by confusing the external with the internal and by confusing the object of an internal state with the state itself.

Theories claiming that thought and language are distinct, but overlapping, must explain the role of language in processing and monitoring mental states. Children think, perceive, feel, and intend. Language provides labels for those processes and a description of the means by which children can infer that these internal states have transpired in themselves and others. Language may also provide children with a set of beliefs about the nature and consequences of mental processing. In this way, language is a means by which children can gain access to and discriminate among internal states. Because the language of internal states is not the state itself, language also provides a distinctive mechanism for self-monitoring. Language provides a sufficient tool for self-awareness.

Language is also a context in which metacognitive skills are practiced and refined (Braine & Rumain, 1983; Olson & Torrance, 1987). Note that the examples of pragmatic versus semantic uses and of words with a central versus a peripheral internal state focus come from discourse. In text analysis, readers, who must monitor the author's cognitive processes, learn something about their own.

Understanding mental-state language

A review of the literature on the internal-state lexicon suggests that its development reflects the differentiation of mental from nonmental uses. Our own research implicates the role of language and conversational context in that differentiation. We will focus on two internal-state categories, cognitive and perceptual words.

Comprehension tasks

Macnamara, Baker, and Olson (1976) report that children have some understanding of cognitive internal-state words as early as the fourth year of life. This finding is corroborated by Johnson and Maratsos (1977), who studied young children's understanding of *think* and *know* in a story format. Three-year-olds could not understand the words, but by 4, young children began to understand the critical distinction between thinking and knowing. Thinking involves hypotheses, but knowing involves truth. This research suggests that young children can distinguish real and mental events, use words to express mental events, and use *think* and *know* to express their understanding.

A similar conclusion was reached by Miscione, Marvin, O'Brien, and Greenberg (1978), who studied young children's knowledge of *know* and *guess*. Children were tested using a task involving knowing versus guessing an object's location. Three-year-olds, but not older children, used an outcome-based strategy in which knowing was equated with guessing correctly, and guessing with making the wrong choice. They used external, not internal, states to differentiate between the words.

Wellman and his colleagues obtained similar results in several investigations. In the first of these (Johnson & Wellman, 1980; Wellman & Johnson, 1979), children's understanding of cognitive words, especially *remember, know, forget,* and *guess,* was tested. As in other research the children judged word meaning on the basis of whether they made the right choice, not on internal criteria. By 4 years of age children distinguish *know* from *think* and *guess,* but even 8-year-olds have difficulty in differentiating between *think* and *guess* (Moore, Bryant, & Furrow, 1989).

Shatz, Wellman, and Silber (1983) and Bretherton and Beeghly (1982) analyzed children's conversations in order to determine when children first used language that referred to mental states. The first use of this language was pragmatic, not semantic. First semantic uses appear as children approach their third birthday.

Levels of meaning

By and large the research we have been discussing has dealt with the ability to distinguish among words like *know*, *guess*, and *think*. The underlying assumption is that such words have a single meaning. In addition, there has been little attempt to assess how the language environment might affect the acquisition of metacognitive language. Hall, Scholnick, and Hughes (1987) suggest that the mental versus nonmental distinction is perhaps an oversimplification. They developed a taxonomy of uses of cognitive words that range in "internality." They also claim that perceptual and cognitive words may have several meanings. Although a given word may be used primarily at one level, it may be extended to other levels.

They report research in which audiotaped recordings were obtained from 36 children who differed in ethnicity (black or white) and social class (working class or professional). The children were taped at least once in each of three situations: free play, directed activity at school, and dinner. The protocols of the children's conversations were coded in order to isolate words that referred to the processes of perceiving, attending, thinking, choosing, or deciding. Each word was categorized into one of the following six levels of meaning on the basis of utterance context. The category scheme begins with the use of these words to refer to external, perceptual data. The categories then move toward increasing internalization and depth of processing of input. The higher levels are increasingly metacognitive and epistemological.

(1)   *Perception* words describe immediate sensory input. The speaker reports the act of perception or draws attention to the speaker or the utterance – for example, "*Watch* me draw" or "I *heard* your story."

(2)   *Recognition* words describe the process of relating input to past experience in order to determine whether that input has been encountered before. The speaker makes a judgment of familiarity or lack of it – for example, "I've *seen* that before" or "I *remember* his face."

(3)   *Recall* describes the actual retrieval of past input. The speaker refers to specific factual information that she recalls or uses a word in a "test question" to elicit factual information. Thus, when the speaker asks, "Do you *know* his name?" or "Do you *remember* the last time we went to a museum?" to cue recall of specific facts, those cognitive words belong in this category.

(4)   *Understanding* describes the referral of knowledge to a semantic network. The speaker refers to conceptual relations, frameworks, or reasoning, as in "I know *why* he did that" or "I *see* what you mean."

(5)   *Metacognitive* words describe the speaker's stepping away from the act to describe awareness of the process, not the product of thinking, as in "*Pretending* can be fun" or "I'm using my *imagination*."

(6)   *Evaluation* occurs when the speaker uses the word to contrast or evaluate messages in terms of whether they imply true observations, contrary to fact propositions, or uncertainty. The speaker refers to suppositions about the truth of statements – for example, "He *guessed* the answer, but I *know* it." This level has been the focus of many experimental studies of cognitive language, but our claim is that children could understand something about cognitive language, but not yet grasp distinctions about contrasting suppositions.

The conversations were analyzed for frequency and diversity of use of cognitive words at different levels of meaning. Overall, both at home and at school, the adults' production of a cognitive state vocabulary was approximately double that of the children. But children's language was correlated with that of adults, so there was a strong relation between the amount of cognitive language the child heard and the child's own production. In addition, the diversity of adult speech that each child heard predicted the overall variety of the child's cognitive internal-state words. Unlike analyses of syntactic learning, adult input affected the children's learning of labels for cognitive states.

This is not surprising, because children cannot invent a communicative vocabulary to refer to mental states, and the elusive, private nature of mental states makes them hard to grasp. When parents provide them with a rich lexicon for labeling mental states, children are faced with an important task. They must distinguish words from one another so as to understand and use the appropriate label. Perhaps the process of making such distinctions enables them to distinguish among perceiving, thinking, understanding, and evaluating. Parents may also use different words within the same sentence frame, such as "I *know, am sure, observed* that the circus is coming." This may provoke children to think about the interconnections among events. Moreover, some sentence frames provide a mental event structure for children. They describe what usually happens when one *thinks*, or *plans*, or *pretends*. Not only do parents tell children the object of thought, but they may also tell them the causes and consequences of some states. So language may have an important influence on a child's theory of mind, because the child is exposed to others' theories of mind.

Developmental differences in the size of the internal-state lexicon precluded direct comparisons of the ways in which children and adults used these words. Instead, scores were converted to proportions in order to ascertain the proportion of words in the lexicon used at each level of meaning. Adults devote a smaller proportion of their lexicon to perceptual meanings than do children and more of their lexicon to metacognitive meanings than do children. But for each age group, the greatest variety of words describes perceptions (Level 1), followed by recall (Level 3), and metacognition (Level 5).

We assumed that Levels 4 through 6 express more advanced understanding of cognitive processes. Although 36% of the child's cognitive lexicon was used to express these three levels, 57% of the adult's cognitive words were at these levels. Children who hear adults using the higher levels of meaning also use more of their available cognitive vocabulary to express those three levels of meaning, r (34) = .62, $p < .05$. Although most preschool children do use the range of cognitive levels, an important conclusion is that they do not use the deeper levels of meaning with abundance. However, this is but a preliminary finding, because the data were restricted to the spontaneous speech of $4\frac{1}{2}$ to 5-year-olds in unstructured situations. A fuller examination of a wider age range might shed light on the origins and course of development.

Studies of comprehension may bring us closer to validating the stronger claims of our analysis, that the deeper levels of usage are more demanding conceptually. Hughes and Hall (1987) tested these claims by using both comprehension and production tasks for the word *know*. They found support for the prediction that children would understand the more concrete levels of meaning before they understood the more abstract ones. The six meaning levels of *know* moved from the perceptual as the most basic understanding to evaluation as the most complex. A strong developmental effect underlies this upward progression (Figures 11.1 and 11.2).

However, the research raised problems about the nature of the semantic progression and the differentiation of cognitive state words. Hall et al.'s (1987) semantic analysis of cognitive internal-state words referred to six increasingly complex levels of processing. They assumed that as meaning levels increased in difficulty, the frequency of words used at those levels should decline. However, neither their research nor Hughes and Hall's (1987) study completely supported the claim. Recognition, a theoretically easy level, was rarely used,

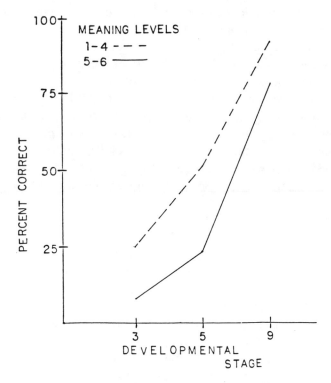

Figure 11.1. Comprehension of *know* at different meaning levels at three ages.

and the relative difficulty of the two highest levels, metacognition and evaluation, was not clearly distinguished.

These discrepant findings led Frank and Hall (1989) to make three changes in the sequence. First, *recognition* and *recall* were merged into one level organized around the broader process of memory. This change standardized the breadth of distinctions marked by each level. Second, *evaluation* preceded *metacognition*. This change was based on the fact that whereas metacognition always refers to abstract content, evaluation may apply to a continuum of referents ranging from the concrete to the abstract and thus, in certain instances, may require less internal processing than metacognition. Last, the range of cognitive activities was extended to include *planning*, which was thought to be the most integrative form of cognitive activity. These changes resulted in the following sequence: awareness, memory, understanding, evaluation, metacognition, and planning.

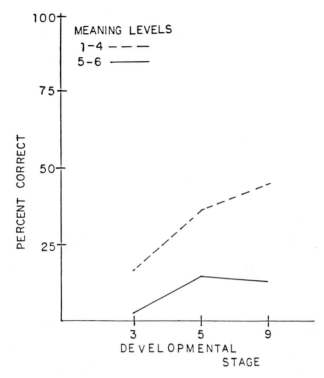

Figure 11.2. Production of *know* at different meaning levels at three ages.

In order to compare the original and the revised semantic sequences, Frank and Hall analyzed the frequency of usage of two polysemous, cognitive internal-state words, *know* and *think*, in the transcribed protocols described earlier. The data in Table 11.1 indicate that the new sequence most closely captures the reality of levels of internal processing. With the revised model, when *know* and *think* are considered together, the frequency of usage of each successive meaning level decreases in the predicted order, except for the *evaluation* level. This finding suggests that restructuring the semantic analysis sequence by merging recognition and recall, changing the ordering of metacognition and evaluation, and adding the level of planning solves one of the problems inherent in the original model.

However, the data raise a second problem. Although *know* and *think* considered together fit the revised sequence closely, the words

Table 11.1. *Comparative level of use of* know *and* think

Process	know		think	
	Adult	Child	Adult	Child
Perception	28.25	14.58	1.28	0.19
Memory	11.58	4.00	2.06	0.33
Understanding	2.36	2.61	1.25	0.08
Evaluation	0.03	0.00	9.72	1.28
Metacognition	0.03	0.03	1.72	0.22
Planning	0.00	0.00	0.53	0.11

Note: Figures indicate mean uses per speaker.

do not fit the model in identical ways. *Know* provided a perfect fit; *think* did not. It is therefore probable that *know* and *think* considered together produce a different frequency distribution among levels than would some other combination of cognitive internal-state words or all cognitive state words considered as an aggregate. In fact, the anomalous ranking of the *evaluation* level may result from the sample of words selected. Consequently, before expressing full confidence in the new sequence, two further tests should be made. First, the results of this study should be compared with an analysis of the entire set of cognitive words in the available transcribed protocols. If the new ordering is indeed valid and our assumption that the meaning levels reside in the aggregate of cognitive internal-state words is veridical, then this analysis should provide a perfect fit to the new sequence. Further, in recognition of the possibility that factors other than difficulty level might be affecting frequency of usage, an experimental study using comprehension and production of meaning levels as the dependent measure should be implemented.

The contrast between *think* and *know* has developmental implications. The two words, although polysemous, have different meanings. The sources of our knowledge are perceptions, learning (encoded in memory), and the implications of understanding. Although it can be argued that the sources of thought are the same, thinkers do not regard their thoughts as firm belief. Each cognitive word may have a prototypical meaning level. Words with prototypes at the less complex levels may be learned earlier, and when words at higher levels are initially learned, they may first be used at lower meaning levels.

Conclusion

All representation beyond infancy is symbolic. Representation beyond this point in the life cycle does not depend on the physical presence of stimuli (Bjorklund, 1989). Word meanings also shift away from the here and now (Nelson, 1985). Piaget (1969) argued that the shift to abstract, conceptual thought occurs because of children's acquisition of hypothetical deductive reasoning, which equips them to acquire concepts, integrate them, and reflect upon them. For Piaget language was merely a useful means by which knowledge is expressed, and not the source of concepts. Vygotsky (1962) and Luria (1976) took a different position. Both argued that language plays a pivotal role in directing thought and that the roles of language and thought change developmentally. The following essential questions underlie the formulations of Piaget, Vygotsky, and Luria: What shall a thing be called? How do we come to call a group of things or actions by one name? What is the primary motivation underlying this activity? These questions are difficult to answer, particularly when they are posed globally. In the metacognitive realm, neither language nor thinking can account exclusively for development. The content of thought need not be verbal, and thinking can occur even when we are unaware of it and cannot label it. Labeling something a thought may not change the nature of thought content. However, language is a means by which we gain access to thinking, and it is a means by which we can refine our awareness of mental states, even if we do not necessarily do so. We argue that language provides children not only with a tool to make thinking accessible for analysis, but also with a context in which they work out the difference between the mental and the physical worlds. Parents use words to describe processes and epistemological suppositions. When children test word meaning, the proving ground is not just the external world of objects, but the conversational context.

Thus, children gain knowledge of their own cognitive states by listening to language using cognitive verbs and also by using and listening to language that expresses cognition. Although mental-state verbs appear in vocabulary by the third year, sentences containing adverbial clauses introduced by subordinating conjunctions such as *before*, *after*, *when*, and *until*, and the causal and logical connectives *because*, *so*, and *if*, appear somewhat later. Their full implications may not be understood until well into the elementary school years.

These words, which are the tools of reasoning, may also provide insight into the relation of language and thinking.

Subordinating conjunctions

The meaning of subordinating conjunctions

Supposition. Cognitive words refer to internal states directly. Subordinating conjunctions like *if, although,* and *because* implicitly convey the speaker's supposition about the truth of a sentence. They also express the nature of the connection between the subordinate and main clauses. In the latter capacity they may cue a set of inferences (Bates, 1976; Bowerman, 1986; Wing & Scholnick, 1981).

Some cognitive verbs and subordinating conjunctions signal the speaker's beliefs about the truth of an utterance. Although beliefs vary along a continuum of "hypotheticality" (Comrie, 1986), we will divide suppositions into three categories: factuals, counterfactuals, and uncertainty expressions (see Bates, 1976; Wing & Scholnick, 1981). The speaker of "I *know* Mary is here" is convinced of the fact of Mary's presence. "I'm *pretending* she is here" implies the opposite. The counterfactual *pretend* signals that the speaker is merely imagining an event. "I *guess* he is here" expresses the speaker's uncertainty (Wing & Scholnick, 1986). Similarly, *because* and *although*[1] connote a belief that the events described in the clauses headed by those conjunctions are true. Upon hearing "*Because* it is raining, the ground is wet," we expect to see drizzle and a muddy lawn. The combination of *if* or *unless* with an indicative verb conveys uncertainty or possibility. "*If* it rains, the ground will get wet" implies that the speaker is uncertain about the weather.[2] The same two conjunctions are counterfactual when they are combined with a subjunctive verb as in "*If* it were raining, the ground would be wet."

The appropriate use of these subordinating conjunctions requires an understanding of the conceptual distinctions between truth and speculation. In addition, the listener must operate on two levels, literal interpretation of the sentence and supposition. Like cognitive internal-state verbs, the appropriate use of these conjunctions requires either self-reflection or insight into the reflections of others.

Clause relations. The subordinating conjunctions heading adverbial clauses can relate the main and subordinate clauses in many ways.

Most of these conjunctions can express more than one connection. *If* will be used as an illustration. "*If* it rains, the ground will be wet" expresses causality; the event in the subordinate clause produces the event in the main clause. Sometimes, the condition in the subordinate clause does not produce the event in the main clause, but the *if* clause simply describes a condition that must be satisfied if the action or event in the main clause is to occur. An example of a circumstantial *if* is, "*If* he is 21, he can vote." In definitions, the object in the *if* clause is a member of the class of objects described in the main clause, as in "*If* it has four right angles, it is a rectangle." But not all *if* clauses describe preconditions or contingencies. Sometimes the main clause contains the precondition, as in "*If* he bought beer, he must be 21." In other cases, the two clauses are noncontingent, as in "*If* you are looking for the newspaper, it is on the table." The interpretation of *if* sentences requires knowledge of the direction of influence between the conditions in the main and subordinate clauses and discrimination of different kinds of influence such as causality.

Deduction. When these subordinating conjunctions imply contingent relations between the clauses that they conjoin, they can cue deductions (see also Byrnes, Chapter 10, this volume). *If* is a constituent of syllogisms used to test conditional reasoning. The typical first premise of a conditional syllogism contains an adverbial antecedent *if* clause and a consequent main clause. The sentence usually supposes uncertainty, and most often the semantic relation between the clauses is circumstantial. An example of such a first premise is "*If* it is a holiday, my school is closed."

Two additional premises complete a syllogism. The uncertainty of the initial premise is resolved by a second premise that either affirms or denies the truth of the antecedent *if* clause or the consequent main clause in the first premise. The third premise contains an inference about the content of the remaining clause.

In formal logic, the proposition in the consequent clause always follows from the proposition in the antecedent *if* clause, but the reverse is not true, because the contents of the main clause can follow from other antecedents. Schools always close on holidays, but there can be other reasons for closing. Therefore, there are only two ways of reasoning from the first premise to reach a valid and certain conclusion: *modus ponens* and *modus tollens* arguments. However, there are three other ways reasoners proceed from an initial premise to a conclusion. Examples of the five patterns of reasoning follow.

In a *modus ponens* argument, the second premise affirms the truth of the *if* clause (the antecedent), and the third premise affirms the main clause (the consequent):

If it is a holiday, my school is closed.	(First premise)
It is a holiday.	(Affirms antecedent)
So my school is closed.	(Affirms consequent)

The second premise of *modus tollens* arguments denies the truth of the consequent, and the conclusion denies the antecedent:

If it is a holiday, my school is closed.	(First premise)
The school is open.	(Denies consequent)
So it must not be a holiday.	(Denies antecedent)

Indeterminate conclusions are permitted by the rules of formal logic. The indeterminacy reflects the asymmetry of the first premise, which states what happens when the antecedent is affirmed but says nothing about what happens when the antecedent is denied. Two different second premises can produce this uncertainty: denial of the antecedent or affirmation of the consequent:

If it is a holiday, my school is closed.	(First premise)
It is not a holiday.	(Denies antecedent)
Schools may or may not be open.	(Indeterminate conclusion)

or

If it is a holiday, my school is closed.	(First premise)
The schools are closed.	(Affirms consequent)
It could be a holiday or a teachers' meeting.	(Indeterminate conclusion)

Ordinary reasoners rarely produce conclusions based on material implication. Instead, they use *biconditional* reasoning when the antecedent is denied or the consequent is affirmed. They draw a definite conclusion due to a mistaken assumption that *if* describes a symmetrical relation between the antecedent and consequent clause. If the antecedent is denied, so is the consequent; if the consequent is affirmed, so is the antecedent. Biconditionals are often implied in threats, bribes, and promises (Braine, 1978; Fillenbaum, 1986):

If it is a holiday, I won't go to school.	(First premise)
It is not a holiday.	(Denies antecedent)
So you'd better go to school.	(Denies consequent)

Refutations focus on the validity of the semantic relation between clauses rather than further implications of the sentence. In a refutation the reasoner denies that the antecedent always leads to the consequence mentioned in the initial premise, and cites an exception:

If it is a holiday, your school is closed.	(First premise)
It is a holiday.	(Affirms antecedent)
But my school is staying open.	(Denies consequent)

Supposition

Language and thinking

What is the role of language and thinking in appreciating the distinctive beliefs that these conjunctions signal and the inferences conditional sentences permit? We shall argue that both language and thought are implicated in the understanding of supposition. We begin with the role of language.

Language as supportive context. In order to learn the suppositions subordinating conjunctions express, children must first learn to make the distinctions and then learn that these distinctions can be expressed indirectly. Language may provide a supportive, meaningful context for comprehending the fuzzy distinctions between truth and hypothesis and between the possible and impossible.

Children's understanding of supposition has often been measured by asking them to make judgments. Meaningful sentences facilitate judgments. In a series of studies (Scholnick & Wing, 1982, 1983; Wing & Scholnick, 1981) listeners had to evaluate sentences like "*If* this animal has humps, it is a wug." Then they were asked, "Does the speaker believe it is a wug? or has humps?" In these tasks, 6-year-olds discerned factuals; 8-year-olds detected counterfactuals, but only preadolescents or older listeners judged that *if* and *unless* could indicate the speaker's uncertainty about the animal's identity. However, when the sentence content describes familiar animals, appreciation of uncertainty appears much earlier (see also Jorgensen & Falmagne, 1988). Meaning plays the role of supportive context. Familiar material is easier to encode than unfamiliar material. Meaningful material may also make it possible to bypass one component of judging suppositions. Listeners consult their own beliefs about the material as the basis for evaluating the speaker's beliefs.

The supportive role of meaning is particularly apparent in analyses of children's conversations. Suppositions are used more maturely in conversation than in experimental settings. In an experiment, children must make explicit judgments of supposition, but in spontaneous speech, these judgments are implicit and supported by the situation. On experimental tasks, young children rarely understand that *if* conveys uncertainty, but in their conversations 4-year-olds use *if* and *when* to contrast suppositions, and *if* is used primarily to express speaker uncertainty (Reilly, 1986). Children show more mastery of supposition in conversation than in laboratory tasks because they voice their own beliefs about sentence content or because they can respond to familiar speakers in familiar settings. The meaningful content and the focus on personal beliefs simplify the choice of supposition and enhance accuracy.

Conversation also supplies certain pragmatic props for processing supposition. Some situations are marked for an exchange of opinions or pretending, making the choice of supposition implicit and easy. Moreover, in conversation it is sometimes appropriate to admit uncertainty or disbelief. In contrast, experimental tasks require children to be explicit about an unfamiliar speaker's beliefs. Children assume that in tests, people are expected to appear definite and competent. They may be reluctant to say that the speaker is unsure and be afraid that a judgment of uncertainty implies that they are also uncertain.

Perhaps because familiar material helps children judge the underlying attitude of the speaker, familiar material may also enable them to acquire the very concepts of supposition that subordinating conjunctions convey. The linguistic context helps by providing direct reference so that children can judge whether the speaker's statement is true, or false, or merely possible. French and Nelson (1985) claim that children's first use of conditionals and first conceptions of the alternative outcomes that conditionals imply occur in the context of scripts. Eventually, children may be able to abstract the framework defining supposition and use it with unfamiliar material.

Speakers also act as models and tutors. Scholnick and Wing (1991) found that parents' use of supposition predicts their children's usage. Once they have introduced topics with *if*, parents may also elaborate the possibilities and uncertainties, and also explain their criteria for distinguishing certainty from uncertainty.

Language as modulator. Language, in the role of modulator, may also influence the ease of encoding or expressing suppositions. Few concepts have a single means of expression. There are many ways to express beliefs about the truth of a statement, and some means of expression may be easier to understand than others. Children's encounters with either simpler or more complicated forms of expressing the same idea may influence their extraction of meaning. This is what we mean by *modulator*.

Children who try to grasp the uncertainty of *if*, or the factual belief implied by *because*, already have experience with these distinctions. They have merely to apply previous learning to the mastery of new terminology. A simpler lexicon is available for expressing speakers' beliefs and notions of truth, falsehood, and uncertainty. All judgments of word meaning involve decisions about truth, contradiction, and ambiguity (Macnamara, 1986). So long before the process of judgment is referred to explicitly, children are deciding whether they believe an object can be described by a particular linguistic term. That is, they know language use involves truth and belief judgments. Children gain control of two other systems of expressing certainty and uncertainty before acquiring skill with subordinating conjunctions, modal verbs, and cognitive verbs (Byrnes & Duff, 1989). The acquisition of cognitive verbs like *know, pretend,* and *guess* may help children realize that speakers can signal their underlying beliefs because cognitive verbs refer explicitly to the mental processes of the individual who holds the belief. Cognitive verbs are also simpler to interpret because they do not simultaneously convey diverse semantic relations between clauses. Not surprisingly, Wing and Scholnick (1986) found that children made more accurate judgments of speakers' beliefs expressed by cognitive verbs than by subordinating conjunctions. Children who can use *pretend* to signal a discussion of imaginary events may link that understanding to a new form of counterfactual, *if* (Bates & MacWhinney, 1987). There is even a construction that couples cognitive verbs with *if*: "I don't know *if*," or "I wonder *if*."

Cognitive contributions. In the preceding paragraphs we have argued that features of the linguistic environment may produce, facilitate, and provide the context for learning to evaluate the speaker's beliefs by calling attention to mental processes and providing terminology and contexts for discussing mind and belief before acquisition of *if, because,* or *unless.* However, it is doubtful that language is the only source of understanding suppositions. Cognition may provide some prerequisite knowledge and a supportive context in which notions of truth and uncertainty, belief, and disbelief are worked out. These notions may then provide the framework for linguistic expression. Long before children make judgments of linguistic reference, infants make predictions that are confirmed or disconfirmed. The simple problems of everyday life provide a fertile field for building the notions of necessity, possibility, and impossibility that language expresses (Pieraut-Le Bonniec, 1980).

There are also nonlinguistic sources of children's ability to detect these beliefs in others. Flavell, Green, and Flavell (1989) note that during the preschool period (which is the time when these subordinating conjunctions emerge in speech to mark presuppositions), children begin to distinguish their visual perspective from those of others and begin to discriminate between appearances and reality. They suggest that perspective taking and appreciation of the appearance–reality distinction are based on children's understanding that people hold beliefs that may conflict with those held by others and conflict with reality. These cognitive advances may support linguistic development.

Moreover, just as language can refine children's understanding of criteria for judging truth, cognitive advances can enrich linguistic expression. Take the case of uncertainty. Older children detect more situations than younger children in which there is insufficient information to make judgments. Five- and 6-year-olds know that a hint that applies to two choices is ambiguous (Somerville, Hadkinson, & Greenberg, 1979), but older children realize that rules that predict equally probable outcomes are ambiguous, too (Byrnes & Overton, 1986; Pieraut-Le Bonniec, 1980; Scholnick & Wing, 1991).

Wing and Scholnick (1986) asked listeners to judge what speakers had in mind when using *if* or *unless*. Preadolescents suggested these conjunctions implied that speakers did not know whether an event would occur. Adolescents suggested that these conjunctions also indicated that alternative causes could account for the same event. Pieraut-Le Bonniec (1980) has suggested that the construction of a single logical framework encompassing notions of necessity, possibility, and impossibility increases appreciation of the suppositions that subordinating conjunctions convey.

Thus, language and conceptual development may each contribute to the use of subordinating conjunctions to distinguish suppositions. They may provide different sources of understanding and mutual enrichment. Perhaps each provides alternative and interacting routes to growth in the child's understanding. Further study of the links between conceptual and linguistic understanding of uncertainty is warranted (e.g., Scholnick & Wing, 1982).

Conditional reasoning

Language and thought

Discussion of the relative contributions of language and thought to the emergence of conditional deduction has been particularly heated. In general, debates about the interplay of language and cognition are complicated by the fact that language and cognition are multifaceted. This is nowhere more evident than in the case of the conditional deductions that often follow sentences containing *if*. These sentences have reference, a syntax, an implicit supposition, and a pragmatic function. Which of these attributes influences deduction? *If* is also polysemous. It appears in adverbial clauses and in complement clauses, too. *If* can be counterfactual or uncertain, and sometimes even factual depending on the context. Although traditional syllogisms employ *if* to express a conditional relation, not all uses of *if* resemble the first premises of syllogisms. Therefore, it is unclear whether any aspect of *if* language, aside from reference, can be a reliable guide to deduction, and those who claim that *if* is a reliable guide to inference emphasize different aspects of *if*.

Yet another source of controversy is the characterization of deduction itself (Scholnick, 1990). Inferences can be produced in different ways. A reasoner may draw conclusions based on knowledge of the world, some of which is encoded linguistically. The reasoner determines whether the conclusion always holds or whether there are counterexamples. Alternatively, the reasoner may invoke a set of logical rules to generate valid conclusions or to evaluate whether conclusions follow legitimately from particular premises. In conditional logic, an antecedent (e.g., snow) is always paired with a consequent (school closing), but that consequent can be paired with other antecedents (a teachers' strike).

Theories differ in the extent to which they posit that ordinary reasoners use a set of abstract inferential rules to produce and evaluate valid arguments. The more these rules are based on an appreciation of argument validity, the more cognition is implicated. The more deduction is defined in terms of reference to the truth of particular statements rather than the use of logical procedures, the more language plays a decisive role in reasoning. There is a middle position – that children begin by reasoning referentially – but other aspects of *if*, aside from the referential content of the sentence, may guide them toward the construction of a mature set of abstract logical rules.

Judgment by reference. Johnson-Laird (1983) favors semantic reference as the basis for inference and denies the existence of content-free logical rules used to draw inferences from statements. He also denies that people reason by using *if* to cue deductions, because *if* is not a reliable indicator of conditional relations. Not all *if*s are conditionals, and not all conditional statements are *if*s. *If* appears in sentences with complement clauses, in indirect questions, and in one-clause subjunctive sentences such as, respectively, "I don't know *if* that is true," "Ask him *if* it's true," and "*If* only it were true!" In the sentence "*If* you want to reach me, I'll be at home," the speaker will be at home regardless of the addressee's wants. In "*If* he voted, he must be 21," the consequent clause is a prerequisite for the main clause, rather than the opposite sequence typifying most conditional syllogisms.

Johnson-Laird claims that people reason by building a model of the events described in an inferential problem to see if their experience matches or contradicts the model. Since language can be used to encode and generate event representations, language enables people to make inferences; however, other methods of generating event representations are available. Because reasoners rely on understanding specific word meanings and use simple processes like retrieval and detection of contradiction, abstract formal logic is unnecessary in explaining deduction. Invalid conclusions arise from processing overload, inexhaustive search, or inadequate retrieval strategies, not logical error.

Syntactic cuing. Braine takes the opposite view and proposes that language is merely the context for inference. Braine (1978, 1990; Braine & Rumain, 1983) contends that people reason by invoking an assortment of innate primary inference schemes, or formulas enabling them to make inferences from particular logical arguments. Those schemes enable them to integrate information and comprehend spoken discourse. Thus, inferential schemes work on linguistic input. Perhaps the schemes are innate, but children must learn to access them. Inference schemes are cued by the presence of particular subordinating conjunctions. One inference scheme incorporates the simplest form of conditional argument, *modus ponens*. Given an adverbial-clause *if* sentence as a major premise and a second premise affirming the antecedent *if* clause of that sentence, the reasoner supplies the missing affirmed consequent clause. Braine argues that reasoners can make *modus ponens* inferences because such inferences are encoded in the meaning of *if*, namely, that the consequent always follows from the antecedent.

Children acquire *if*'s meaning the same way they learn the meaning of any word, through feedback. They are warned, "*If* you throw that glass, it will break." When a child ignores the warning and hurls the container, the parent looks at the shattered glass and says, "See, you threw it and it broke." In this sentence, *if* means that the antecedent leads to the consequent, so *if* implies *modus ponens* reasoning. Hence, the child learns the meaning of *if* by paying attention to sentence reference and then maps the meaning of *if* onto a content-free logical rule.

Braine discusses a second role for language, as context. Western schooling promotes an analytical use of language, and with it the ability to learn new inference schemes that are not part of children's initial capacity. In this way, language plays the same role in logic that it does in metacognition, to produce analytical awareness.

Language plays a third role, as modulator of competence. In the following two examples, the linguistic context hampers accurate deduction. First, sentences describing inducements invite erroneous biconditional inferences. The threat "*If* you don't do your homework, you will fail your exam" implies that doing the work will guarantee a good grade. But failure can arise for other reasons, such as a particularly difficult test. Second, conditionals can be expressed in many syntactic forms. "*If* it is a triangle, it has three sides" is logically equivalent to "All triangles have three sides," but the latter is easier to use in deduction (O'Brien et al., 1989).

Clause relations. Whereas Braine describes how children's acquisition of adverbial-clause *if*s eventually leads to a *modus ponens* rule, Falmagne (1988, 1990) emphasizes the impact of particular *if*-clause relations on broader deductive competence. She posits two roles for language, as providing a context for abstracting inference rules and as evidence of abstractive ability in inference.

Language exerts its influence through the different clause relations *if* expresses. *If* can describe causal and temporal sequences. Even before using *if* deductively, children understand many causal concepts. They know what rain does to the soil, and that mud can be caused by other sources of moisture. They also know that sentences express causation. For example, actors cause actions. Armed with knowledge about rain and about the potential for language to express causality, children can interpret sentences such as "*If* it rains, the ground gets wet," even when they do not know what *if* means. That knowledge enables them to extract the meaning of *if* and to make the appropriate inferences when told the ground is dry, that is, that it has not rained recently. When children hear other *if* statements expressing causation, reference to the real world will enable them to comprehend *if* and to make deductions, too. Eventually, they will abstract the rule that *if* sentences express causes, so that even when novel content is introduced, they will assume that causation is implied and make the appropriate inferences. Thus, children build upon an early understanding of sentence reference and causation to construct rules for generating and evaluating causal inferences.

The same "semantic bootstrapping" occurs for temporal relations. Knowledge of specific temporal contingencies in daily life enables children to understand *if* sentences describing such contingencies and to make appropriate inferences. Eventually, children form an abstraction. When *if* presents temporal contingencies, certain deductions are valid. Next they coalesce the causal and temporal schemes into conditional logic and use that logic to generate inferences when the content and clause relations are unfamiliar. Falmagne (1988, 1990) also reasons by analogy. Children's ability to abstract syntactic and thematic relations in language suggests the availability of a second powerful abstraction mechanism – for constructing and using deduction.

Language as context and modulator. Piaget's (1969) stance, which we cited earlier, is at the opposite end of the continuum from Johnson-Laird's. Byrnes and Overton (1988, pp. 195–196) echo his position on the meaning of *if* and its close link to logic. "Connectives such as 'if' . . . do not refer to particular objects, but to a *set* of permissible instances. . . . If a subject had knowledge of which instances are permissible and which are impermissible for a given propositional concept (as expressed by its appropriate connective), then the subject can be said to have acquired that concept." Thus, conditional reasoning is not tied to the meaning of a single sentence. Conditional logic is one manifestation of the coordinated structure underlying all propositional thought.

Propositional thought arises from the individual's overt operations on objects, leading to the formation of conceptual relations, subsequent symbolization of those relations, and eventual reflection on the necessary (logical) integration of those relations. Language is an outgrowth of the capacity for symbolic representation that arises late in the sensorimotor period. Language is not independent of its cognitive origins. Piaget (1969) claims that for a while language and thinking pursue independent developmental paths, and it is not until children begin to use formal operations that they are coordinated. At that time, when deductive thought flowers, language serves as a medium for the operation of logic. Verbal propositions and propositions that are contrary to fact (counterfactual) become the object of propositional thinking.

Language helps to refine logic by serving as a means of monitoring thought and repairing errors. Communication also offers the opportunity for corrective feedback. Language becomes a context for the operation of logic. Piaget argues that, as such, language may be a necessary component of logical thought, but not a sufficient one, because deduction originates in earlier intellectual accomplishments. A well-known finding in the research on deduction is that even adults have difficulty with reasoning when the content of the problem is abstract and unfamiliar. As Overton's (Byrnes & Overton, 1986; Overton et al., 1985; Overton, Ward, Noveck, Black, & O'Brien, 1987) programmatic research shows, providing meaningful and familiar sentences facilitates deduction, but only among adolescents and adults, who presumably have constructed an intellectual structure supporting propositional thought. Language is necessary, but not sufficient, for the development of logic. Linguistic reference deals with truth, the match between a symbol and a concept, whereas logic deals with validity or necessity. It is easier to find necessary relations among meaningful concepts.

This summary of conflicting views on the role of language and cognition in deduction illustrates our argument. Braine, Falmagne, and Piaget differ in their descriptions of deduction and in the role of language as producer, interacting partner, or simply modulator. They also target different aspects of language that affect deduction. Braine

428   E. K. Scholnick and W. S. Hall

focuses on lexical meaning in a particular syntactic format, Falmagne on the semantic relations between clauses, and Piaget on language as representation. Which description fits the data on deduction?

Children's conversations

There is extensive research on the way children reason with *if* (Braine & Rumain, 1983). Children entering school can make *modus ponens* deductions. Other kinds of conditional reasoning are at best fragile even into adulthood; performance is very dependent on the nature of the verbal material employed. In contrast, in conversation 4-year-olds use *if* to express a wide variety of suppositions and clause relations (e.g. Bowerman, 1986; McCabe, Evely, Abramovitch, Corter, & Pepler, 1983; Reilly, 1986). However, the linguistic and cognitive data are not derived from the same child, so there is no way of determining whether children who appear to use *if* fluently are also skilled in deduction.

Unlike Johnson-Laird, both Braine and Falmagne posit that the type of *if* usually found in syllogisms is prevalent in adult and child speech. It provides a basis for learning the meaning of *if*, and possibly the deductions *if* permits. However, we lack data on parent and child language to test those claims. Therefore, in order to find out how *if* is used spontaneously, and whether conversation reveals deduction and has an impact on deduction, Scholnick and Wing (1989) examined the conversations of 39 $4\frac{1}{2}$-year-old children. These children were recorded twice in six home and four school situations (Hall, Nagy, & Linn, 1984). This is a more extensive analysis of the corpus described in the study of cognitive internal-state words. Although the data are drawn from children at just one age, they provide an extensive sample of child and adult use of *if* and of spontaneous inferences from *if* sentences.

Syllogistic speech. One purpose of the analysis was to compare adult and child use of *if* and to determine whether adults and children ever speak "syllogistically," producing sentences resembling the first premises of syllogisms and then reasoning from them. A potential premise is *"If it rained, then he went to the movies."* *If* appears in an adverbial clause providing information for the listener and specifying the circumstance that served as a precondition for the event in the main clause. The speaker expresses uncertainty about the weather. In order to ascertain the frequency of such forms, we coded every *if* that was not a false start and that was spoken in a context that was sufficiently complete for us to ascertain the supposition, syntax, entailment, and pragmatic use of *if*. From the 2,431 *ifs* so coded, we selected the 1,742 sentences produced by three sets of speakers: the target children who were recorded, their parents and grandparents, and their teachers. The data were adjusted in order to equate speakers for the number of conversational turns that they produced. Each speaker's score was the mean number of *ifs* the speaker produced in 100 of the conversational turns.

Four analyses of variance were performed. In each, the dependent variable was *if* rate, the average number of codable *ifs* produced by a speaker per 100 of the speaker's conversational turns, and there were two independent variables: the speaker (parent, child, and teacher) and linguistic category. We expected higher *if* rates for adults and for categories of *if* use that characterized the initial premise of syllogisms.

Table 11.2 presents the *if* rates for each speaker. Each analysis produced a similar pattern of data. "Syllogistic" use of *if* predominated. The most frequently used supposition expressed uncertainty. Most *ifs* appeared in adverbial clauses, and those clauses typically described the circumstances under which the event in the main clause occurred. Parents and children used *if* mainly in information statements but teachers used *if* most often in directives. Speaker differences were usually confined to the predominant category of usage. In that category, teachers produced higher *if* rates than parents, who in turn used *if* more often than the children. Thus, there is a prototype *if*, used in an adverbial clause to inform the listener of the circumstance under which the main-clause event occurred. The prototype *if* also expresses uncertainty. These are the kinds of *ifs* most often found as initial premises in syllogisms. Children used *if* less frequently than adults, and speaker differences were most pronounced for the prototype category.

However, although there were absolute differences in the absolute frequency of use of the dominant category of *ifs*, the proportion of each speaker's *ifs* that fell into that category was similar. For example, uncertainty *ifs* accounted for .78 of the children's *ifs*, .81 of the parent's *ifs*, and .87 of the teacher's *ifs*. Similarly, the proportion

Table 11.2. *Child, parent, and teacher if rates in each linguistic category*

Category	Speaker		
	Child	Parent	Teacher
Supposition			
Uncertainty[a]	0.71	1.63	2.82
Counterfactual	0.08	0.19	0.26
Factual	0.09	0.15	0.22
Syntax			
Adverbial clause[a]	0.68	1.60	2.44
Noun and one-clause	0.20	0.38	0.85
Clause relations[b]			
Cause/definition	0.17	0.32	0.43
Circumstance[a]	0.44	1.11	1.83
Other	0.07	0.18	0.18
Pragmatic functions			
Information[a]	0.48	1.04	1.00
Directive	0.25	0.70	1.71
Question	0.15	0.24	0.58

Note: Data are number of *if*s per 100 of the speaker's turns.
[a]Usually found in conditional syllogisms.
[b]Clause relations are unambiguous only for adverbial-clause *if*s.

of *if*s appearing in adverbial clauses was .72 of the children's *if* sentences, .73 of the teachers' *if*s, and .79 of the parents' *if*s.

The normative *if* is used "syllogistically." The syntax and clause relations employed in children's speech typifies the sentence structure of syllogisms. The pragmatic function of parent and child *if* sentences also resembles the style of syllogisms. *If* has a structure that resembles many prototype classes. So if children can learn the content of other prototype categories, they can certainly learn the meaning of *if*. Thus, there is support for the claim that conversation can provide a semantic context for understanding *if*.

Moreover, correlational evidence suggests that children's production of *if* is influenced by their language environment. Stepwise multiple regression analyses were performed to determine whether children's use of specific forms of *if* was correlated with the speech of adults in their environment. The dependent variable was the child's *if* rate in a given coding category. Two types of predictors were in-

Table 11.3. *Stepwise multiple regressions predicting child* if *rate in different linguistic categories*

Dependent variable	Significant predictors	R
Supposition		
Uncertainty	Teacher true generalization	$R(37) = .43^{**}$
Counterfactual	Teacher uncertainty, parent uncertainty	$R(36) = .50^{**}$
Factual	None	
Syntax		
Adverbial clause	Parent adverbial clause	$R(37) = .42^{**}$
Noun and one-clause	None	
Clause relations		
Cause/definition	Parent cause/definition	$R(37) = .40^{**}$
Circumstance	Parent cause/definition	$R(37) = .44^{**}$
Other	Teacher other	$R(37) = .51^{*}$
Pragmatics		
Information	Teacher information	$R(37) = .43^{**}$
Question	Parent question	$R(37) = .34^{*}$

$^{*}p < .05; ^{**}p < .01.$

cluded in each regression equation: direct and indirect. The direct predictors were parent and teacher *if* rate for the same coding category – for example, parent and teacher use of *if* in information statements to predict child use of *if* in information statements. Because adult speech in a coding category can provide the child with models of a particular kind of *if*, adult use of specific forms of *if* should be correlated with child use. Indirect predictors were also included in the regression equation. These were parent and teacher *if* rates for the other coding categories along the same dimension (questions and directives). For example, a parent who uses *if* in questions may elicit *if* in information statements in reply.

There were 11 stepwise multiple regression equations predicting child use of the three categories of supposition, three categories of clause relations, two categories of syntax, and three categories of pragmatic function. Table 11.3 summarizes the outcomes of the analyses. Five equations revealed significant direct influences.[3] The frequency of parental use of *if* in adverbial clauses predicted child use of *if* in adverbial clauses, too. Child causal/definitional *if* rate was predicted by use of the same category in parents. Child *if* rate for the miscellaneous clause relation category was predicted by teacher use of the same category, and frequent parental use of *if* in questions was associated with high use of the same pragmatic function for *if* in children. High teacher use of *if* in information statements was associated with high use of *if* in similar statements by their pupils.

Three equations revealed indirect influences. The parents' rate of using causal and definitional *ifs* predicted not only the child's use of the same category, but also the child's use of circumstantial *if*-clause relations. Two categories of supposition also revealed indirect influences on the child's speech. The child's *if* rate for counterfactuals was significantly predicted by a combination of the teacher's and parents' rate of use of uncertainty *ifs*. The child's use of uncertainty *ifs* was predicted by the teacher's rate of *ifs* as factuals. Thus, there appeared to be an association between adult speech and the children's general use of adverbial-clause *ifs* and particular use of specific clause relations.

Deductions

Children and adults speak the kind of *ifs* that resemble the initial premises of syllogisms, and children exposed to an environment rich in *if* use also produces many *ifs*. Thus, the language environment is ripe for the use of *if* for deduction, and indeed there were many instances of deduction. When we examined the entire corpus, not just the speech of the parents, children, and teachers, there were 185 instances in which there was an *if* sentence, followed by an affirmation or denial of one clause of the sentence, and then a conclusion.

One analysis focused on the author of the concluding premise containing the inference (Table 11.4). Both adults and children produced *modus tollens* deductions and indeterminate inferences, although both types of reasoning were rare. However, adults and children differed in the kinds of inferences they made. The five kinds of arguments can be reduced to two categories, *relational* and *elaborative*. In both *modus ponens* and refutation arguments, the second premise affirms the antecedent. The conclusion is based on whether the reasoner accepts the initial premise stating a contingency between the antecedent *if* and consequent clause. Acceptance leads to

Table 11.4. *Number of arguments concluded by different speakers*

	Speaker of conclusion	
Argument	Child	Adult
Modus ponens	17	12
Refutation	37	25
Biconditional	29	45
Modus tollens	5	8
Indeterminate inference	1	6
Total	89	96

Note: Fourteen of the inferences were made by older children. The distribution of inferences was similar across the two age groups, so the data were pooled.

a restatement of the initial contingency between clauses (*modus ponens*). A failure to accept the contingency leads the reasoner to contradict it. Because these two arguments deal with evaluating the validity of the initial *if–then* relation, they are called *relational* arguments. In the other arguments, the reasoner accepts the hypothesized contingency and produces implications using material that is not stated in the original premise. These arguments *elaborate* on the initial premise. A greater proportion of child arguments than adult arguments were relational (.61 vs. .39, $z = .61$, $p < .05$).

Children and adults also differed in the discourse structure producing inferences. Each argument was categorized by whether or not all premises were produced by the same speaker. Adults were more likely than children to produce all three premises in an argument (.48 vs. .23, $z = 2.35$, $p < .02$). Elaborative arguments were more likely to have a single author than were relational arguments (.59 vs. .07, $z = 4.79$, $p < .001$). Even within elaborative arguments, adults were more likely than children to be the author of every premise ($z = 3.75$, $p < .001$). Children may be very reliant on the kind of linguistic environment adults provide for the material from which to draw inferences. This leads to an important question: Does adult language have an impact on child speech?

In order to determine influences on children's production of arguments, stepwise multiple regression analyses were performed. The dependent variable was the number of arguments the target child concluded. In the first regression equation, the predictors were the number of arguments the child's teachers and parents concluded and the *if* rates of the child, parents, and teachers. Just the rate of parental *if* production significantly predicted child deductions, $R(37)$ = .44, $p < .005$. Four subsequent regression equations examined whether frequent use by teachers and parents of particular syntactic constructions, suppositions, clause relations, and pragmatic functions was associated with a higher production of arguments by the target children. The target children's inferences were predicted by four facets of parental production: rate of production of adverbial *if* clauses, $R(37) = .48$; rate of use of causal *ifs*, $R(37) = .57$; rate of use of counterfactuals, $R(37) = .51$; and rate of use of *ifs* in questions, $R(37) = .46$, all *ps* < .003.

Developmental researchers have hotly debated young children's deductive capacities. In the context of meaningful conversations, young children can make the most elementary deductions. In addition, they understand the invited inferences of discourse since they also produce biconditionals. We do not claim that children have abstract inferential skills tightly integrated into a propositional structure. They may, indeed, be arguing only on the basis of semantic reference. But they possess the seeds from which abstract inference can grow. Language supplies a supportive context for deduction.

In summary, as Falmagne argues, children may learn skills in argumentation in a conversational context. Parents provide models of *if* use that resemble premises in syllogisms. Children seem more mature as linguistic and cognitive processors in conversational contexts. Falmagne argues that if children can extract word meaning, they can also use conversations to extract and abstract logical rules. Our data show that by 4 years of age children are able to make logical inferences and judgments of supposition. The data also show the central role of parental input in the emergence of deductive skill.

However, some important information is missing. The developmental history of conversational deductions must be traced. In addition, ancillary independent measures of children's deductive and linguistic competence should provide essential data to buttress interpretations of children's skill and the process of decontextualization of competence referred to by Falmagne.

Conclusion

Language and thought are each means of symbolic representation. To what extent does the acquisition of one form of representation refine or substitute for the other? We have argued that the language of internal states and of reasoning is very complicated. The same cognitive relation or mental process can be described in many ways. Words like *if* and *know* have many meanings, some of which do not convey mental states or contingent relations. In this respect, internal-state language and subordinating conjunctions probably do not differ from other words. Clark (1983) argues that meanings are discriminated by contrast. In the case of words for things, the contrast can be between one labeled object and another object with its distinctive name. Contrasts are also provided by the content of discourse. Clearly, both labels and discourse context can enable children to understand metacognition and conditional logic.

However, language may do much more. Mental processes are inferred to some extent. It is hard to learn their names by ostensive definition. Language provides accessibility to thought, and conversation may provide a set of frames in which remembering, pretending, or voicing opinions may occur. In addition, in conversations parents may model and label mental processes since there is a relation between what parents say and the diversity of the child's vocabulary to describe mental phenomena. In the case of *if*, language may provide an integrative frame unifying the diverse instances that exemplify conditional contingencies. Parents provide both a model for *if* use and a supportive context for using *if* deductively. We have also argued that meaningful conversation supports inference, because within that context children appear more logically competent and linguistically competent than in experimental tasks. Finally, language is a training ground, in that the same suppositions are expressed directly and the simpler forms may give rise to later, more complex ones. Conversation is also a medium in which to practice the use of metacognition and deduction.

Is linguistic ability necessary and sufficient for the acquisition of mental-state terms and subordinating conjunctions? Because we studied the acquisition of two lexicons, linguistic skill is an inherent prerequisite. Is language sufficient for progress? Probably not entirely. There has to be thought for there to be a term to monitor it. Validation is certainly a cognitive process, and if conditional logic involves more than *modus ponens*, there must be some cognitive integration. If there is some overlap between the processes of abstraction and verification in language and in concepts, then cognition is integral to each domain. We have argued elsewhere (Scholnick, 1990) that abstraction, mapping, validity evaluation, monitoring, and deduction are so central to human functioning that they would underlie information processing in many domains. Each domain could provide unique but also overlapping sources of information, and when there is overlap there would be a form of bootstrapping that would enhance development. Here we argue that because accessibility to mental acts and mental products is complex and indirect, language plays a particularly vital role as tutor, scaffold, and signal.

Notes

1. In some cases *if* is used as a synonym for *whenever*, and so it also expresses a factual belief, as in the generalization "*If* it rains, we get wet."
2. Even when *if* is used as a synonym for *whether*, it conveys uncertainty, as in "I don't know *if* it is raining" or "Ask *if* it is raining in Boston."
3. Parent and teacher total *if* rate singly or in combination did not predict child *if* rate, so the correlations do not reflect an overall predisposition to use *if*.

References

Bates, E. (1976). *Language and context.* New York: Academic Press.

Bates, E., & MacWhinney, B. (1987). Competition, variation, and language learning. In B. MacWhinney (Ed.), *Mechanisms of language acquisition* (pp. 157–193). Hillsdale, NJ: Erlbaum.

Bjorklund, D. F. (1989). *Children's thinking: Developmental function and individual differences.* Belmont, CA: Brooks-Cole.

Bowerman, M. (1986). First steps in acquiring conditionals. In E. C. Traugott, A. ter Meulen, J. S. Reilly, & C. A. Ferguson (Eds.), *On conditionals* (pp. 285–307). Cambridge University Press.

Bowerman, M. (1988). Inducing the latent structure of language. In F. S. Kessel (Ed.), *The development of language and language researchers: Essays in honor of Roger Brown* (pp. 23–49). Hillsdale, NJ: Erlbaum.

Braine, M. D. S. (1978). On the relation between the natural logic of reasoning and standard logic. *Psychological Review, 85,* 1–21.

Braine, M. D. S. (1990). The "natural logic" approach to reasoning. In W. F. Overton (Ed.), *Reasoning, necessity, and logic: Developmental perspectives* (pp. 135–158). Hillsdale, NJ: Erlbaum.

Braine, M. D. S., & Rumain, B. (1983). Logical reasoning. In P. H. Mussen (Ed.), *Handbook of child psychology: Vol. 3. Cognitive development* (4th ed. pp. 266–340). New York: Wiley.

Bretherton, I., & Beeghly, M. (1982). Talking about internal states: The acquisition of an explicit theory of mind. *Developmental Psychology, 18,* 906–921.

Brown, R. (1973). *A first language: The early stages.* Cambridge, MA: Harvard University Press.

Byrnes, J. P., & Duff, M. A. (1989). Young children's comprehension of modal expressions. *Cognitive Development, 4,* 369–388.

Byrnes, J. P., & Overton, W. F. (1986). Reasoning about certainty and un-certainty in concrete, causal, and propositional contexts. *Developmental Psychology, 22,* 793–799.

Byrnes, J. P., & Overton, W. F. (1988). Reasoning about logical connectives: A developmental analysis. *Journal of Experimental Child Psychology, 46,* 194–218.

Case, R. (1985). *Intellectual development: A systematic reinterpretation.* New York: Academic Press.

Clark, E. V. (1983). Meanings and concepts. In P. H. Mussen (Ed.), *Handbook of child psychology: Vol. 3. Cognitive development* (4th ed., pp. 787–840). New York: Wiley.

Comrie, B. (1986). Conditionals: A typology. In E. C. Traugott, A. ter Meulen, J. S. Reilly, & C. A. Ferguson (Eds.) *On conditionals* (pp. 77–99). Cambridge University Press.

Falmagne, R. J. (1988). *Is language a constitutive factor in logical knowledge?* (Cognitive Science Laboratory Technical Report No. 28). Princeton, NJ: Princeton University.

Falmagne, R. J. (1990). Language and the acquisition of logical knowledge. In W. F. Overton (Ed.), *Reasoning, necessity, and logic: Developmental perspectives* (pp. 111–134). Hillsdale, NJ: Erlbaum.

Fillenbaum, S. (1986). The use of conditionals in inducements and deterrents. In E. C. Traugott, A. ter Meulen, J. S. Reilly, & C. A. Ferguson (Eds.), *On conditionals* (pp. 179–196). Cambridge University Press.

Flavell, J. H. (1972). An analysis of cognitive-developmental sequences. *Genetic Psychology Monographs, 86,* 279–350.

Flavell, J. H., Green, F. L., & Flavell, E. R. (1989). Young children's ability to differentiate appearance-reality and level 2 perspectives in the tactile modality. *Child Development, 60,* 201–213.

Frank, R. E., & Hall, W. S. (1989, April). *Polysemy in "know" and "think."* Paper presented at the biennial meeting of the Society for Research in Child Development, Kansas City, MO.

Frederiksen, C. H. (1975). Effects of context-induced processing operations on information acquired from discourse. *Cognitive Psychology, 7,* 139–166.

French, L. A., & Nelson, K. (1985). *Young children's knowledge of relational terms: Some ifs, ors, and buts.* New York: Springer.

Gordon, D. & Lakoff, G. (1971). *Conversational postulates.* Paper presented at the seventh regional meeting of the Chicago Linguistic Society.

Hall, W. S., & Nagy, W. E. (1986). Theoretical issues in the investigation of words of internal report. In I. Gopnik & M. Gopnik (Eds.), *From models to modules* (pp. 26–65). Norwood, NJ: Ablex.

Hall, W. S., & Nagy, W. E. (1987). The semantic–pragmatic distinction in internal state words: The role of the situation. *Discourse Processes, 10*(2), 169–180.

Hall, W. S., Nagy, W. E., & Linn, R. (1984). *Spoken words: Effects of situation and social group on oral word usage and frequency.* Hillsdale, NJ: Erlbaum.

Hall, W. S., Scholnick, E. K., & Hughes, A. T. (1987). Contextual constraints on usage of cognitive words. *Journal of Psycholinguistic Research, 16,* 289–310.

Hughes, A. T., & Hall, W. S. (1987, April). *A hierarchical model of the acquisition of word meanings.* Paper presented at the biennial meeting of the Society for Research in Child Development, Baltimore.

438   E. K. Scholnick and W. S. Hall

Huxley, A. (1962). Words and their meanings. In M. Black (Ed.), *The importance of language* (pp. 1–12). Englewood Cliffs, NJ: Prentice-Hall.

Johnson, C. N., & Maratsos, M. P. (1977). Early comprehension of mental verbs: *Think* and *know*. *Child Development, 48,* 1743–1747.

Johnson, C. N., & Wellman, H. M. (1980). Children's developing understanding of mental verbs: Remember, know, and guess. *Child Development, 51,* 1095–1102.

Johnson-Laird, P. N. (1983). *Mental models: Towards a cognitive science of language, inference, and consciousness.* Cambridge, MA: Harvard University Press.

Jorgensen, J. C., & Falmagne, R. J. (1988). *Aspects of the meaning of* if: *Hypotheticality, entailment, and suppositional processes.* Unpublished manuscript.

Kintsch, W. (1974). *The representation of meaning in memory.* Hillsdale, NJ: Erlbaum.

Kosslyn, S. (1981). The medium and the message in mental imagery: A theory. *Psychological Review, 88,* 46–66.

Luria, A. (1976). *Cognitive development: Its cultural and social foundations.* Cambridge, MA: Harvard University Press.

Macnamara, J. (1986). *A border dispute.* Cambridge, MA: MIT Press.

Macnamara, J., Baker, E., & Olson, C. (1976). Four-year-olds' understanding of *pretend, forget,* and *know*: Evidence for propositional operations. *Child Development, 47,* 62–70.

McCabe, A. E., Evely, S., Abramovitch, R., Corter, C. M., & Pepler, C. J. (1983). Conditional statements in young children's spontaneous speech. *Journal of Child Language, 10,* 253–258.

Miscione, J. L., Marvin, R. S., O'Brien, R. G., & Greenberg, M. T. (1978). A developmental study of preschool children's understanding of the words "know" and "guess." *Child Development, 49,* 1107–1113.

Moore, C., Bryant, D., & Furrow, D. (1989). Mental terms and the development of certainty. *Child Development, 60,* 167–171.

Nelson, K. (1985). *Making sense: The acquisition of shared meaning.* New York: Academic Press.

O'Brien, D. P., Braine, M. D. S., Connell, J. F., Noveck, I. A., Fisch, S. M., & Fun, E. (1989). Reasoning about conditional sentences: Development of understanding of cues to quantification. *Journal of Experimental Child Psychology, 48,* 90–113.

Olson, D., & Torrance, N. (1987). Language, literacy, and mental states. *Discourse Processes, 10,* 157–168.

Overton, W. F. (in press). The structure of developmental theory. In P. Van Geert & L. P. Mos (Eds.), *Annals of theoretical psychology* (Vol. 6). New York: Plenum.

Overton, W., Byrnes, J. P., & O'Brien, D. P. (1985). Developmental and individual differences in conditional reasoning: The role of contradiction training and cognitive style. *Developmental Psychology, 21,* 692–701.

Overton, W. F., Ward, S. L., Noveck, I., Black, J., & O'Brien, D. P. (1987). Form and content in the development of deductive reasoning. *Developmental Psychology, 23,* 22–30.

Piaget, J. (1969). Language and intellectual operations. In H. Furth (Ed.), *Piaget and knowledge* (pp. 121–130). Englewood Cliffs, NJ: Prentice-Hall.

Piatelli-Palmerini, M. (1980). *Language and learning: The debate between Jean Piaget and Noam Chomsky.* London: Routledge & Kegan Paul.

Pieraut-Le Bonniec, G. (1980). *The development of modal reasoning: Genesis of necessity and possibility notions*. New York: Academic Press.

Reilly, J. S. (1986). The acquisition of temporals and conditionals. In E. C. Traugott, A. ter Meulen, J. S. Reilly, & C. A. Ferguson (Eds.), *On conditionals* (pp. 309–331). Cambridge University Press.

Scholnick, E. K. (1990). The three faces of If. In W. F. Overton (Ed.), *Reasoning, necessity, and logic: Developmental perspectives* (pp. 159–182). Hillsdale, NJ: Erlbaum.

Scholnick, E. K., & Wing, C. S. (1982). The pragmatics of subordinating conjunctions: A second look. *Journal of Child Language, 9*, 461–479.

Scholnick, E. K., & Wing, C. S. (1983). Evaluating presuppositions and propositions. *Journal of Child Language, 10*, 639–660.

Scholnick, E. K., & Wing, C. S. (1988). Knowing when you don't know: Developmental and situational considerations. *Developmental Psychology, 24*, 190–196.

Scholnick, E. K., & Wing, C. S. (1991). Speaking deductively: Preschoolers' use of if in conversation and in conditional inference. *Developmental Psychology, 27*, 249–258.

Shatz, M., Wellman, H. M., & Silber, S. (1983). The acquisition of mental verbs: A systematic investigation of the child's first reference to mental state. *Cognition, 14*, 301–321.

Slobin, D. I. (1979). *Psycholinguistics* (2d ed.). Glenview, IL: Scott-Foresman.

Somerville, S. C., Hadkinson, B. A., & Greenberg, C. (1979). Two levels of inferential behavior in young children. *Child Development, 50*, 119–131.

Vygotsky, L. S. (1962). *Language and thought*. Cambridge, MA: MIT Press.

Wellman, H. M., & Estes, D. (1987). Children's early use of mental verbs and what they mean. *Discourse Processes, 10*, 141–156.

Wellman, H. M., & Johnson, C. N. (1979). Understanding of mental process: A developmental study of *remember* and *forget*. *Child Development, 50*, 79–88.

Wing, C. S., & Scholnick, E. K. (1981). Children's comprehension of pragmatic concepts expressed in *because, although, if*, and *unless*. *Journal of Child Language, 8*, 347–365.

Wing, C. S., & Scholnick, E. K. (1986). Understanding the language of reasoning: Developmental, cognitive, and linguistic factors. *Journal of Psycholinguistic Research, 15*, 383–401.

12. Parent–child collaboration in young children's understanding of category hierarchies

MAUREEN A. CALLANAN

Current views of conceptual development assume that children actively construct mental categories. In this sense, the field owes much to the insight of Piaget. Although many researchers in the field of cognitive development have rejected Piaget's claims about qualitative stage changes in development, we almost take for granted his insight about children's active role in organizing and interpreting their experiences. Within the field, there is another growing trend toward considering the construction of knowledge not just as a pursuit of the individual, but as a social process. Much of this work has been inspired by Vygotsky's ideas. Piaget's and Vygotsky's approaches may seem at first to be at odds with one another, but in fact they are quite complementary. By combining these two approaches we may better understand the interaction between (a) children's expectations about category structure and word meaning and (b) the way that parents use language to structure the world for young children. Considerable attention is now focused on a third approach, which emphasizes not only the separate roles of parents and children, but also the convergence process by which parents and children construct shared meanings for words and concepts.

The notion that language is situated within social interaction and that conversational partners converge on the meanings of words within conversation has its roots in Vygotsky's (1962, 1978) work and has been elaborated recently in Rogoff (1990), Bruner (1984, 1987),

The writing of this chapter and the research reported in it have been supported in part by funds from National Institute of Mental Health Grant MH42708, National Institute of Child Health and Human Development Grant HD26228, faculty research grants from Lehigh University and the University of Texas, and research funds from the Institute for Research on Learning. I am grateful to Margarita Azmitia, Sandra Waxman, James Byrnes, and Susan Gelman for helpful comments on an earlier version.

H. Clark (1985), and others (see Bruner & Haste, 1987). Vygotsky (1962, 1978) described cognitive development as a process of internalizing patterns of social interaction (see Wertsch & Stone, 1985). In activity theory (developed by Vygotsky's follower Leontev, 1981) and in more recent arguments about situated cognition (e.g., Lave, 1988; Pea, 1989), the focus has been on the way concepts continue to be constructed within social interaction throughout life. Taking these arguments as a point of departure, we might suggest that parents and children work collaboratively to determine the meanings of words and that these word meanings remain open to revision depending on the goals and the context of each interaction. Though these ideas are compelling, taking the approach seriously requires that we face the considerable challenge of specifying how this social convergence process works and of explaining how it can be combined with more traditional accounts of the understanding of concepts and word meanings by individuals. Studying everyday interactions among social partners is an essential element of this approach. But deciding on the kind of empirical data that will support and constrain the theory is less obvious. If we wish to take a developmental perspective, we have an additional challenge: to explain how such collaborations figure in the more global developmental changes that occur in children's understanding of words and concepts. In other words, the developmental questions force us to assess not only how speakers converge on meanings within conversations, but also how these conversations affect the understanding that the speakers take away from each situation and carry into subsequent interactions.

My aim in this chapter is to face these challenges by working out a social convergence account of one particular domain of conceptual development: the problem of how children learn hierarchical systems of category names for common objects. To do this, I will examine converging data from several sources and various methodologies. In my work I have conducted observational studies of children and parents interacting, as well as experimental studies to test hypotheses about how children make use of information in parents' speech. I will argue that such a combination puts us in a better position to study each of the essential components of the social convergence approach: children's developing understanding of words and concepts, parents' strategies for talking about objects and categories, and the mechanisms by which parents and children converge on word meanings within conversations.

In this chapter, I will discuss each of these components in turn. I will begin by outlining what we know about what children bring to the task of learning category names, paying special attention to the recent research proposing constraints on children's expectations about word meanings. I will next focus on the role of parents' language as data relevant to theories of conceptual development. In particular, I will describe four different approaches to studying parental input, each with different implications for a general theory of conceptual development. Next I will take on the central task of trying to connect children's and parents' contributions, by discussing research on parents' labeling strategies in speech to children in conjunction with research on how children make use of the information in parents' speech. Finally, I will draw some conclusions about the role of parent–child collaboration in the development of categories and word meanings and propose some directions for future work.

Research on children's understanding of categories and labels

In reviewing the research on children's developing knowledge of object categories, I will focus on three important issues that children must face and that theories of conceptual development must explain. First, children must find a way into the task of mapping words to categories. Second, once they have made their initial interpretations of words, children must often revise these interpretations to better match the adult interpretations of the same words. Third, children must come to understand the inclusion structure of conceptual hierarchies and the related fact that individual objects can be named and categorized in several different ways.

One of the most puzzling problems of development is how children get started on learning the meanings of words in their language. Within the domain of object categories, it is clear that children have some ability to form categories before learning any words. There is some controversy over whether these early categories enjoy the same status as those formed by older children and adults (Cohen & Younger, 1983; Mandler, 1988; Nelson, 1988). Regardless of how this controversy is settled, it seems plausible that there is a connection between infants' perceptual object categories and the categories that begin to be mapped onto the earliest labels for objects.

In asking how children make word–category mappings, the focus has been on the enormous ambiguity problem with which children are faced when trying to interpret the meanings of words heard in conversation (Markman, 1989). Children seem to learn much of their early vocabulary through ostensive definition, or pointing and labeling (Ninio, 1980; Ninio & Bruner, 1978). It is not a trivial problem, however, for children to resolve the ambiguity of this type of reference. As Quine (1960) and Wittgenstein (1953) have argued, there is nothing in the environment that restricts ostensive labeling to refer to the whole object rather than to some attribute or part of the object, or to its relation to other objects. And yet very young children do quite an impressive job of learning nouns and apparently using them to refer to categories of objects. Several research projects on infants' sensitivity to the connection between words and nonverbal cues such as pointing and gaze have begun to help us understand how this process begins (Baldwin & Markman, 1989; Scaife & Bruner, 1975). There also seem to be constraints on children's hypotheses about the kinds of categories that words encode, which may help explain how children disambiguate words that are used in ostensive reference.

One proposal that has received some support is that children are likely to interpret nouns to refer to whole objects rather than parts or attributes of the object (Macnamara, 1972; Mervis & Long, 1987; Ninio, 1980). Markman and Hutchinson (1984) proposed another constraint that would help solve the ostension problem for children. They argue that young children expect single nouns to refer to object categories rather than to thematically related objects, that is, that children expect a word like *dog* to refer to objects that are similar to one another rather than to objects that are related in other ways (such as a dog and a bone). Markman and Hutchinson provide evidence that while young children often pay more attention to thematic relations among objects (e.g., pairing a dog with a bone in an oddity task), the presence of a novel word leads them to focus instead on similarity among members of the same taxonomic category (e.g., pairing a dog with a cat). In a study of production of object labels during the single-word period, Huttenlocher and Smiley (1987) provided further evidence that children's early object labels refer to categories rather than to thematic or complexive relations. Similarly, Waxman and Gelman (1986) have found that the presence of an unfamiliar noun helps 3- and 4-year-olds to sort objects taxonomically.

The whole-object constraint and taxonomic word constraint together would considerably reduce the ambiguity of the word-learning situation for children. Even with these constraints, however, some ambiguity remains, because any object can be categorized at several different levels in a hierarchy. For example, suppose a child hears the word *feline* used to label a cat. The whole-object and taxonomic assumptions would allow the child to rule out many possible interpretations for the word ("furry," "cat's paw," "cat and its milk") but would leave open several taxonomic interpretations ("cat," "Siamese cat," "mammal," "animal"). How do children decide which hierarchical level is being picked out by a new word? One possible solution is an even more specific constraint, namely, that children expect novel words to refer to basic-level categories. Rosch and her colleagues (Rosch, 1978; Rosch, Mervis, Gray, Johnson, & Boyes-Braem, 1976) have shown that basic-level categories are preferred by both adults and children, making this a reasonable hypothesis. In fact, this basic-level constraint is sometimes assumed without being tested. Indirect evidence appears in two studies in which children were taught artificial categories at different hierarchical levels (Horton & Markman, 1980; Markman, Horton, & McLanahan, 1980). Although the two studies used quite different procedures, in both cases simple labeling of pictures or objects led the children to infer that a basic-level category had been indicated. However, the children in these studies needed more than pure ostension in order to learn superordinate categories.

In preliminary work with 3-, 4-, and 5-year-old children, Repp, McCarthy, and I have tested the basic-level expectation hypothesis more directly. We first pretested children so that we could ensure that some words were familiar to them and some were unfamiliar (see Table 12.1 for a list of the items used). A puppet then introduced new words – for example, pointing to a poodle and saying, "This is a quadruped." We tested children's interpretation of the words by asking them to choose from a set of pictures all those with the same name as the target picture (e.g., "Find all of the quadrupeds"). The data from this study did not support a strict basic-level constraint hypothesis (Callanan, Repp, & McCarthy, 1989). In fact, the cases in which the children were most likely to expect novel words to refer to basic-level categories were those in which they already knew the basic-level term and could translate the novel term as a synonym. When the children knew both the subordinate and

12.1 *Items used in the Callanan, Repp, and McCarthy (1989) study*

Picture	Label taught
I. Familiar subordinate label– familiar basic label	
Poodle	Quadruped
Rose	Vegetation
Owl	Raptor
Rocking chair	Artifact
II. Unfamiliar subordinate label–familiar basic label	
Fedora-type hat	Apparel
Monarch butterfly	Lepidopteron
Sedan-type car	Conveyance
Whiptail lizard	Saurian
III. Unfamiliar subordinate label–unfamiliar basic label	
Router	Exscinder
Bar clamp	Binder
Plumose anemone	Coelenterate
Manta ray	Ichthyo

basic labels for an item, their interpretations of the novel word were split between those two levels. When they knew no word for an item, most 3-year-olds interpreted the novel word at the subordinate level, whereas older children's interpretations were divided among the subordinate, basic, and superordinate levels. (Three-year-olds' choices do not seem to result from a conservative preference to stick to the target picture, because most children were willing to extend the label to other pictures from the same subordinate category as the target.) This pattern of findings is somewhat surprising given previous research showing that children tend not to interpret a new word as a synonym for a familiar word (Markman & Wachtel, 1988; Taylor & Gelman, 1989), so we must be cautious about drawing firm conclusions. These results do suggest, however, that 3-year-olds may not have a strong expectation that nouns refer to basic-level categories.

Should these findings hold up under further scrutiny, how can they be explained? One possible explanation is that children start out with a basic-level constraint, but that by 3 years of age it has been abandoned. This hypothesis cannot be addressed by our data and should be tested with younger children. If the basic-level constraint weakens with age, however, one might predict a developmental trend away from a basic-level expectation; instead, we found that basic-level interpretations were more likely among 4- and 5-year-old children than among 3-year-old children.

Another possible interpretation of this finding is that children's initial word–category mappings do not exactly match the mappings reflected in adults' basic-level categories. We know that the majority of their early words are basic-level nouns (E. V. Clark, 1983; Markman, 1989), but this does not guarantee that these words map onto (adult) basic-level categories for children. The level at which infants form perceptual categories may not be the adult basic level. Instead, as Mervis (1987) argues, children may start out carving the world into "child-basic" categories and only later revise their initial categorizations to match the adult-basic level. Mervis reports evidence that the child-basic level may be either more general (*car* for any four-wheeled vehicle) or more specific (*duck* for only yellow ducks) than the adult basic-level category for the corresponding term. She argues that as children become more experienced with the intended functions of artifacts and the place of natural categories in the world, they revise their organization schemes. By adulthood, though individual differences and flexibility in conceptual organization remain (Barsalou, 1987), there is much more agreement about which things are referred to by which words. Rather than a starting point for children's word–category mappings, then, the basic level may be seen as the *result* of the social convergence process. Mervis's child-basic proposal has a great deal of merit, particularly in the way it draws connections between early perceptual categorization and the first word–category mappings. Notice, however, that it is difficult to derive principled predictions about how the child-basic level will differ as a function of the knowledge domain, the situation, and the child's knowledge.

In sum, the situation is much more complex than children expecting nouns to refer to basic-level categories. There is clearly a range of possible interpretations for words from which even very young children can choose. Even if there is no basic constraint, however, there may be a constraint that excludes superordinate categories from the set of hypotheses that young children consider when interpreting a new word applied to an individual object. In our study (Callanan et al., 1989), it was very rare for 3-year-old children to interpret a new word at the superordinate level (though older children sometimes showed evidence of superordinate interpretations for the most unfamiliar items). Mervis (1987) found evidence for child-basic categories that were more general than the basic level, but they were still categories based on perceptual features. The similarities among different four-wheeled vehicles may be more perceptually salient to a young child than the similarities in size and shape that determine the boundaries among cars, trucks, vans, and buses. But a category like *vehicle,* which includes airplanes and boats and is based on more abstract functional features (Tversky & Hemenway, 1984), is not likely to be children's first guess about a word's meaning.

The notion that it is superordinate categories (rather than basic categories) that are distinctive from categories at other levels has appeared in several guises in the literature (see Markman, 1989, for a review). Data from several studies support the idea that superordinate categories include groups of objects whereas basic (and subordinate) categories include individuals. For example, Wisniewski and Murphy (in press) found that in written text, basic labels most often refer to individuals, whereas superordinate labels most often refer to groups of objects or classes of objects. In addition, young children sometimes interpret superordinate categories as referring to groups or collections, that is, interpreting the word *toy* as referring to a group of different toys, but not to a single toy (Callanan & Markman, 1982; Macnamara, 1982; Markman, 1989; Markman et al., 1980). Similarly, adults are faster at categorizing objects as superordinate category members when they are shown as part of a scene rather than in isolation (Murphy & Wisniewski, 1989).

Shipley's (1989) work suggests an interesting account of these differences between the superordinate level and other levels. She makes an important distinction between *class-inclusion hierarchies,* which contain categories of individuals, and *kind hierarchies,* which contain categories of categories. Shipley reports evidence that preschool children think of basic-level categories as categories-of-individuals, but that they think of superordinate categories as categories-of-categories. For example, Shipley (1989) found that children who were asked to "tell me two dogs" were likely to mention two individual dogs ("Ruffy and Kristen"), but when the same children were asked to "tell me two animals," they were likely to mention two categories of animals (e.g., "giraffe and monkey"). Although it is logically possible for superordinate categories to be thought of as categories-of-objects, it may be more natural to think of them as categories that include several distinct subcategories. Shipley argues that this kind hierarchy or category-of-categories structure has important implications for children's developing inferential abilities. For our present purposes, however, this work provides another strand of support for the claim that young children are not likely to consider a superordinate category interpretation for a novel word applied to a single object.

In light of these arguments, I propose that children expect that category labels refer to categories-of-objects as distinct from categories-of-categories. Rather than a constraint to expect basic-level labels, this expectation would exclude superordinate category interpretations. It would imply not that children cannot learn superordinate categories, but that they would not interpret them as names for individuals. Hence, children's knowledge of broad ontological categories such as *animal* (Carey, 1985; Keil, 1979) would not be inconsistent with this view, as long as these were categories-of-categories rather than categories-of-individuals. I will return to this proposal later in the chapter, once I have discussed some related data on parents' strategies for labeling objects at different levels.

Thus far was have discussed the problems of how children interpret a new word that they hear adults use and how they revise child-basic categories so that they are closer to adult-basic categories. At some point children are faced with another set of problems: learning that objects can be categorized and labeled at multiple levels and learning the inclusion relations among the categories at different levels. Markman has proposed that there is another constraint, the mutual exclusivity assumption, which simplifies the task of word learning by leading children to maintain nonoverlap among the word meanings they acquire (Markman, 1989; Chapter 3, this volume; Markman & Wachtel, 1988). Merriman and Bowman (1989) have argued that instead of guiding children's initial attempts at word learning, the mutual exclusivity bias comes in well after children have begun to learn words. In either case, however, this mutual exclusivity bias would make it difficult for children to learn the names of objects at different hierarchical levels. If children assume that objects have only one name, then once they have learned a name for an object (e.g., the basic-level name), they should resist learning additional names, including those subordinate and superordinate to the known label.

The inclusion relation itself, though perhaps not as difficult as

Piaget's class-inclusion work suggested, also seems to present some difficulty to young children (Blewitt, 1989; Markman & Callanan, 1984; Smith, 1979). We now have impressive evidence that 2-year-olds can simultaneously use category labels at different hierarchical levels (Blewitt, 1989; Taylor & Gelman, 1989; Waxman, 1990; Chapter 4, this volume). Even in these cases, however, we do not have unambiguous evidence that the inclusion relation is clearly understood. There are examples in the literature where children use labels at different levels but understand them in nonhierarchical ways. Some examples involve atypical subordinate labels; many children for example use *duck* and *bird* as contrastive rather than hierarchically related category labels (E. V. Clark, 1983). Even when the extensions of two hierarchical terms appears to match that of adults (e.g., *animal* and *dog*), this fact alone does not guarantee that the inclusion relation and its implications are understood. In particular, appreciation of the hierarchical status of categories entails knowledge about the asymmetry of the inclusion relation and the resulting asymmetry of the inferences that can be made from one category level to another. There is some evidence that 4-year-old children can make inductive and deductive category inferences (Blewitt, 1989; Gelman, 1988; Gelman & Markman, 1986, 1987; Smith, 1979). Before age 4, however, children have difficulty with some types of inferences (Blewitt, 1989), and even after age 4, their performance on inference tasks is not consistently strong (Smith, 1979). Thus, coming to understand the implications of hierarchical organization may be a gradual process; the comprehension and production of words at different category levels may mark the beginning of the process.

This brief review of the conceptual development literature has pointed out three problems that face young children: (a) getting started on the task of mapping words to categories, (b) revising child-basic categories to more closely match the adult-basic distinctions and learning the conventional names for these categories, and (c) learning the inclusion structure of hierarchies, especially the relation between the basic level and the superordinate level. We know that children solve all three problems within a fairly short time. In order to understand how they succeed in doing so, we will now examine how parental input may help children to solve these problems. Constraints on children's understanding of category labels (e.g., the taxonomic assumption, that nouns refer to taxonomic categories) have been proposed as part of the solution to the puzzle of how children learn word meanings with very little guidance. These issues are discussed in at least three chapters of the present volume (Clark, Chapter 2; Markman, Chapter 3; Waxman, Chapter 4). Data on parent–child interaction is likely to help clarify our understanding of where these constraints come from, how they come to be relaxed, and how they interact with other factors in the everyday interactions during which word learning takes place. In the next section I will discuss the ways that parents' speech may be used as evidence within a theory of conceptual development. In a later section, I will return to the three problems I have just posed and consider more specifically how parent–child collaboration may help account for the developmental data on these important issues.

Parents' role in children's understanding of categories and labels

Beginning with Brown's (1958) account of the "original word game," researchers have long acknowledged the importance of the social situation in which children begin to learn words. Pointing and labeling objects seems to account for a large proportion of parents' speech to very young children, and children's earliest words are largely nouns that name classes of objects. At least in Western middle-class culture, parents and young children spend a great deal of time on games of naming objects, pictures, and body parts. These sorts of games may help children to learn the referential function of words as well as the meanings of particular words (Ninio & Bruner, 1978; Snow & Goldfield, 1983).

Despite this long-standing concern with parents' labels for objects as an important factor in semantic acquisition, the place of parental input data in current theories of development has not yet been well articulated. A simplistic view is that input data are needed to resolve the nature–nurture debate. Any discussion of parents' effects on children's development brings to mind the age-old controversy of nature versus nurture. At first glance, an emphasis on the study of parental input may connote an environmental account of language development. Indeed, Skinner's initial account of the language acquisition process relied on reinforcement and correction by parents (though this view was strongly contradicted by the data, e.g., Brown & Hanlon, 1970). Further, the research on the "motherese hypothesis" was motivated by a fundamental disagreement with Chomsky's claims about an innate language acquisition device (e.g., Snow & Ferguson, 1977). Though some imitation is certainly necessary for learning language (as in the case of phonology), we need not always interpret parental input data as evidence of a nurturist position (Kuczaj, 1986). It is clear by now that neither a strong nature position nor a strong nurture position can provide a full explanation of language development and that the study of parental iput does not lead to such quick and easy answers as "It's there from the beginning" or "It's learned or taught." Instead, there seems to be an interaction between what children bring to the task of learning language and what parents provide in the way of guidance. The difficult and challenging question is precisely how to characterize the nature of that interaction. What do particular patterns of parental input tell us about the process of conceptual development?

In studies of parents' influence on cognitive development, it is often difficult to determine the status of parental input as evidence relevant to a theory of cognitive or conceptual development. For example, the finding that basic-level labels are the first used by young children (e.g., Rosch et al., 1976) is often mentioned together with the finding that basic-level labels are also used most frequently by parents, especially when they are speaking to young children (e.g., Blewitt, 1983; Lucariello & Nelson, 1986; Shipley, Kuhn, & Madden, 1983). However, it is not clear how to describe the relation between these two effects or their implications for children's conceptual development. Sometimes children's and parents' use of basic-level words are taken as two lines of independent evidence for the notion that the basic level is primary. These two forms of evidence are clearly not independent, however. It could be that children use basic-level labels only because those are the words they hear in parents' speech. This is unlikely, but much more must be said about the interaction between the two findings. In this section, I will describe and illustrate four different approaches to the study of parental input data. I will try to spell out the theoretical assumptions underlying those approaches and discuss their implications for the social convergence view of conceptual development.

Identifying mismatches between parent and child

Researchers sometimes examine parental input in order to rule out parental teaching as a competing hypothesis for their claims about changes within children. For example, Huttenlocher, Smiley, and

Ratner (1983) identified a pattern of developmental change in children's use of verbs. They then looked at parents' use of the same verbs in order to determine whether the children's pattern could be accounted for by their imitation of changes in parents' speech. The children's pattern of verb use was not found in parents' speech in this case, giving strength to the researchers' claims about a cognitive developmental trend within children to account for the change. Similarly, Goldin-Meadow and Mylander (1984) described a gesture system in a group of deaf children of hearing parents. Again, in order to rule out imitation as an explanation for the children's signs, the authors studied the parents' gestures and demonstrated clear differences between the parents' and the children's systems. A mismatch between the patterns of word use or systems of organization used by parent and child, then, suggests to us that children have created an interpretation of their own.

Since in this approach, input is taken mainly as negative evidence for developmental change, no clear theoretical claims are made about the role of parents in cognitive development. Instead, claims are usually made about a particular developmental change as instigated by the child, and input must be checked in order to rule out a less interesting possibility. In fact, when a mismatch does not occur, this strategy gives us no help in determining what our theory should be. For example, consider the basic-level finding mentioned earlier: Children use predominantly basic-level labels in their early speech. When we check the input, however, we find that parents also use predominantly basic-level labels when they speak to young children. The input data do not rule out the imitation hypothesis, but neither do they provide strong support for the imitation model. There are several possible interpretations of this pattern in the data, and the mismatch approach does not allow us to decide among them.

Patterns of input as potential data for children

A second approach to the study of parents' speech is exemplified by much of the "motherese" research that began in the 1970s. The idea here is to identify patterns or strategies in parents' speech and then to postulate ways in which these patterns might affect children's acquisition. This approach has been used in most of the research on parents' influences on language development and, more recently, on conceptual development. The theoretical assumptions underlying this approach are that parents' systematic input can be noticed, understood, and used by children. In some sense this approach looks for "matches" between parents and children (as opposed to the mismatches sought in the preceding approach). But notice that it is a matter not of finding identity matches, but of testing hypotheses about particular patterns of input that can have beneficial effects on children's learning.

Consider the motherese literature (e.g., Snow & Ferguson, 1977), which emerged in response to the question of how children acquire syntax. Because of certain features of parents' speech to children, the argument went, the problem of learning syntax is greatly simplified and we need not postulate so much in the way of innate language-learning devices. The evidence that parents' speech to children is different from speech to adults is strong and consistent. However, it has been more difficult to find strong evidence for the claim that these differences have a causal role in children's language acquisition. Despite various methodological problems, however, there have been some demonstrations of connections between input and syntax acquisition (Hoff-Ginsberg & Shatz, 1982).

More recently, in the field of conceptual development, several researchers have conducted studies of parents' speech to children with a related focus in mind (e.g., Blewitt, 1983; Callanan, 1985; Lucariello & Nelson, 1986; Shipley et al., 1983; Wales, Colman, & Pattison, 1983; White, 1982). The goal here is to understand how children learn the meanings of words, given the ambiguity of ostensive reference. By identifying the nature of the linguistic data base from which children are actually able to draw, we may be able to construct a clearer picture of the way they solve the problem. Further, the structure of parents' speech to children may itself constrain the task of word learning. For example, if parents used only basic-level terms in their speech to young children, children could avoid, for awhile, the problem of coordinating the meanings of multiple labels for the same object. A clearer picture of what the child has to work with should help us to determine the kinds of understanding and abilities children must bring to the task.

Scaffolding strategies as mechanisms for developmental change

Another major approach to the study of parental input involves more microscopic analysis of conversations between parents and children as they engage in various tasks. The goals of this approach are to understand the dynamic process by which parents assess children's understanding and offer guidance and to look for evidence that children use the guidance to progress in the task. Many researchers have been struck by the fine-tuning used by some parents and teachers to provide an ideal balance of support, on the one hand, and encouragement of independence, on the other (e.g., Kaye, 1982; Rogoff, 1990; Rogoff & Wertsch, 1984; Wood, Bruner, & Ross, 1976). Children might make use of this sort of guidance not only to solve the problem at hand but also to learn how to solve such problems in the future.

Wood et al. (1976) introduced the term *scaffolding* to describe the strategies they observed adults using to help children solve a puzzle. The tutor, or parent, seems to take account of the child's abilities and successes at each step of the task and to change the level of guidance offered as a function of the child's needs. This idea is related to Vygotsky's (1978) notion of the "zone of proximal development" in that, through scaffolding techniques, a skilled tutor will find the appropriate zone in which to help the child progress in a task. The claim is that these scaffolding patterns play an important role in children's learning. The parent is, in a sense, modeling the thought processes that the child might use in solving the problem. By internalizing these strategies, Vygotsky would argue, children are better equipped to deal with similar problems on their own.

Wood's (1980) analysis suggests that the most successful tutoring involves (a) finding the child's zone of sensitivity and (b) making the type of guidance contingent on the child's performance on the preceding step. The *zone of sensitivity* is defined as the level of support at which a child is most likely to produce a successful move. The optimal strategy, Wood argues, is to reduce the guidance by a small amount each time the child completes a successful step and to increase the guidance by a small amount with each failure.

This strategy for measuring scaffolding assumes a task with a clear solution. In fact, much of this research has used "schoollike" problems such as puzzle tasks (e.g., Pratt, Kerig, Cowan, & Cowan, 1988; Renshaw & Gardner, 1987; Rogoff, Ellis, & Gardner, 1984; Rogoff & Gardner, 1984; Wertsch, Minick, & Arns, 1984). In fact, much of the research that focuses on scaffolding uses this type of task (see

Azmitia & Perlmutter, 1989, for an excellent review and analysis of this literature). The focus of this chapter, the task of learning the meanings of words, is much more ill-defined, and it is more difficult to define the steps that one should take in providing optimal guidance. Though classification tasks have been used to study parents' scaffolding techniques (Rogoff et al., 1984), it is not clear how to draw parallels from such tasks to naturally occurring situations. It is hard to know the exact point at which children understand the meaning of a word (in the sense that we know the point at which a puzzle has been solved), and there is some controversy over whether it makes sense to talk about people having consistent mental representations of word meanings across situations (Barsalou, 1987; Greeno & Stucky, 1990).

The scaffolding metaphor may be applied to the study of the development of word meaning, however, if broader strokes are used to define the levels of scaffolding. Ninio and Bruner's (1978) longitudinal study of a single parent–child pair showed that parents' demands on children in book-reading exchanges can be fine-tuned in such a way that children are provided with guidance to succeed in vocabulary learning. For example, before this child's production of labels, his mother seemed to accept nonlexical verbalizations as acceptable turns. After the child had begun to produce labels, however, she often responded to such vocalizations with questions like "What's that?" therefore demanding a more well formed label (see also Miller, 1982). Notice that making the level of guidance contingent on their previous performance means something quite different in helping children learn word meanings than in helping them solve puzzles. The time course is different than in the problem-solving tasks, and changes in children's performance and in parents' guidance are much more subtle. According to Ninio and Bruner, the child's increasing role as a partner in the redundant and restrictive structure of the book-reading routine is the basis for learning the relationship between words and the objects to which they refer (see also Snow & Goldfield, 1983). It is likely that children also learn about word meanings and about hierarchical inclusion during everyday activities other than book reading; in less routinized activities, it may be even more difficult to know how to apply the scaffolding approach.

456 M. A. Callanan

Identifying cultural attitudes regarding parents' role in development

A fourth way to study input is to look at the more deliberate and
global strategies of parents. In the culture of middle-class families
in the United States, for example, tutoring strategies appear in very
early interactions between parents and children. Heath (1983) has
shown us, however, that these strategies are by no means universal;
they do not even hold true within subcultures in the United States.
She found in one of the Appalachian communities she studied that
parents did not think it reasonable to ask a child questions to which
they already knew the answer. The games of "What's that?" that
are so prevalent in middle-class families, and that we take for granted
as part of language learning, may be culturally specific. Overall assumptions that parents have about their own role in children's cognitive development are certain to influence the kinds of interactions
that occur, and we must keep these cross-cultural considerations in
mind as we formulate theories about the kind of input that is required for conceptual development (see Rogoff, 1990). I will return
to these issues later in the chapter.

Summary

These four approaches to the study of parents' speech make quite
different assumptions about parents' role in conceptual development. The identifying mismatches approach considers input mainly
as a competing hypothesis. The cultural-attitudes approach is an essential direction for future research, but not much attention has so
far been paid to such cross-cultural concerns. Most of the research
in this field takes either the patterns-of-input approach or the scaffolding approach. In principle, these two approaches could provide
complementary ways to study the same data. The patterns approach gives us a broad overview of the pattern of parents' speech
that children hear, whereas the scaffolding approach gives us a means
of studying the detail of particular interactions as they unfold. In
practice, however, there tends to be a confound between approach
and task, such that scaffolding studies focus on problem-solving tasks,
whereas patterns-of-input studies focus on more ill defined tasks
such as language acquisition. One goal of future work might be to
coordinate the two approaches for a more balanced view.

Our goals in developing a social convergence account of conceptual development are to explore the ways that parents and children work together to understand concepts and word meanings and to find means of testing causal hypotheses about how these interactions influence development. It is often difficult to test causal hypotheses. In the patterns approach the results tend to be correctional, leading to problems in inferring the direction of causality (Newport, Gleitman, & Gleitman, 1977). In the scaffolding approach, parent and child are studied in the same analysis, and it is often difficult to avoid circular reasoning about cause and effect. For example, if increased scaffolding leads to more improvement, this could be because children who begin the task doing poorly receive more scaffolding and also have more room for improvement.

In my own work I have tested causal hypotheses by combining observational and experimental methods. First I have identified patterns in parents' speech through observational studies; then I have conducted experimental studies to test children's sensitivity to these patterns. In the next section, I will review data on parents' strategies for labeling objects and on the way children use these strategies, paying special attention to ways in which we can draw causal conclusions either about scaffolding effects or about how children use the information in the patterns of parents' speech.

Social convergence: Interaction between constraints and parental strategies

Three questions were formulated on the basis of my earlier review of the conceptual development data with children: (a) How do children get started on the mapping between words and objects? (b) How do children come to revise their initial attempts at categorization so that their categories begin to resemble the more conventional adult categories? (c) How do children learn to use multiple labels for objects and to understand hierarchical inclusion relations among categories? In this section, I will discuss these three questions in turn, considering examples of research programs that attempt to characterize the role of parental input in children's solutions to these problems. First, I will discuss the proposal that constraints on word meanings allow children to begin the word-learning process and the suggestion that parents' labeling practices can help us to determine the origin of such constraints. Second, I will discuss Mervis's data on parents' role in category evolution.

Finally, I will discuss my research on parents' role in children's acquisition of hierarchical systems of category names.

Parents' labels and children's expectations

In recent discussions of constraints on word meanings it has been suggested that parental input data should help us to determine the origin of these constraints (e.g., E. V. Clark, 1989; Nelson, 1989). The appropriate way to approach this question would presumably be to use the identifying mismatches approach described earlier. If parents' labeling practices do not match children's expectations about labels, these expectations are likely to be innate, or to originate from the child. It should already be clear, however, that the data provide us with several cases of "matches" between parents' labeling strategies and children's proposed constraints. As I argued earlier, this pattern of data leaves us uncertain about the relative roles of parent and child in the phenomenon under study. One might argue, on the one hand, that parents adjust their input to match children's preexisting expectations or, on the other hand, that parents' systematic labeling strategies lead children to formulate an expectation. A brief review of the relationship between specific constraints and relevant parental input will illustrate the problem and help us to make suggestions about further study of this issue.

For several of the constraints proposed for children, there are analogous patterns in parents' speech. The whole-object constraint, which leads children to expect labels to refer to whole objects rather than to parts or attributes, is supported by parents' labeling strategies. Ninio (1980) found that parents' ostensive definitions label whole objects 95% of the time. When parents name parts of objects, they signal to the child that a different kind of thing is being named by including a reference to the whole object before labeling the part (e.g., "Here is a train; here are the wheels." "These are the girl's eyes." "Look, what a lovely doll; where is the doll's nose?"). Ninio (1980) asks "whether mothers are aware that this practice fosters an expectation on the part of the child that ostensive definitions always refer to the whole object pointed to" (p. 566). This quotation suggests a view that children's expectations result from patterns in the input. Although this is indeed possible, it seems equally likely that children guide parents to use these strategies. For example, parents might start out labeling parts ostensively, but if children mistakenly interpret such utterances as references to the whole object, the parents might alter their labeling strategies. Another possible alternative is that both mother and child start with the same expectation that labels refer to whole objects. Although we have data showing that children interpret nouns as referring to whole objects rather than to parts (Mervis & Long, 1987), it is difficult to decide among these possible reasons for the effect.

Similarly, children's expectations that nouns refer to taxonomic categories and to categories at roughly the basic level may be influenced by parents' labeling. Parents' tendency to use basic-level labels as names for objects when speaking with children is strong and consistent (Adams & Bullock, 1986; Anglin, 1977; Blewitt, 1983; Callanan, 1985; Shipley et al., 1983), although more recent data have shown that this effect can be altered somewhat by the degree of contrast among the surrounding objects (Adams & Bullock, 1986; Callanan & Weed, 1990) and by the kind of activity in which parent and child are engaged (Lucariello & Nelson, 1986). In picture-book reading, parents' use of syntactic frames such as "That's an X" involve predominantly basic-level category names (Ninio, 1980; Callanan & Weed, 1990). Further, parents honor the mutual exclusivity constraint by using special strategies to introduce superordinate and subordinate labels (Blewitt, 1983; Callanan, 1985; Callanan & Weed, 1990; Shipley et al., 1983). Parents are probably not very self-conscious about these labeling strategies; it is most likely that their emphasis on basic-level labels reflects their own conceptual structure, as well as their attempt (conscious or not) to speak in concrete terms to young children.

Parents do not always use their own knowledge as a guide when labeling objects for children, however. Mervis's (1984, 1987) work on the child-basic level demonstrates that parents often accept very young children's incorrect labels (e.g., *car* for a truck; *kitty* for a lion). Mervis (1984) has further interesting data showing that parents of Down syndrome children are less likely to accept their children's child-basic labels. Presumably parents of disabled children view the correction of mistakes as a more important kind of input than do parents of normal children. Parents are clearly adjusting their input as a function of their perception of the children's abilities and needs. It is interesting that Mervis used her data from parents of Down syndrome children to argue that child-basic categories originate within the child; both Down syndrome and normal children develop child-basic categories, despite the fact that parents of Down syndrome children do not encourage their children's child-basic forms.

In short, although it does not seem likely that parents teach children constraints on word meaning, we do have evidence that parents and children use similar strategies to map words to categories from very early on. It is difficult to discern where the causal links might be between these two sources of data. Perhaps Mervis (1986) is correct in stating that children start out with some fundamental principles such as "Look for form–function correlations" and "Pay attention to patterns in parents' input." Within the structure of parent–child routines of labeling objects (which begin very early in infancy) the constraints may then be constructed in a collaborative manner. This hypothesis should be tested in research with very young children and their parents.

Although direct effects between parental input data and constraint data have not been tested, there are some promising avenues for future research. For the remaining two topics, however, explicit attempts have been made to explore the ways in which children make use of the information in parents' labeling strategies.

Parent–child conversations and children's category evolution

In her work on category evolution, Mervis (1986, 1987; Banigan & Mervis, 1988; Mervis & Mervis, 1988) has taken an approach that emphasizes testing the connection between parents' input and children's thought. As mentioned earlier, she has found that children often start out with a concept different from the conventional one, because they focus on different form–function correlations than adults do. These child-basic categories must eventually evolve into adult-basic categories. Mervis has also found that parents of very young children often accept the child-basic labels offered by their children. She has recently studied in more detail the kinds of strategies parents used to help children with this realignment.

Mervis and Mervis (1988) point out that researchers often assume that parents' corrections of children's overextensions or child-basic labels lead children to realign their category boundaries. They argue, however, that this type of labeling feedback is not likely to be as helpful to very young children as feedback that focuses more explicitly on the form–function correlations that children's initial classifications have ignored. They propose two kinds of input that would serve this function for children: Verbal descriptions of the relevant form–function correlations and demonstrations of the form–function correlations. For very young children, actual demonstrations of functions were expected to be much more useful than verbal descriptions. Mervis and Mervis (1988) tested their claims in a longitudinal study that combined observations of parents' and children's speech during spontaneous play with comprehension and production tests of the children's knowledge of the target words (*kitty, car,* and *ball*). Mervis and Mervis looked for evidence that parents' demonstrations of important form–function correlations preceded children's first comprehension of the relevant word. They found that when a child included a child-basic object in the adult-basic category during one of their comprehension tests, it was extremely likely that earlier in that session the child's mother had provided a demonstration of a relevant form–function correlation for that object. For example, many of these cases involved parents' providing a label and an appropriate sound for an animal that the child had been calling a cat (e.g., *roar* for lion). They also found that demonstrations were followed by earlier comprehension than were non-demonstration attempts at correction.

In another study, Banigan and Mervis (1988) went a step further and experimentally tested the effects of demonstration and verbal description of form–function correlations compared with merely providing the correct label. Children in the condition where the label was accompanied by both a description and a demonstration were most likely to learn the adult-basic label. Children who heard only the label were least likely to learn it. If only one kind of additional information accompanied the label, demonstration was more effective than description.

Mervis has provided us with an example of separate research strategies converging on conclusions about the relative contribution of parent and child to an aspect of lexical development. I have used a similar approach in studying children's learning of hierarchical category names, which I will discuss next.

Labeling objects at multiple levels: Children's understanding of hierarchies

At some point parents begin to label objects at multiple levels. In my work, I have asked whether parents' strategies for introducing

Table 12.2 *Examples of labeling strategies used by parents*

Strategy	Description	Example
Ostension	Point and label	This is a porcupine
Anchor	Label same object at two levels	This is a mixer; it's also called a machine
Inclusion	Make explicit statement of inclusion relation	A mixer is a kind of machine
Multiple referent	Label group of objects	These are all vehicles

Source: Callanan (1985).

non-basic-level labels differ from their strategies for introducing basic-level labels. Particularly with superordinate labels, there is evidence that parents mark these words in some ways that may be helpful for young children. Since the data differ for superordinate and subordinate categories, I will treat each in turn.

Superordinate labels. In one set of studies (Callanan, 1985), mothers were asked to teach words at different levels to their 2-, 3-, and 4-year-old children. For each item, the mothers were given a word and four pictures (e.g., *vehicle*: car, bus, truck, boat; *porcupine*: four porcupines) and told to use whatever strategies seemed natural to them. When mothers taught basic-level categories (e.g., *porcupine*), they tended simply to use the label as the name for an object (or picture), as if they assumed that children were guided by a basic-level constraint. Typically, once the label had been mentioned the mothers seemed satisfied that children had learned the concept and that it was time to go on to the next category.

When mothers taught superordinate categories (e.g., *vehicles, furniture*), however, they did not simply point to an object and label it with the superordinate name. Several labeling strategies differentiated superordinate categories from basic categories (Table 12.2). First, mothers were likely to label the same picture at both the basic and superordinate levels, as the following excerpt illustrates:

M: What do you think a machine is?
C: Maybe it looks like a bacuuming thing.
M: Yeah. There's lots of different kinds of machines, though, don't forget. There's . . . some machines type.
C: Yeah.

M: The typewriter is a machine. And some machines clean.
C: Yeah.
M: The vacuum cleaner is a machine, you're right. And some, uh, what else do some machines – the lawnmower is a kind of machine.
C: Yeah! It vacuumings the, um, grass!
M: It does! Yeah, it does vacuum the grass. It cuts the grass too. And then it throws it to the back.
C: Yeah.
M: You know, there's lots of kinds of machines. Machines, machines do work for us usually.

Notice in this excerpt that the mother never says, "This is a machine." Instead, she labels each item at the basic level first and then uses the superordinate label. In fact, mothers used more basic labels than superordinate labels, on the average, though the superordinates were the ones they had been asked to teach. I have called this strategy *anchoring* at the basic level; it is similar to a finding reported by Blewitt (1983) and Shipley et al. (1983). Anchoring, then, is one strategy that may be a signal for children that a superordinate term is being used. Another strategy mothers used with superordinate labels is also illustrated in the excerpt just presented: explicit statements of the inclusion relation. Notice that this mother not only mentioned the basic- and superordinate-level labels, she also explicitly mentioned the inclusion relation between the two levels (e.g., "The lawnmower is *a kind of* machine"). This is something that 71% of the mothers did when they were talking about superordinate categories; in contrast, none of the mothers talked about the inclusion relation when they taught basic categories (even if they were discussing relatively unfamiliar animals and could have said, "A koala is an animal").

A third superordinate strategy that mothers used, the multiple-referent strategy, consisted of providing a label for a group of objects rather than just one object. For example, one mother asked: "What are all those pictures of? The car, and the submarine, and the Skylab, and the, um, what was the other one? The tank. They're all vehicles." Mothers labeled multiple referents much more often with superordinate than with basic labels. This finding has been replicated in several other studies (e.g., Shipley et al., 1983; White, 1982).

More recently, we conducted a picture-book-reading study (Callanan & Weed, 1990) in order to look at parents' labeling in a more open-ended task. We found that parents used very few superordinate labels, even on pages where several members of the same superordinate category were pictured (several kinds of tools). Though preliminary analyses show some evidence of the anchoring and multiple-referent strategies, parents in this study used virtually no inclusion statements, even when speaking to children as old as 6 years. It is likely that the nature of the task is responsible for this difference. In the teaching study, parents were specifically asked to focus on superordinate terms, whereas the picture-book study was left open-ended. Several other studies using open-ended picture and picture-book tasks have revealed infrequent use of superordinate terms by parents (Blewitt, 1983; Shipley et al., 1983).

Lucariello and Nelson (1986) explored parents' label use with 2-year-olds in three different contexts: free play with a variety of toys, routine caregiving (such as eating lunch or getting ready for bed), and a novel play situation in which a castle toy was presented to the dyad. Superordinate labels were used less often than other labels, and this did not differ by context. Lucariello and Nelson did find, however, that some parents used the anchoring and multiple-referent strategies with superordinate labels. In the future, it will be important to explore the range of tasks, especially more naturally occurring ones, in which parents are likely to talk about superordinate category membership and to see how parents' strategies for introducing superordinate terms vary with task goals.

Taken together, these results suggest that, at least in some situations, parents use strategies that could help children to determine the hierarchical level of a new word. Parents tend not to use simple ostensive reference with superordinate terms. When they do use superordinate terms, they introduce them in special ways. Clearly, the next step was to find out whether these strategies influenced children's interpretations of new words. In a set of experimental studies (Callanan, 1989), a puppet taught new words to children, using the strategies that mothers used. The children were then given a set of pictures and asked to find all of the things that are labeled by the word they had just learned. This task allowed me to investigate whether different strategies lead children to interpret words at different hierarchical levels.

In one study, a puppet taught new words to 3- and 5-year-old children by pointing to a picture and labeling it with a nonsense label (e.g., "terval"). The children's job was to help the puppet find, for example, all of the "tervals." In four different conditions, the

Table 12.3 *Examples of labeling strategies in four conditions*

Study 1
Ostension with one picture
This is a terval. [Point to picture of car]
Inclusion with one picture
This is a wug. A wug is a kind of terval. [Point to picture of car]
Ostension with two pictures
This is a terval. [Picture of car]
This is another terval. [Picture of truck]
Inclusion with two pictures
This is a wug. A wug is a kind of terval. [Picture of car]
This is another kind of terval. [Picture of truck]
Study 2
Ostension
This is an amphibian. [Point to picture of frog]
Inclusion
This is a frog. A frog is a kind of amphibian. [Point to picture of frog]

Source: Callanan (1989).

puppet used labeling strategies modeled on some of the actual strategies that parents used.

The four conditions resulted from crossing Labeling Strategy (label vs. inclusion) with Number of Pictures Labeled (one vs. two). Examples of the labeling strategies used in this study are shown in Table 12.3. In the label–one-picture condition, the puppet pointed to a picture (e.g., a car) and labeled it ("This is a terval"). This is analogous to the strategy mothers used with basic-level category labels. In the inclusion–one-picture condition, the puppet labeled the same object in the context of an inclusion statement ("This is a wug. A wug is a kind of terval"). This is analogous to mothers' inclusion strategy with superordinate labels. Two other groups of children heard the new label applied to two objects (e.g., a car and a truck) instead of one. This was a test of the multiple-referent strategy. There was a label condition with two pictures ("This is a terval. This is another terval") and an inclusion condition with two pictures ("This is a wug. A wug is a kind of terval. This is another kind of terval").

After hearing the new label, the children were asked to find all of the "tervals" from an array of pictures. The picture sets were constructed so that we could determine whether the children interpreted the word at the subordinate, basic, or superordinate level or whether they had some other interpretation. They were shown 12 pictures: 3 from the same subordinate category as the labeled picture (3 sedans), 3 from the same basic-level category (station wagon, volkswagon, sportscar), 3 from the same superordinate category (truck, tractor, boat), and 3 unrelated pictures. Notice that if one interprets "terval" at the subordinate level, one should pick only the sedans; if one interprets it at the basic level, one should pick all the sedans and all of the other cars; if one interprets it at the superordinate level one should pick all of the vehicles (which includes the subordinate, basic, and superordinate pictures). No category interpretation should lead one to pick the distractors.

The proportion of children whose means matched the different kinds of interpretations (subordinate, basic, superordinate, other) varied by condition. The multiple-referent strategy clearly had an effect on the children's interpretations of the novel words. The children who saw one picture when they heard the label were most likely to interpret the word at the basic level; 57% of these children had a basic-level interpretation, whereas 18% had a superordinate-level interpretation. In contrast, the children who saw two pictures were most likely to interpret the word at the superordinate level; 26% of these children had a basic interpretation, whereas 52% had a superordinate interpretation.

The inclusion strategy had no effect in this study. Children who heard the label within an inclusion statement were no more likely to induce a superordinate category than those who heard the label alone (36 and 34% superordinate interpretations, respectively). It may be, however, that the use of nonsense words made this an unfair test of children's ability to use the inclusion strategy. Actually it would be somewhat surprising if children could use inclusion information in the context of two novel labels. It is likely that hearing "A cat is a mammal" would tell children much more about mammals than hearing "A platypus is a mammal" if they did not know the word *platypus*.

This interpretation was supported by the findings of a second study, in which the inclusion strategy was tested again using unfamiliar English words. Further, an attempt was made to choose at least some items for which the children would know the basic-level term. The items were constructed as in the preceding study, except that the labels children heard were English words such as *utensil* or *amphibian* (see Table 12.3). Half the children were in a label condition ("This is a utensil") and half were in an inclusion condition ("This is a spoon; a spoon is a kind of utensil"). In this study, children in the inclusion condition *were* more likely to interpret the novel word at the superordinate level (50% of the children) than children in the label condition (31%).

Together, these studies suggest that children can use the inclusion and multiple-referent strategies to alter their hypotheses about a new word. Since these are strategies that children are likely to hear parents use, at least in some situations, this work gives us information about how children may figure out the categories that nouns name. I am currently testing children's ability to use the anchoring strategy of labeling an object at two levels without explicit mention of the inclusion relation. Preliminary results suggest that this strategy may be less effective than the others in signaling to children that a superordinate label is being used. This is not surprising given that it is a much more subtle strategy. On the basis of these results, I would argue (as have Adams & Bullock, 1986) that there is a collaboration process going on, in which parents and children constrain the task in different ways, some more effective than others, and work toward a shared system of conceptual organization.

One particularly promising aspect of the approach outlined here is the combination of observational and experimental methods. The research strategy involves drawing hypotheses from rich natural observations, which can then be tested rigorously in an experimental paradigm. This combined method provides us with converging evidence and helps to diminish the inherent limitations of each method alone. It also allows us to begin to draw causal conclusions about the relation between parents' speech and children's interpretations of words. Further, the approach may help us to solve some of the mysteries of how children begin to understand and use language. Experimental studies of children under the age of 2 have always been very difficult. Perhaps observations of natural interactions between young children and their parents will lead us to formulate new hypotheses and new experimental paradigms about children's earliest word meanings.

Subordinate labels. Whereas parents make clear distinctions in their use of basic and superordinate category terms, their uses of subordinate and basic terms are not very different. In general, it seems clear that parents use more subordinate labels than superordinate labels (Blewitt, 1983; Lucariello & Nelson, 1986). In another teaching study (Callanan, 1985), I have explored how mothers introduce subordinate labels. These mothers taught basic and subordinate categories to their children. As in the study described earlier, they were given four pictures and a word (*monkey wrench*: four monkey wrenches; *thermometer*: four thermometers). Here a very different pattern emerged. There were no clear differences between the strategies mothers used to label objects at the subordinate and at the basic level. They rarely used the inclusion or multiple-referent strategies. They tended to use simple ostensive definition: subordinate ostension when teaching subordinate categories ("This is a monkey wrench") and basic ostension when teaching basic categories ("This is a thermometer"). This seemed to leave the children without much help in distinguishing between subordinate and basic category labels.

In several other studies, including the picture-book study we conducted (Callanan & Weed, 1990), there is evidence that parents anchor subordinate terms at the basic level (see also Blewitt, 1983; Lucariello & Nelson, 1986). That is, when using a subordinate label such as *collie* or *dachshund*, the majority of parents sometimes *also* labeled the same picture at the basic level (*dog*). This could help children to differentiate between basic and subordinate labels. Another clue might lie in the fact that many subordinate labels contain the basic-level word (e.g., *monkey wrench, bluebird*). Waxman's (1990; Chapter 4, this volume) data suggests that these sorts of labels may lead children to look for subordinate categories (see also Clark, Gelman, & Lane, 1985). In summary, there may be some information in parents' labeling strategies that will help children to learn the relation between subordinate and basic labels, though it is certainly less explicit than the information at the superordinate level.

Adams and Bullock (1986) present some interesting work on how mothers introduce subordinate labels to young children. When reading a picture book depicting various types of animals, atypical category members (e.g., penguin) were more likely to be labeled at the subordinate level, whereas typical category members (e.g., robin) were more likely to be labeled at the basic level (i.e., *bird*). In looking at the way labeling changed with age of the child and across the two sessions of their study, however, they found a very clear shift in the contribution of mother and child to labels at different levels.

When children are 14 months old, mothers provide most of the labels at all levels, but by 38 months children produce more basic labels than do their mothers and an almost equal number of atypical subordinate labels as do their mothers. Further, when children are 38 months old, mothers begin to use many more typical subordinate labels. Adams and Bullock suggest a scaffolding-type explanation such that parents introduce the new, more complex type of label only when they believe that the child has become proficient with the earlier and simpler type of label. Perhaps most interesting, Adams and Bullock mention some strategies that the mothers used to justify their use of a label at a particular level. For example, they sometimes used hedges ("A penguin is a funny kind of bird") or mentioned features or functions that explained the subordinate category membership of the item (e.g., "A zebra is a horse with stripes"). Adams and Bullock do not present detailed analyses of the use of these strategies, and their examples seem to focus on the atypical cases. It would be very interesting to know how the strategies differ for the typical and atypical subordinate labels and to explore how such strategies may help children to figure out the hierarchical inclusion relation between the basic and subordinate levels. Perhaps helping children to accept the inclusion of atypical subordinate items (which already have a clear identity in another category) into the basic category is an important first step in their understanding of hierarchical inclusion.

Summary. In sum, there may be very useful information about the hierarchical status of categories in parents' speech to children. Further, the differences between subordinate and superordinate labeling strategies seem to be very important. Subordinate labels are used much more often as names for objects (Blewitt, 1983; Lucariello & Nelson, 1986; Shipley et al., 1983). In the teaching task (Callanan, 1985) and the picture-book task (Callanan & Weed, 1990) described earlier, it is striking that the parent seems to single out the superordinate level. In the teaching task, special labeling strategies were used for superordinate terms, whereas in the picture-book task superordinate labels were seldom used as names for objects at all. Recall my earlier argument (based on Shipley's, 1989, claim) that children may see superordinate terms as labels for categories-of-categories rather than for categories-of-objects. The parental input data presented here seem to support such an interpretation. The strategies parents used to label superordinate categories focus on groups of objects or subclasses rather than individual objects. In using the multiple-referent strategy, parents refer to a group of objects. The inclusion strategy states the relation between classes at two hierarchical levels ("A mixer is a kind of machine") rather than labeling an individual as a member of the superordinate category.

Open questions and future directions

The problem of context

The emphasis on parent–child interaction as a context for development is part of a larger concern with the particular contexts in which learning takes place. Studying cognition in the context of real-world activity is an important goal. *Context*, however, is a term that is used in many different ways. In studies of cognitive and language development, it can mean such diverse things as the linguistic frame of the utterance in which a word is found, the perceptual scene in which an object appears, the type of activity in which the parent and child are engaged, and the broad cultural framework within which people are socialized. Indeed, as Nelson (1985) points out, what counts as context is a figure – ground problem, that is, whatever is not being studied is part of the context. This catch-all use of *context* makes it virtually impossible to make useful predictions about how context affects word learning. Careful theoretical and empirical work is needed to solve the problem of studying cognition in context.

Several analyses of context have produced taxonomies made up of microanalytic and macroanalytic layers of context (Leontev, 1981; Nelson, 1985). For example, Leontev argued that the same action can be analyzed at three different levels: operations (particular strategies used by participants), actions (the tasks or goals of the participants), and activities (the larger cultural framework of the participants). As we have seen, most of the research on parent–child interaction as a context for conceptual development has focused on the interaction of middle-class parents and children during unstructured play or picture-book-reading tasks (see Nelson, 1985; Rogoff, 1990). By working within a narrow range of tasks and subject populations, we are, in general, exploring neither the action nor the activity level in Leontev's scheme (Renshaw & Gardner, 1987). Although the available data will serve as an important foundation for

future work, a commitment to the study of cognition in context requires that we broaden our perspective, both by looking at different
settings for parent–child interaction within a culture and by considering how the larger cultural context affects parent–child interaction.

Researchers in this field have, however, begun to recognize the
importance of analyzing a situation. For example, Rogoff et al. (1984)
found that parents gave different kinds of guidance to children on
a "homelike" classification task (putting groceries on the appropriate shelves in a kitchen) than on a "schoollike" task (classifying pictures into the appropriate superordinate categories). Lucariello and
Nelson (1986) found differences in parents' use of labels depending
on the type of activity they were engaged in. Most of the research,
however, has focused on the free play and picture-book reading as
natural settings in which parents' and children's labeling of objects
is easily observed. There are several advantages to these as contexts
for looking at children's acquisition of word meaning. There are,
however, potential disadvantages (beyond the obvious fact that we
may be limiting ourselves to only a few types of situations). Researchers have often used artificially constructed books or carefully
chosen toys for the purposes of controlling what the parent and
child have to talk about. These choices may not reflect the kinds of
objects and pictures that children are apt to find available in natural
situations. More subtly, reading and playing, though natural activities in our culture, may be situations in which language is used
more reflectively than in other settings. In fact, Nelson (1988) has
argued that our theoretical focus on pointing and labeling may be
an artifact of the types of activities we have studied. She argues that
this focus may be inappropriate because this type of input is not
representative of most of what children hear. In the dyadic tasks on
which we have focused, parents may be much more self-conscious
about teaching words to children than they usually are (see also
Rogoff, 1990). It is important to continue to expand the kinds of
tasks within which parent–child conversations are observed, and
especially to use routine tasks in which parents name objects not
for the sake of naming them, but for the sake of saying something
about them. Jeff Shrager and I and Myers and Mervis (1989) have
independently chosen baking as a natural activity in which this type
of language can be observed. Lucariello and Nelson's (1986) choices
of eating meals and getting ready for bed are also situations of this

type. By comparing labeling practices across the kinds of situations that children ordinarily engage in, we are sure to come up with a clearer picture of the ways that parents and children construct word meanings and category systems.

The studies reviewed also tell us little about the ways in which parents' strategies differ across socioeconomic and cultural groups. The subjects in most of these studies were middle-class families in the United States. They were reasonably well educated and had whatever qualities lead parents to volunteer for research. There is therefore no reason to expect that they are representative of other populations of parents. I would certainly expect cultural differences in parents' strategies, and there is in fact evidence that those differences exist. Shipley (1987) has data on object labeling by inner-city black mothers, and she finds that those mothers talk less about inclusion relations than do white middle-class mothers. There are also anthropological data (e.g., Sharp, Cole, & Lave, 1979) suggesting that taxonomic categories are not equally preferred in all cultures and that their use is correlated with amount of schooling. Finally, Heath's work (1983) suggests that parents in different cultural groups may have very different ways of talking with children about names for things.

A very useful framework for understanding such cultural differences was provided by Newport et al. (1977) in their discussion of motherese. If some aspect of language or cognition is nonuniversal, it is very likely that input will have a strong effect on children's learning of that aspect of the system. Something that children seem to learn without any help (e.g., basic-level categories) should not be highly influenced by variations in parental input. But for something that does vary from language to language or culture to culture, parents and other adults are likely to play a very important role in acquisition. Although hierarchical systems of category terms are present in most languages, there seem to be cross-cultural differences in the emphasis placed on hierarchical classification and in the levels in a hierarchy that are named (see Waxman, Chapter 4, this volume). Applying Newport et al.'s view to these observations, one would expect to find variability in parents' strategies for discussing hierarchical inclusion relations and to find that those variations have important effects on children's understanding of inclusion. We know about some such differences in input, but the important question of how they affect children's development remains unanswered.

Beyond labels: Parents' descriptions and explanations

Just as we need to expand the range of situations in which we study parent–child interaction, it is important that we expand our study of input beyond parents' labels for objects. As already shown by several studies reviewed here, parents are most likely to help children understand something new about categories and words when they provide some sort of explanation or description of properties of objects. This may include demonstrations of important functions (Mervis & Mervis, 1988), explanations of how atypical category members fit into a category (Adams & Bullock, 1986), and explanations of the inclusion relation between two category levels (Callanan, 1985).

There has been a shift in the field of conceptual development away from the study of category structure per se and toward the study of how categories generate inferences (Blewitt, 1989; Gelman, 1988; Shipley, 1989) and how they are embedded in causal theories (Carey, 1985; Keil, 1989; Kremer & Gelman, 1989; Murphy & Medin, 1985). For example, not only do children learn that a robin is a bird, they also learn what birds do, where one sees them, why they engage in certain behaviors, how they differ from or are similar to other kinds of animals, and so on. In the same way, we need analyses of parents' descriptions of objects and explanations of how they are organized into categories. In two recent studies, I have begun to explore parents' descriptions of objects and explanations in conversations with children.

Object descriptions are a potential data base for children who are learning to use categories to make inferences. We have learned a great deal from several recent studies of young children's inferential abilities, for example, by Carey (1985), Gelman (1988), Gelman and Markman (1986, 1987), and Keil (1989). One of the mysteries of induction was articulated by Goodman (1973) among others: How do children keep from inferring that every property of an object can be generalized to other objects of the same kind? For example, how do children come to know that eating worms is a property of birds that may be expected to generalize to other birds, whereas being sick is not such a property? Solutions to this problem range from suggestions that children start out predisposed to generate certain kinds of hypotheses rather than others (Peirce, 1960) to suggestions that children base their inductions on how often a predicate or category has been involved in induction in the past (Goodman, 1973). As in the study of constraints on word meanings, one important step in deciding among such alternatives is to characterize the structure of information children encounter in the environment.

I have begun to look at the way parents describe properties of objects for evidence that they use strategies that may be helpful for children in making inferences (Callanan, 1990). Using the transcripts from the teaching tasks described earlier, in which mothers taught their 2- to 4-year-old children about concepts at different hierarchical levels, I have analyzed mothers' descriptions of objects. These data suggested several ways in which parents may help children to limit inferences. First, the mothers had a tendency to spend most of their time talking about the kinds of properties that are most generalizable within the category. When teaching basic and subordinate categories, they were likely to mention perceptual features and parts, whereas when teaching superordinate categories they were more likely to mention functions. For example, while talking to their children about camels (a basic-level category), mothers were likely to mention little more than the humps. But while teaching the superordinate category of *vehicles*, mothers were likely to mention little more than the fact that they are things to ride in.

In addition to teaching children about the content of valid inferences, parents may provide more abstract information about the kinds of inferences that can be valid. There is an asymmetry in mothers' presentation of functions at different hierarchical levels, such that higher-level functions are "anchored" at the lower level. For example, in the following excerpt one of the mothers in the study discusses the general function of machines (they help you do work) in the context of the more specific subfunctions of different kinds of machines (mixers help you make scrambled eggs, etc.):

M: Do you know what kind of machine this is?
C :   Coffee machine.
M: No, it's not a coffee machine; it's a mixing machine.
C :   (*laughs*) Mixing.
M: Show me how you do egg beater with your hands. (*Child pretends to stir with hand.*)
M: That's right. And what if you had to do that all day and make scrambled eggs for your whole class? Would you get tired of making so many scrambled eggs?
C :   Yeah.
M: Well, if you put scrambled eggs in a machine like that and then you just go "ping" and then they go "whirr" and then you'd give the scrambled eggs to your class.

M: OK, same thing here, see, look at this machine. See that floor-polishing machine?

C: Mm hm.

M: You wanna clean the floor, would it be easier to get down on the floor with a rag and rub the floor, or would it be easier to have a big machine like that?

C: Big machine like that.

M: Maybe, yeah. Cause see, machines can help you do work. Right?

Just as in the case of anchoring with basic-level labels, this strategy could have the effect of teaching children about the asymmetrical nature of hierarchies and the resulting asymmetry of deductive inference. I am currently developing a more detailed coding scheme that will distinguish more carefully among the kinds of properties parents and children discuss (actions, locations, perceptual features, etc.). Future experimental work will determine how children make use of the information parents provide in these object descriptions. The data certainly suggest some potential ways in which children's inferences may be guided by such conversations.

Finally, let me turn to the question of how parents' explanations in response to "why" questions may inform the developing theories in which concepts are embedded. Children not only learn that objects have properties, but formulate intuitive theories about *why* such properties exist. Lisa Oakes and I have been exploring ways in which parents guide the development of such causal theories. We collected diary reports of children's spontaneous "why" questions from parents of preschoolers. In our sample, 3- to 5-year-old children produced the following questions: "Why do some saws have so many teeth and why are some of the teeth bigger than others?" "Do cow babies come from eggs?" "Why don't kitties have hands?" "How does bamboo make more plants?" "Who makes tennis shoes?" and "Why do cows have milk in them?" (Callanan & Oakes, 1989). Although few of the questions in our corpus are explicitly about word meanings or category structure, these examples reflect a conscious attempt by young children to organize the knowledge they have about particular domains and to understand how and *why* categories are related to one another in particular ways. The questions serve as a reminder that children's concepts are embedded in larger knowledge structures or theories about how the world works (Carey, 1985; Murphy & Medin, 1985; Wellman, 1988). We are also exploring these question–explanation exchanges in cooking and book-reading data I am collecting with Jeff Shrager and Carol Capelli. The explanations that parents provide in answer to such questions are a potential source of further insight into the complex social process by which children learn about language and concepts.

Summary and conclusions

In general, I have proposed that children and parents collaborate to produce the developmental changes we see in conceptual and semantic knowledge. I have identified three central problems for children (beginning the mapping process, revising initial mappings, learning the inclusion structure of hierarchies) and four approaches to the study of input. The goal, however, is to put together what we know about the child and the parent and to develop a social convergence account of conceptual development. We are not yet at a point where we can formulate such a theory, but I will now briefly sketch an outline of a model and some suggestions about where future research must fill in the gaps.

With regard to the initial word–category mapping problem, we cannot yet determine the relative contributions of parent and child. The similarity in the patterns of parents' speech and children's expectations are striking, but they leave unanswered the questions about the direction of causality. In further exploration of constraints on word meaning, I think we would benefit from developing techniques for finding clues in very early interactions as to when and how these constraints appear and whether they are developed collaboratively by parent and child. It is possible that it will be difficult to disentangle the relative roles of parents and child even if we look at very young infants, both because of methodological difficulties inherent in studying such young infants and because of the truly collaborative nature of these interactions. As with any nature–nurture debate, our question will most likely change into one about *how* parent and child influence one another rather than *whether* they do.

I suspect, however, that at least some constraints are innate. As Huttenlocher and Smiley (1987) argue, children may start with gestalt notions of what an object category is, and these early categories may be the primitives from which other categories and category systems are built. Although these initial categories are probably not equivalent to adult-basic-level categories (Mervis, 1987), they seem to be categories-of-objects and to fall roughly in the range of the basic level. These are likely to be the categories to which words are initially mapped. Parents' tendency to use basic-level names in their simple labeling strategies meshes well with children's expectations and ensures a shared understanding of labels that gives children a way into the language of object labels. My guess, however, is that parents' labeling does not cause children to have these expectations.

Yet the child's task of building category systems from these initial categories does seem to be strongly influenced by parent–child conversations. Parents' labeling strategies seem to provide guidance for children when their initial expectations do not match the structure of the material to be learned. Two examples of this type were discussed here in some detail: (a) revising initial categories so that they are more closely aligned with the conventional adult categories and (b) learning the hierarchical structure of inclusion and the multiple labels that refer to the categories at different levels. In both of these cases, there is clear evidence not only that parents provide potentially helpful information, but that young children are able to make use of the information. Mervis's work (Banigan & Mervis, 1988; Mervis & Mervis, 1988) shows that 2-year-old children can use parents' demonstrations of new form–function correlations to learn the adult-basic categorization of an object that they had initially included in a child-basic category. My work on children's interpretations of category labels (Callanan, 1989) shows that the kinds of strategies that parents use to label superordinate categories can help children to overcome their initial expectations about the meaning of a novel word and to interpret it at the superordinate level. In addition to these two cases, several other examples have been mentioned of parents providing input that seems to help children to get beyond their initial expectations, such as Ninio's (1980) data on parents' strategies for talking about parts of objects and Adams and Bullock's (1986) data on parents' use of subordinate terms.

The study of conversations between parents and children has provided a rich source of data that must be accounted for in any complete theory of conceptual development. An important question that remains unanswered has to do with the mechanisms by which children make use of parents' guidance. Mervis's predictions about how parents' demonstrations help children to revise child-basic categories are based on the fact that young children appreciate actions more than words. She argues that physical actions accompanied by language are more likely to be informative for children than is speech alone. In my work on hierarchical organization, I have argued that children use regularities in parents' speech to interpret the meanings of words. We know, for example, that very young children are sensitive to the way that subtle syntactic changes (such as the presence or absence of the word *the*) can affect meaning (Gelman & Taylor, 1984; Katz, Baker, & Macnamara, 1974), although where this competence comes from is still something of a mystery. This kind of sensitivity might allow children to use the syntax of parents' strategies to decide on the level of a particular category term. For example, they might notice the use of a plural label or the phrase *is a kind of* as different from the standard labeling strategy, which might lead them to look for another interpretation. In this way, parents' labeling strategies might teach children not only the meanings of particular words, but the nature of hierarchical relations among categories. To understand such mechanisms fully, however, we must combine the patterns-of-input approach I have used with some of the other techniques (e.g., scaffolding) for analyzing the dynamic interactions within which parents and children negotiate the meanings of these words.

We are, unfortunately, still a long way from having a theory of how word meanings arise collaboratively between parent and child. The four approaches to input that I have outlined will provide four strands of data that will fit into a social convergence theory: (a) The mismatch approach tells us about aspects of development in which parents' speech does not account for developmental changes. (b) The patterns approach has given us some important evidence of how children make use of global patterns in parents' speech as they construct word meanings and systems of categories. (c) The scaffolding approach must be modified so that it can be applied more directly to data on the way word meanings are understood in everyday interactions. These techniques hold promise for analyses of minute-by-minute negotiations of word meanings. (d) The cross-cultural approach will tell us how the findings from the other approaches generalize across social class, ethnic, and cultural groups. We need more data in all four approaches before we can put them together to form a complete theory of social convergence.

I have argued that we need to consider a balanced view in which the child's and the parent's conceptual structures, the parent's knowledge of the child's conceptual structure, and the social convergence that occurs during the conversation are all taken into account. The importance of looking at real-life activities should, by now, be quite clear. As Nelson (1985) and others have argued, children's initial word meanings seem to be deeply embedded in the events in which they were learned (see Ninio & Bruner, 1978; Snow & Goldfield, 1983). Traditionally, we have understood this to be a developmental phase from which children go on to learn more stable word meanings. Current views about adult concepts and word meanings lead us to question this assumption (Barsalou, 1987; Greeno & Stucky, 1990). Instead, word meanings may be constantly renegotiated within the contexts in which they are spoken. In either case, however, studying the development of word meanings within particular events is essential. In real-life situations, parents label objects and provide information about categories in the context of ongoing interaction. Children play a very active role in these conversations, as illustrated by the examples of "why" questions mentioned earlier. Children's willingness to realign category boundaries or to accept new subordinate and superordinate labels is dependent not only on their attention to cues in parents' speech, but on their rich existing knowledge base about particular domains. Incorporating children's explanatory mechanisms and their knowledge of language and of category structure into our understanding of how development takes place within social interactions is a difficult goal, but one toward which we have taken some important initial steps.

References

Adams, A. K., & Bullock, D. (1986). Apprenticeship in word use: Social convergence processes in learning categorically related nouns. In S. A. Kuczaj II & M. D. Barrett (Eds.), *The development of word meaning* (pp. 155–197). New York: Springer.

Anglin, J. (1977). *Word, object, and conceptual development.* New York: Norton.

Azmitia, M., & Perlmutter, M. (1989). Social influences on children's cognition: State of the art and future directions. In H. W. Reese (Ed.), *Advances in child development and behavior* (Vol. 22, pp. 89–144). New York: Academic Press.

Baldwin, D. A., & Markman, E. M. (1989). Establishing word–object relations: A first step. *Child Development, 60,* 381–398.

Banigan, R. L., & Mervis, C. B. (1988). Role of adult input in young children's category evolution: II. An experimental study. *Journal of Child Language, 15,* 493–504.

Barsalou, L. (1987). The instability of graded structure: Implications for the nature of concepts. In U. Neisser (Ed.), *Concepts and conceptual devel-*

480 M. A. Callanan

opment: Ecological and intellectual bases of categorization (pp. 101–140). Cambridge University Press.

Blewitt, P. (1983). "Dog" vs. "collie": Vocabulary in speech to young children. *Developmental Psychology, 19,* 602–609.

Blewitt, P. (1989). Categorical hierarchies: Levels of knowledge and skill. *Genetic Epistomologist, 17,* 21–30.

Brown, R. (1958). How shall a thing be called? *Psychological Review, 65,* 14–21.

Brown, R., & Hanlon, C. (1970). Derivational complexity and order of acquisition in child speech. In J. R. Hayes (Ed.), *Cognition and the development of language* (pp. 11–53). New York: Wiley.

Bruner, J. (1984). Vygotsky's zone of proximal development: The hidden agenda. In B. Rogoff & J. V. Wertsch (Eds.), *Children's learning in the "zone of proximal development"* (pp. 93–97). San Francisco: Jossey-Bass.

Bruner, J. (1987). The transactional self. In J. Bruner & H. Haste (Eds.), *Making sense: The child's construction of the world* (pp. 81–96). London: Methuen.

Bruner, J., & Haste, H. (Eds.). (1987). *Making sense: The child's construction of the world.* London: Methuen.

Callanan, M. A. (1985). How parents label objects for young children: The role of input in the acquisition of category hierarchies. *Child Development, 56,* 508–523.

Callanan, M. A. (1989). Development of object categories and inclusion relations: Preschoolers' hypotheses about word meanings. *Developmental Psychology, 25,* 207–216.

Callanan, M. A. (1990). Parents' descriptions of objects: Potential data for children's inferences about category principles. *Cognitive Development, 5,* 101–122.

Callanan, M. A., & Markman, E. M. (1982). Principles of organization in young children's natural language hierarchies. *Child Development, 53,* 1093–1101.

Callanan, M. A., & Oakes, L. (1989, April). *Parent–child collaboration in the development of category inferences and causal theories.* Paper presented at the biennial meeting of the Society for Research in Child Development, Kansas City, MO.

Callanan, M. A., Repp, A., & McCarthy, M. (1989, April). *Children's hypotheses about word meaning: Is there a basic level constraint?* Paper presented at the biennial meeting of the Society for Research in Child Development, Kansas City, MO.

Callanan, M. A., & Weed, S. (1990). *Parent–child conversations in picture book reading.* Unpublished data.

Carey, S. (1985). *Conceptual change in childhood.* Cambridge, MA: MIT Press.

Clark, E. V. (1983). Meanings and concepts. In J. H. Flavell & E. M. Markman (Eds.), *Cognitive development* (Vol. 3, pp. 787–840 of P. H. Mussen [Ed.], *Handbook of child psychology*). New York: Wiley.

Clark, E. V. (1989, April). *Discussant: The case for "constraints" on lexical development.* Presented at the biennial meeting of the Society for Research in Child Development, Kansas City, MO.

Clark, E. V., Gelman, S. A., & Lane, N. M. (1985). Compound nouns and category structure in young children. *Child Development, 56,* 84–94.

Clark, H. H. (1985). Language use and language users. In G. Lindsay &

E. Aronson (Eds.), *Handbook of social psychology* (3rd ed., pp. 179–231). New York: Random House.

Cohen, L. B., & Younger, B. A. (1983). Perceptual categorization in the infant. In E. Scholnick (Ed.), *New trends in conceptual representation: Challenges to Piaget's theory?* (pp. 197–220). Hillsdale, NJ: Erlbaum.

Gelman, S. A. (1988). Children's inductive inferences from natural kind and artifact categories. *Cognitive Psychology, 20,* 65–95.

Gelman, S. A., & Markman, E. M. (1986). Categories and induction in young children. *Cognition, 23,* 183–209.

Gelman, S. A., & Markman, E. M. (1987). Young children's inductions from natural kinds: The role of categories and appearances. *Child Development, 58,* 1532–1541.

Gelman, S. A., & Taylor, M. E. (1984). How two-year-olds interpret proper and common names for unfamiliar objects. *Child Development, 55,* 1535–1540.

Goldin-Meadow, S., & Mylander, C. (1984). Gestural communication in deaf children: The effects and non-effects of parental input on early language development. *Monographs of the Society for Research in Child Development, 49* (3–4, Serial No. 207).

Goodman, N. (1973). *Fact, fiction, and forecast* (3rd ed.). Indianapolis, IN: Bobbs-Merrill.

Greeno, J. G., & Stucky, S. U. (1990). *Using words to count.* Unpublished working paper, Institute for Research on Learning, Palo Alto, CA.

Heath, S. B. (1983). *Ways with words: Language, life, and work in communities and classrooms.* Cambridge University Press.

Hoff-Ginsberg, E., & Shatz, M. (1982). Linguistic input and the child's acquisition of language. *Psychological Bulletin, 92,* 3–26.

Horton, M. S., & Markman, E. M. (1980). Developmental differences in the acquisition of basic and superordinate categories. *Child Development, 51,* 708–719.

Huttenlocher, J., & Smiley, P. (1987). Early word meanings: The case of object names. *Cognitive Psychology, 19,* 63–89.

Huttenlocher, J., Smiley, P., & Ratner, H. (1983). What do word meanings reveal about conceptual development? In T. R. Seiler & W. Wannenmacher (Eds.), *Reader: Concept development and the development of word meaning* (pp. 210–233). Berlin: Springer.

Katz, N., Baker, E., & Macnamara, J. (1974). What's in a name? On the child's acquisition of proper and common nouns. *Child Development, 45,* 469–473.

Kaye, K. (1982). *The mental and social life of babies.* Chicago: University of Chicago Press.

Keil, F. C. (1979). *Semantic and conceptual development: An ontological perspective.* Cambridge, MA: Harvard University Press.

Keil, F. C. (1989). *Concepts, kinds, and cognitive development.* Cambridge, MA: MIT Press.

Kremer, K., & Gelman, S. A. (1989, April). *Children's causal explanations of the origins and structure of natural kinds and artifacts.* Paper presented at the biennial meeting of the Society for Research in Child Development, Kansas City, MO.

Kuczaj, S. A. (1986). Discussion: On social interaction as a type of explanation of language development. *British Journal of Developmental Psychology, 4,* 289–299.

Lave, J. (1988). *Cognition in practice.* Cambridge University Press.

Leontev, A. N. (1981). The problem of activity in psychology. In J. V. Wertsch (Ed.), *The concept of activity in Soviet psychology* (pp. 37–71). Armonk, NY: Sharpe.

Lucariello, J., & Nelson, K. (1986). Context effects on lexical specificity in maternal and child discourse. *Journal of Child Language, 13,* 507–522.

Macnamara, J. (1972). Cognitive basis of language learning in infants. *Psychological Review, 79,* 1–13.

Macnamara, J. (1982). *Names for things: A study of human learning.* Cambridge, MA: MIT Press.

Mandler, J. (1988). How to build a baby: On the development of an accessible representational system. *Cognitive Development, 3,* 113–136.

Markman, E. M. (1989). *Categorization and naming in children: Problems of induction.* Cambridge, MA: MIT Press.

Markman, E. M., & Callanan, M. A. (1984). An analysis of hierarchical classification. In R. Sternberg (Ed.), *Advances in the psychology of human intelligence* (Vol. 2, pp. 325–365). Hillsdale, NJ: Erlbaum.

Markman, E. M., Horton, M. S., & McLanahan, A. G. (1980). Classes and collections: Principles of organization in the learning of hierarchical relations. *Cognition, 8,* 561–577.

Markman, E. M., & Hutchinson, J. E. (1984). Children's sensitivity to constraints on word meaning: Taxonomic vs. thematic relations. *Cognitive Psychology, 16,* 1–27.

Markman, E. M., & Wachtel, G. F. (1988). Children's use of mutual exclusivity to constrain the meanings of words. *Cognitive Psychology, 20,* 121–157.

Merriman, W. E., & Bowman, L. L. (1989). The mutual exclusivity bias in children's word learning. *Monographs of the Society for Research in Child Development, 54* (3–4, Serial No. 220).

Mervis, C. B. (1984). Early lexical development: Contributions of mother and child. In C. Sophian (Ed.), *Origins of cognitive skills* (pp. 339–370). Hillsdale, NJ: Erlbaum.

Mervis, C. B. (1986). *Operating principles and personal theories: Their roles in early lexical development.* Paper presented to the New England Child Language Association, Cambridge, MA.

Mervis, C. B. (1987). Child-basic object categories and early lexical development. In U. Neisser (Ed.), *Concepts and conceptual development: Ecological and intellectual bases of categorization* (pp. 201–233). Cambridge University Press.

Mervis, C. B., & Long, L. M. (1987, April). *Words refer to whole objects: Young children's interpretation of the referent of a novel word.* Paper presented at the biennial meeting of the Society for Research in Child Development, Baltimore, MD.

Mervis, C. B., & Mervis, C. A. (1988). Role of adult input in young children's category evolution. I. An observational study. *Journal of Child Language, 15,* 257–272.

Miller, P. J. (1982). *Amy, Wendy, and Beth: Learning language in South Baltimore.* Austin: University of Texas Press.

Murphy, G. L., & Medin, D. L. (1985). The role of theories in conceptual coherence. *Psychological Review, 92,* 289–316.

Murphy, G. L., & Wisniewski, E. J. (1989). Categorizing objects in isolation and in scenes: What a superordinate is good for. *Journal of Experimental Psychology: Learning, Memory, and Cognition, 15,* 572–586.

Myers, N. A., & Mervis, C. B. (1989). A case study of early event representation development. *Cognitive Development, 4,* 31–48.

Nelson, K. (1985). *Making sense: The acquisition of shared meaning.* New York: Academic Press.

Nelson, K. (1988). Constraints on word learning? *Cognitive Development, 3,* 221–246.

Nelson, K. (1989, April). *Discussant: The case for "constraints" on lexical development.* Presented at the biennial meeting of the Society for Research in Child Development, Kansas City, MO.

Newport, E., Gleitman, H., & Gleitman, L. R. (1977). Mother, I'd rather do it myself: Some effects and non-effects of maternal speech style. In C. Snow & C. Ferguson (Eds.), *Talking to children: Language input and acquisition* (pp. 109–149). Cambridge University Press.

Ninio, A. (1980). Ostensive definition in vocabulary teaching. *Journal of Child Language, 7,* 565–573.

Ninio, A., & Bruner, J. S. (1978). The achievement and antecedents of labelling. *Journal of Child Language, 5,* 1–15.

Quine, W. V. O. (1960). *Word and object.* Cambridge, MA: MIT Press.

Pea, R. D. (1989). *Distributed intelligence and education.* Unpublished working paper, Institute for Research on Learning, Palo Alto, CA.

Peirce, C. S. (1960). *Collected papers of Charles Sanders Peirce* (C. Hartshorne & P. Weiss, Eds.) (4th ed., Vols. 1 & 2). Cambridge, MA: Harvard University Press.

Pratt, M. W., Kerig, P., Cowan, P. A., & Cowan, C. P. (1988). Mothers and fathers teaching 3-year-olds: Authoritative parenting and adult scaffolding of young children's learning. *Developmental Psychology, 24,* 832–839.

Renshaw, P. D., & Gardner, R. (1987, April). *Parental goals and strategies in teaching contexts: An exploration of "activity theory" with mothers and fathers of preschool children.* Paper presented at the biennial meeting of the Society for Research in Child Development, Baltimore, MD.

Rogoff, B. (1990). *Apprenticeship in thinking.* New York: Oxford University Press.

Rogoff, B., Ellis, S., & Gardner, W. (1984). Adjustment of adult–child instruction according to child's age and task. *Developmental Psychology, 20,* 193–199.

Rogoff, B., & Gardner, W. (1984). Adult guidance of cognitive development. In B. Rogoff & J. Lave (Eds.), *Everyday cognition* (pp. 95–116). Cambridge, MA: Harvard University Press.

Rogoff, B., & Wertsch, J. V., Eds. (1984). *Children's learning in the "zone of proximal development."* San Francisco: Jossey-Bass.

Rosch, E. H. (1978). Principles of categorization. In E. H. Rosch & B. B. Lloyd (Eds.), *Cognition and categorization* (pp. 27–48). Hillsdale, NJ: Erlbaum.

Rosch, E. H., Mervis, C. B., Gray, W., Johnson, D., & Boyes-Braem, P. (1976). Basic objects in natural categories. *Cognitive Psychology, 3,* 382–439.

Scaife, M., & Bruner, J. S. (1975). The capacity for joint visual attention in the infant. *Nature, 253,* 265–266.

Sharp, D., Cole, M., & Lave, C. (1979). Education and cognitive development: The evidence from experimental research. *Monographs of the Society for Research in Child Development, 44* (1–2, Serial No. 178).

Shipley, E. F. (1987). *Parents' speech to children: Information on category terms and category relations.* Unpublished manuscript, University of Pennsylvania, Philadelphia.

Shipley, E. F. (1989). Two types of hierarchies: Class inclusion hierarchies and kind hierarchies. *Genetic Epistomologist, 17,* 31–39.

Shipley, E. F., Kuhn, I. F., & Madden, E. C. (1983). Mothers' use of superordinate category terms. *Journal of Child Language, 10,* 571–588.

Smith, C. L. (1979). Children's understanding of natural language hierarchies. *Journal of Experimental Child Psychology, 27,* 437–458.

Snow, C. E., & Ferguson, C. (1977). *Talking to children: Language input and acquisition.* Cambridge University Press.

Snow, C. E., & Goldfield, B. A. (1983). Turn the page please: Situation-specific language acquisition. *Journal of Child Language, 10,* 551–569.

Taylor, M., & Gelman, S. A. (1989). Incorporating new words into the lexicon: Preliminary evidence for language hierarchies in two-year-old children. *Child Development, 60,* 625–636.

Tversky, B., & Hemenway, K. (1984). Objects, parts, and categories. *Journal of Experimental Psychology: General, 113,* 169–193.

Vygotsky, L. S. (1962). *Thought and language.* Cambridge, MA: MIT Press.

Vygotsky, L. S. (1978). *Mind in society: The development of higher psychological processes.* Cambridge, MA: Harvard University Press.

Wales, R., Colman, M., & Pattison, P. (1983). How a thing is called: A study of mothers' and children's naming. *Journal of Experimental Child Psychology, 36,* 1–17.

Waxman, S. R. (1990). Linguistic biases and the establishment of conceptual hierarchies: Evidence from preschool children. *Cognitive Development, 5,* 123–150.

Waxman, S. R., & Gelman, R. (1986). Preschoolers' use of superordinate relations in classification and language. *Cognitive Development, 1,* 139–156.

Wellman, H. M. (1988). First steps in the child's theorizing about the mind. In J. W. Astington, P. L. Harris, & D. R. Olson (Eds.), *Developing theories of mind* (pp. 64–92). Cambridge University Press.

Wertsch, J. V., Minick, N., & Arns, F. J. (1984). The creation of context in joint problem-solving. In B. Rogoff & J. Lave (Eds.), *Everyday cognition* (pp. 151–171). Cambridge, MA: Harvard University Press.

Wertsch, J. V., & Stone, C. A. (1985). The concept of internalization in Vygotsky's account of the genesis of higher mental functions. In J. V. Wertsch (Ed.), *Culture, communication, and cognition: Vygotskian perspectives* (pp. 162–179). Cambridge University Press.

White, T. (1982). Naming practices, typicality, and underextension in child language. *Journal of Experimental Child Psychology, 33,* 324–346.

Wisniewski, E. J., & Murphy, G. L. (in press). Superordinate and basic category names in discourse: A textual analysis. *Discourse Processes.*

Wittgenstein, L. (1953). *Philosophical investigations.* New York: Macmillan.

Wood, D. J. (1980). Teaching the young child: Some relationships between social interaction, language, and thought. In D. R. Olson (Ed.), *The social foundations of language and thought* (pp. 280–296). New York: Norton.

Wood, D., Bruner, J. S., & Ross, G. (1976). The role of tutoring in problem solving. *Journal of Child Psychology and Psychiatry, 17,* 89–100.

13. Beginning to talk with peers: The roles of setting and knowledge

LUCIA FRENCH, MARYLOU BOYNTON,
AND ROSEMARY HODGES

This chapter focuses on the development of young children's communicative abilities as they manifest themselves through talk, that is, the use of language to receive and send messages.[1] From a communicative perspective, the relationship between language and thought can be conceptualized of as one of medium (language) to content (thought). The preschool years are a period of rapid development in the domain of communication as young children establish and expand their knowledge base and language skills, as well as the social skills that are needed for successful interpersonal interactions. Some excellent reviews of the literature on the development of communication processes are available (Garvey, 1984; Mueller & Cooper, 1986; Shatz, 1983). Here we limit ourselves to a consideration of the literature that bears directly on the question guiding our present research: How do 2- and 3-year-old children learn to communicate verbally with one another?

An extensive literature describes early parent–child interactions and argues that such interactions are crucial for early language development (e.g., Bruner, 1983; Snow, 1977, 1979). However, there is very little in the literature that addresses the question of how the young child moves out of the intimate parent–infant exchanges and learns to talk with peers. The literature on parent–infant conversational exchanges documents the parent's expertise as a conversational partner. How do young children, accustomed to conversing with their parents, move into situations in which they must converse with others, particularly with others who, like themselves, are conversational novices? Even conversationally skilled adults find 2-year-olds (particularly those who are not their own children) to be extremely difficult conversational partners. How, then, do conversationally inept 2-year-olds manage to talk with one another? Our

485

hypothesis is that children learning to talk with one another are most successful when they are able to rely on physical contexts that evoke shared knowledge about familiar activities. Our data indicate that familiar physical contexts provide conversational support that is functionally similar to the conversational support provided by parents.

Early communication: Child–adult

The extensive literature on children's early communication tends to focus on adult–child, usually mother–child, interactions. In reviewing the early investigations of mother–infant communicative interactions, Snow (1979) describes three phases of research, each having a different goal. The first phase involved assessing the syntax of adults' infant-directed speech and determining that it was simplified relative to the syntax of adult-directed speech. The second phase involved assessing the content of infant-directed speech and determining that it was adjusted in accord with the infant's knowledge base, focusing on the here-and-now environment, on topics familiar to the child, and so forth. The third phase involved demonstrating that the infant played an active role in determining the mother's syntactic and semantic adjustments, by offering and withdrawing attention, interest, and vocalizations in response to the comprehensibility of the mother's messages.

The earliest forms of parent–child communication are person-to-person exchanges that do not refer to the external environment (e.g., Wells, Montgomery, & MacLure, 1979). The mother tends to "create" conversation between herself and the child by assigning communicative intent to any infant response (e.g., Bates, Camioni, & Volterra, 1979; Bruner, 1981; Garvey, 1984; Snow, 1977). Within the first 12 months of life, these early person-to-person exchanges develop into adult–child shared attention to, and action upon, aspects of a common environment (Bruner, 1983; Wells et al., 1979).

There is now a growing body of literature that describes the form of structured mother–infant interactions such as peekaboo (Bruner, 1983; Bruner & Sherwood, 1976; Hodapp, Goldfield, & Boyatzis, 1984; Ratner & Bruner, 1978) and book reading (DeLoache & DeMendoza, 1987; Ninio & Bruner, 1978; Snow, 1985; Snow & Goldfield, 1983). These interactions typically have four central features: a restricted format, a clear and repetitive structure, defined positions for vo-

calization, and reversible role relations (e.g., Ratner & B
These interactions are guided by the adult so as to g
cessful and ever-increasing participation by the child
research has generally been interpreted in terms of
perspective (Vygotsky, 1978) that focuses on the w
provides communicative support that is calibrated to the cʜɪʟᴅ
of competence. Adults lessen and eventually remove particular forms
of support as the child acquires the ability to operate without support or to glean support from other sources, such as the physical
setting or mental representations (e.g., French, Lucariello, Seidman,
& Nelson, 1985; Lucariello, 1987). Bruner, who captures the temporary and adjustable nature of parental support with the term *scaffolding*, has been one of the leading researchers in this area (Bruner,
1975, 1983; Ninio & Bruner, 1978; Ratner & Bruner, 1978). Wertsch
has discussed his observations of the support mothers offer their
children while jointly solving puzzles in similar terms (e.g., Wertsch,
1979; Wertsch, McNamee, McLane, & Budwig, 1980).

Early communication: Child–child

Typically, children begin to converse with one another after they
have learned to converse with adults. That is, child–child talk is
somewhat delayed relative to child–adult talk. Furthermore, children who spend a great deal of time with other children (e.g., children with twins or older siblings, children residing in institutions)
tend to acquire language more slowly than do children who spend
a greater proportion of time with adults (e.g., Bates, 1975).

Because of a lack of research addressing differences between adult–
child and child–child discourse, there can as yet be no definite explanation for the fact that children are slower to talk with peers than
with adults. However, it is likely that talking to peers is quite a bit
more difficult than talking to adults, because the peer dyad must
somehow initiate and sustain conversation without the conversational "expertise" that adults possess.

In an extensive review of the literature on child–child discourse,
Bates (1975) identifies two factors that she feels may be particularly
important in accounting for the relative delay in language acquisition by those children with a higher proportion of peer input. These
factors are difficulty in establishing shared presuppositions to support communication (which in turn derives from a failure to predict

the listener's knowledge) and difficulty in sending and interpreting feedback cues that indicate the extent to which the listener has understood a message.

Piaget's (1926/1955) observations of child–child talk led him to claim that young children's peer communication is highly egocentric and that peer exchanges can be characterized as collective monologues (turn taking without a shared topic) rather than as contingent and conversational. Subsequent research indicated that young children are generally less egocentric than Piaget suggested, with their verbal exchanges showing evidence of perspective taking and shared topics (e.g., Garvey & Hogan, 1973; Maratsos, 1974; Mueller, 1972; Nelson & Gruendel, 1979; Ochs & Schieffelin, 1976).

Research indicating that children are less egocentric than Piaget suggested is of great theoretical importance in terms of illustrating young children's basic social and communicative competence and motivation to communicate. Nevertheless, investigators challenging Piaget's characterization of children's early communicative competence have neither demonstrated nor claimed that young children have mature communicative skills. Bates's (1975) suggestion that children communicating with one another often experience difficulty in establishing shared presuppositions and in interpreting one another's feedback is compatible with demonstrations that children *sometimes* display these abilities. Our program of research has illustrated that contextual factors may affect the extent and quality of young children's peer communication by affecting the ease with which they establish shared presuppositions and take one another's perspective.

Contextual effects on peer communication

Instead of simply documenting the existence of peer communication, a growing body of research addresses the content and form of peer communication among young children (e.g., Bates, 1976; Brenner & Mueller, 1982; Ervin-Tripp, 1979; Garvey, 1974; Gleason, 1973; Mueller, 1972; Mueller, Bleier, Krakow, Hededus, & Cournoyer, 1977; Mueller & Brenner, 1977; Mueller & Lucas, 1975; Mueller & Rich, 1976; Ochs & Schieffelin, 1976; Shatz & Gelman, 1973). Much of this research can be interpreted as indicating that peer communication is sensitive to contextual factors of various types. For example, Shatz and Gelman (1973) demonstrated young children's sensitivity to the age and communicative status of their conversational partners, whereas Mueller and his colleagues have demonstrated the role that objects play in bringing very young children together (e.g., Brenner & Mueller, 1982; Mueller & Lucas, 1975; Mueller & Rich, 1976).

It is now well established that, contrary to suggestions made by some theorists (e.g., Clark & Clark, 1977), preschool children are quite capable of engaging in displaced reference (talking about topics removed in space and/or time) when the conversational situation supports or demands such reference (e.g., French & Nelson, 1982, 1983; Sachs, 1983; Shugar, 1981). Nevertheless, it is indeed the case that relative to adults and older children preschoolers tend to rely more on the physical setting to guide their verbal and nonverbal interactions with one another. For example, Garvey's (1984) research on 3- to 5-year-old children's peer play indicates that the children's play and language tend to refer to the toys available in the immediate setting.

The influence of the physical setting on young children's peer interactions is not surprising given that preschoolers tend to play with one another rather than discuss their experiences and opinions as do adults and older children. Although children *may* talk about a wide variety of topics while playing, it is *likely* that their talk will refer to their play activities. Their play activities in turn are referenced to the materials, for example the toys, available in the physical setting.

Play takes place in, and is simultaneously supported and constrained by, particular physical settings. That is, any physical setting contains objects that permit certain sorts of play and disallow other sorts. Because the toys with which young children interact are likely to exert considerable influence on the topic of their play, it is likely that they will influence the language that accompanies the play.

Although the physical setting is a central component of preschoolers' peer interactions, it is not, in and of itself, sufficient to enable young children to establish and maintain conversation. That is, there cannot be a direct link between setting and language. Language is mediated by thought, and physical settings can influence language only insofar as they tap into the participants' extant knowledge base. Children's real-world knowledge influences their ability to share ideas and joint action in play. Physical settings that elicit similar knowledge across children are most likely to lead to communicative success, because the shared knowledge provides a presuppositional base to support the sending and interpretation of messages.

Nelson and her colleagues have discussed the role of generalized event representations (sometimes referred to as *scripts*) in supporting children's peer conversations (French et al., 1985; Nelson & Gruendel, 1979; Nelson & Seidman, 1984). Very young children have detailed and well-structured knowledge about events in which they participate regularly, such as bathing, eating lunch, and going to McDonalds (e.g., Nelson et al., 1986). This event knowledge seems to serve a number of purposes (e.g., French, 1985; Nelson & Gruendel, 1981), not the least of which is to enable them to interpret and participate appropriately in the activities of daily life.

Elicited descriptions of events tend to be similar across children, indicating that for many culturally determined activities, event knowledge is to a large extent shared (e.g., Nelson et al., 1986). Just as event knowledge can guide children's behavior and interpretation when they are actual participants in an event, shared event knowledge can also serve as a presuppositional base when events are discussed or when they are enacted in a pretense mode. Elaborated, shared event knowledge allows children to use "language as its own context" (e.g., Hickmann, 1985), such that linguistic signs are used and interpreted with reference to other linguistic signs rather than simply with reference to the nonlinguistic environment.

Although little research has directly examined the role of physical setting on the complexity of children's play and the accompanying language (but see Pellegrini, 1983; Phyfe-Perkins, 1980), it is plausible that those settings that cue and provide the means of enacting shared event knowledge will support more complex interactions and language than settings that do not evoke shared event knowledge. This hypothesis first arose when we examined videotapes (Boynton, 1990) of "preverbal" toddlers' spontaneous interactions during free play. It was supported by a second set of naturalistic observations and is now being tested and refined with a third data base. The highlights of this program of research are described in the next section.

Investigations of peer interaction and communication

Naturalistic observations

The free play of 14 children in a preschool classroom was video-taped twice a week for 5 months. At the time the observations began, the children's mean age was 22 months (range 17 to 37 months). During free play the children had access to large motor equipment such as a climbing gym, a portable slide, and various "push" toys; fine motor toys such as puzzles and stacking toys; an assortment of cars and trucks; dolls; a desk; and a housekeeping corner that was furnished with child-sized kitchen appliances, a table and chairs, an assortment of dishes, a box of dress-up clothes, a doll's bed, and an ironing board.

Although they used language with their teachers, these children rarely used language to communicate with one another at the beginning of the observations. We were therefore able to observe the emergence of peer-directed language. In most of the play areas, the children used early peer-directed language to greet another, to gain a friend's attention, and to bolster struggles over possessions. "Hi!" "Pe'er!" and "Mine!" were occasionally heard. Children often assumed the role of onlooker or engaged in parallel play. Occasionally there were bursts of nonverbal interaction around shared themes such as run-chase or peekaboo (e.g., Boynton, 1990; Brenner & Mueller, 1982). When interaction occurred, it was brief, typically lasting a few seconds.

In contrast, play in the housekeeping area was thematically constrained and comparatively long-lasting (e.g., one episode continued for 10 minutes). Children exchanged dishes, fed each other, put dishes in the refrigerator and on the stove, and peered into the oven. They acknowledged each other and assumed complementary roles such as cook and consumer. Entry into play was usually achieved by performing an act appropriate to the setting (e.g., peering into the refrigerator) or by assuming a posture that implied a situationally defined role (e.g., sitting at the table and waiting to be fed). We have claimed that the primary reason the children found it so easy to interact was that the setting determined and illustrated the theme and provided props for its enactment (Boynton & French, 1983; French et al., 1985).

Over time, the children began to elaborate the meanings they used to communicate. At first they did this by nonlinguistic means. They developed the theme of eating a meal by using exaggerated gestures such as tipping their heads far back to "drink" from their cups, and they "plucked" imaginary cupcakes from a cupcake tin. Protolinguistic comments such as "Mmmmm!" and "Yummm!" were added to these sequences and served to affirm the theme of enjoying a meal. When words first appeared in this play, they further elaborated an established theme. For example, one girl extended a pie plate to another child and said, "Pizza!"; another time a child added the word "cookie" to a plate that was being passed between children. Just as they maintained contact by imitating each others' actions and passing objects, the children repeated each others' words. These words did not alter the discourse or establish a topic. Rather language extended an established theme by refining meaning or making meaning more explicit: The "something to eat" implied by the gesture of plucking became – with labeling – "cookie" or "pizza."

The children's shared knowledge about "kitchen-appropriate" activities enabled them both to perceive and to display to one another their understanding of the interactions permissible in the housekeeping setting. The mutual understanding cued by the environment permitted the sustained contingent interaction in which language could be used to elaborate meanings. This contrasts with the way language was used in other areas of the classroom to gain attention and to exert control over objects.

In a second series of naturalistic observations, free-play sessions were videotaped at a preschool that was just opening and served a mixed-age group of children who were not previously acquainted. Beginning two days after the center opened, 30-minute free-play sessions were videotaped daily for two weeks, then occasionally thereafter.

Three play episodes have been selected to illustrate the types of play and language use that occurred in the classroom. Without making any claims as to their representativeness in terms of frequency or exhaustiveness, we feel that these episodes illustrate a range of possibilities in terms of the interaction between language use and setting. Episode A involves play with trucks and blocks; in this case, language use is very limited, consisting primarily of sound effects to accompany and emphasize activity. Episode B involves an elaborate cooking and eating scenario in the kitchen area; language is used to supplement and extend the activities suggested by the kitchen props. In Episode C, the jungle gym is "transformed" into a car and used to search for missing parents; here language is the primary means of creating and sustaining shared meaning. In each episode, one of the key participants is Eddie, approximately $3\frac{1}{2}$. Jared, approximately $2\frac{1}{2}$, is a key participant in the truck and kitchen episodes. Danielle, 4, is Eddie's partner in the jungle gym episode.

Episode A began when Eddie heard Jared pushing a dump truck in the block corner and went to investigate; it terminated seven minutes later when the teacher asked the children to begin cleaning up. The episode contained several relatively discrete phases. After a brief period during which both boys pushed their trucks around, Eddie sat down on some large blocks in the corner and stayed there for the remainder of the episode while Jared continued to move about. Jared handed Eddie a plow for his dump truck and got one for himself. Eddie began a routine of dumping the plow from the box of his truck and saying "Beep! Beep!" Jared watched as Eddie repeated this routine several times, then also began saying, "Beep! Beep!" alternating his turns with Eddie's. Jared pushed his truck out of the immediate area, and Eddie continued his game alone. When Jared returned, Eddie requested a block, received it, then requested another. As the "load, dump, say 'beep' " routine continued, the boys took turns saying, "Beep! Beep!" and both introduced variation into their vocalizations, producing some longer series of beeps and adding intonational emphasis in the form of exaggerated or prolonged beeps. Jared pushed his truck away again, and Eddie continued the "load, dump, say 'beep' " routine until the teacher called cleanup time.

The transitions from one phase to another were accomplished easily: When Jared left the area, Eddie continued the routine; when Jared returned, Eddie enlisted his participation by requesting blocks. It appeared that the boys had no difficulty in interpreting one another's verbal or nonverbal meanings and that they shared assumptions about the appropriate components of the play. The episode was only weakly thematic, with the boys apparently sharing a definition of the situation as "playing dump truck." For the most part, their language – consisting primarily of "Beep" – was a component of the play with the same status as the actions of pushing and dumping. That is, the language did not extend the meaning of the activity substantially beyond what could be expressed nonverbally; in this sense, "Beep" is similar to "Mmmm" in the interactions among preverbal toddlers described earlier. Although Eddie and Jared's play was almost continuously accompanied by language, the language was syntactically and semantically simple and repetitive.

The establishment of a cyclic routine involving putting an object in the truck, dumping it out, and saying "Beep! Beep!" contains some of the organizational characteristics of the mother–infant interactional formats discussed by Bruner (1983) and others. Once the routine was well established, slight variations were introduced in the form of intonational changes in the boys' beeps. The structural consistency allowed the children to be successful participants in the exchange; the content variations helped to sustain interest in the interaction. A similar elaboration of a routine occurred in Episode C.

Episode B took place in the kitchen area, which contained a child-sized, makeshift stove, countertop, and sink, as well as cooking and eating utensils and a selection of empty spice jars. With various participants moving in and out, continuous play in this setting was maintained for approximately 30 minutes. The episode began immediately after Dana and Naomi, 5-year-old girls visiting from another center, arrived and were introduced to the other children. The girls went to the kitchen area and began mixing imaginary ingredients. Eddie came over and joined the play by asking, "This is making something? What? What are you making?" Naomi replied, "Salad," and Dana asked, "Do you want to play with us?"

Rather than reply directly to Dana's question, Eddie asked, "Do you want to have supper with me?" This question was one of the few explicit goal statements we observed at this center. With Dana's reply, "Yes, we're having supper with you," it might seem that the overall goal guiding subsequent activity had been established, yet several minutes later Dana responded, "Snack," to a teacher's question, "What is everybody making?"

We suggest that in this episode, the physical setting defined the appropriate range of activities and enabled Eddie to articulate an overall theme for joint pretense. However, the actual activities that the children engaged in were guided by the general constraints of the kitchen setting and could be described as adequately by "snack" as by "supper." Here we see relatively sophisticated communication in Eddie's production of a goal statement, but do not see this language having any substantive effect on the play itself.

Jared entered the setting about a minute after the "supper" exchange and found Eddie pretending to eat a wooden apple. He crossed the room to get himself an apple, pretended to bite it, then came back to the other children and announced, "This is apple." This utterance, and subsequent utterances in this episode, were very unusual in the sense that Jared rarely used sentences to accompany his activities. Instead, he typically used sound effects such as "Beep," "Ahh Choo," and "Hee Haw" that were meaningful only in the context of action routines established by others.

In this episode, Jared modeled his participation closely on Eddie's, requesting pop when Eddie requested pop, claiming his pop was all gone when Eddie did so, and so forth. When the girls ignored Jared's bids for attention, Eddie mediated for him. For example, when Eddie announced that is own (imaginary) pop was all gone, Dana took his glass, but when Jared than said his was all gone she simply said, "OK." Jared repeated, "It's all gone," while extending his glass and was again ignored. Eddie, pointing to Jared, then said loudly, "His pop all gone already. Pop all gone." Jared imitated Eddie's sentence form, saying, "Pop all gone already. Pop all gone already," while holding out his glass, which Dana finally took. Jared then extended his apple silently and was ignored. Eddie then pretended, in an exaggerated manner, to eat his apple, and said, "All done my apple. Here my apple," while extending it toward Dana, who took it. Jared then said, "My apple," and it too was taken.

In comparison with Episode A, both boys used more sophisticated language forms and participated more fully in the pretense. As older children, Dana and Naomi could more readily establish and maintain thematic play into which the boys could place their linguistic and behavioral contributions. It seems clear that to some extent this interaction depended on the presence of the older girls and on their engaging in food preparation activities, which permitted the boys to assume the reciprocal role of food consumers.

However, it also seems clear that the setting played a major role in determining the boys' activities and language use. While the girls served as important foils for the boys' display of appropriate language and activities, their actual engagement with the boys was minimal. The girls rarely spoke directly to the boys and barely engaged with Jared at all except to exchange objects. Although the boys attended closely to one another's language (with Jared imitating Eddie's statements and Eddie highlighting Jared's), they did not talk directly to one another.

Successful discourse is typically defined as necessarily involving contingent verbal exchange. Episode B fails to meet this standard – from the boys' perspective at least – since little talk was directed toward either boy. Yet in comparison with their behavior in the block corner the boys talked a great deal in this episode; their contributions were appropriate and interpretable within the general kitchen theme being enacted, and they were important participants in the fantasy that was created.

The physical setting elicited and supported the boy's thematically appropriate actions and language. Their knowledge of kitchen-appropriate activities constituted a "cognitive repertoire" that they could draw on to talk and act appropriately. In addition to suggesting these behaviors and providing the physical props necessary for their enactment, the kitchen setting elicited a set of shared presuppositions among the participants that made the contributions of each participant interpretable by the others.

The apparently competent yet largely noninteractive discourse that occurred during Episode B is interesting from the perspective of the general question of how children manage the transition from talking primarily with adults to talking with other children. In this episode, the physical setting itself provided Eddie and Jared with the conversational support that they did not receive from one another or from the girls. By relying on the meanings conveyed by the physical setting, they were able to talk appropriately without "engaged" conversational partners; this sort of talk may serve as one form of stepping stone toward genuine discourse. The opening goal statement (which, as it turned out, did nothing to guide subsequent activity) is a further example of how physical setting may support the practice of relatively sophisticated language use.

In Episode C, Eddie and Danielle, a 4-year-old, pretended to search for their missing parents. The episode lasted approximately three minutes and terminated when Danielle noticed and became entranced by the videocamera. Using the jungle gym as a car, Eddie and Danielle drove to different imaginary locations, got off the jungle gym to search for their parents, failed to find them, then returned to the jungle gym. There were five rounds in which a child left the jungle gym to search for a parent. This episode is of interest because it involves the creation and maintenance of a shared and relatively abstract fantasy theme with minimal reliance on physical setting. Although activity provided an important accompaniment, language was the primary means through which the two children created and maintained the shared theme.

Eddie initiated the interaction by urging Danielle to join him on the jungle gym. Once she did so, he said, "Drive me my mommy. Drive me home my mommy and daddy, okay? Do that for me." The following dialogue and actions were cyclical and extremely repetitive. For example, at one point Eddie said, "My daddy and mommy not home. My daddy not – my daddy and mommy not home." Soon thereafter, Danielle said, "My daddy ain't home. My daddy ain't home. My daddy ain't home."

Requests for clarification were nonexistent, and the children seemed to have no difficulty understanding one another. So what role might repetition have been playing? In the absence of a physical setting that might elicit a theme, the children were establishing a verbal foundation for their pretense. Repeating something that has just been said offers a means of staying "on topic" and may also serve to confirm or "fix" the topic (Keenan, 1977). Both of these functions would seem to be very important for inexperienced conversationalists who are just beginning to be able to engage in discourse that is not supported by the physical setting.

The cyclic pattern of this episode is again similar to the structure of mother–infant formats described by Bruner (1983). That is, the interaction can be described as consisting of rounds that have a relatively fixed structure yet allow for expansion. Some semantic content, for example, saying "goodbye" when leaving the jungle gym and reporting the parent's absence upon returning, remained relatively constant across the five rounds. However, elaborations were also added across rounds. For example, in one round Danielle said her father was not at home because he was working, and in the next round Eddie expanded on this by suggesting that her father was working at the same place as his mother. In this brief episode, the children both created and then began to expand on the basic format. It is intriguing that they returned to this familiar, well-established form as they extended their language to the new function of creating a relatively decontextualized play theme.

Using language as the *primary* means of creating shared meaning is a very important step in the development of communicative competence. The creation and maintenance of a shared pretense theme primarily through language represents an important advance over the other episodes reported here, in which the joint activity and creation of shared meaning were heavily dependent on the physical setting. However, the leap the children made in terms of being able to create a fantasy without a supportive physical setting was not without its limitations. Both the actions and language contributions were repetitive. In contrast to the kitchen setting, there were no subthemes or branching off of the activity. It is also important that the underlying theme of "missing parent" was not negotiated or communicated in any detail; rather, it seemed that this was a very salient concept for each child (perhaps because they were newcomers to the daycare setting) and once the theme had been introduced by one child, the other child was able to extend it easily. In other words, even in this episode the children were relying in large part on shared knowledge; here this knowledge was elicited verbally rather than through the physical context.

Direct comparisons across Episodes A, B, and C are difficult to make because of the multiple variables involved. However, Eddie's and Jared's behavior across settings supports our central thesis that the types of communicative interactions that young children are able to engage in are influenced strongly by settings and by the extent to which settings tap into shared event knowledge among participants. The interaction between Eddie and Danielle suggests ways that children may begin to have conversational interactions that are not connected to the physical setting in which they find themselves.

Structured observations

Our naturalistic observations in classroom settings have proved to be a rich source of hypotheses (Boynton & French, 1983; French & Boynton, 1984), but such observations inherently involve a lack of control over a number of potentially important variables, such as the number of children participating in an interaction, the length of time they participate, the factors that precipitate their entering and leaving a particular setting, and so forth. Therefore, we have undertaken a more controlled study that maintains many of the features of spontaneous play.

Partner and setting were varied under controlled conditions to determine their independent and joint influence on young children's ability to use language to accompany and guide their play. Sixteen target children (firstborn girls between 30 and 40 months of age) were videotaped for 15 minutes on four occasions in their own home as they played with materials we provided. Each target child played twice with a female friend of approximately the same age and twice with her mother. Each dyad played once with a child-sized model kitchen and once with assorted age-appropriate toys (large and small blocks, a wagon, a shape box, a doll). The order of the sessions was balanced across dyads. In addition, a presession during which the peers[2] played with a different set of toys familiarized the children with the procedure. Transcripts indicating language and activities occurring during each 15-second segment were prepared for each videotape.

The peer interactions of 6 of the 16 dyads are now being analyzed. We have begun working with this subset of the data because 6 dyads offer a sample that is small enough to permit in-depth consideration of the patterns displayed by individual children, yet varied enough to avoid basing conclusions on the idiosyncrasies of a particular dyad or particular child. All 6 dyads participated in the two peer conditions before participating in the mother–child conditions. Three dyads played in the kitchen first, and three played with the assorted toys first. Because data from only 6 of 16 target children are being reported, the results described here must be considered suggestive only. Thus far, the data have been coded along four dimensions:

(1) Level of social engagement of the children with one another, measured by type of interaction
(2) Amount of talk, measured by the number of utterances by each participant
(3) Syntactic complexity of talk, measured by the mean length of utterance (MLU)
(4) Cohesiveness of discourse, measured by the use of endophoric or exophoric reference

An assumption guiding this investigation of the role of setting in young children's communication is that the model kitchen supports interaction by eliciting shared knowledge about appropriate kitchen activities and providing a physical context within which to enact this knowledge in a pretense mode. In light of this assumption, it was predicted that the children would maintain higher levels of engagement in the kitchen than in the toy setting, that there would be more talk in the kitchen setting, and that the language used in the kitchen setting would be more cohesive than that used in the toy setting. Previous literature gives no basis for making predictions about the effect of setting on MLU.

Table 13.1. *Categories for coding level of engagement*

Level	Description
1	Child is unavailable for interaction; includes being absent from the play area, talking to an adult, being unoccupied, or engaging in solitary play
2	Child is aware of, but not interacting with, partner; includes watching the partner or engaging in parallel play (defined as partners playing with similar materials and passively monitoring one another)
3	Children are engaging in disruptive interactions with one another; includes arguments at both the physical and verbal levels
4	Children are engaged in interaction that involves the exchange of objects and verbal discussion, but is not organized around a shared goal; corresponds to Parten's (1932) category of associative play
5	Children are engaged in interaction that involves role differentiation and the joint achievement of a shared goal; corresponds to Parten's (1932) category of cooperative play

Engagement

Engagement refers to the degree to which children involve themselves with one another. It is an important variable in its own right,
as well as a necessary condition for conversational interaction, our
primary interest. Levels of engagement may range from children
merely being aware of and interested in one another to a coordination of their interaction around a shared goal. To code level of
engagement, we adapted a scale developed by Parten (1932) to assess social participation. The five levels of our scale are described in
Table 13.1. The highest level of engagement displayed by each child
was coded for each 15-second time segment. The mean number of
segments falling into each coding category is shown in Table 13.2.

The means shown in Table 13.2 indicate that setting affected the
distribution of Level 1, Level 4, and Level 5 scores. Level 1 scores,
indicating lack of engagement, and Level 4 scores, indicating engagement without a shared goal, were more frequent in the toy than
in the kitchen setting. Level 5 scores, indicating goal-directed engagement, were much more frequent in the kitchen setting than in
the toy setting.

For a somewhat different way of looking at these data, the Level

Table 13.2. *Mean number of observations by setting and engagement level*

	Engagement level				
Setting	1	2	3	4	5
Toy	13.66	7.33	2.91	28.08	4.66
Kitchen	3.25	7.25	3.50	12.16	30.50

Note: These figures are based on the individual coding of each member of the six dyads at 15-second intervals. One dyad was observed for 10 minutes in each setting; all others were observed for 15 minutes.

3 (disruptive engagement) codings were omitted, and the remaining scores were collapsed into *disengaged* (Levels 1 and 2) and *engaged* (Levels 4 and 5) categories. In each setting, the children were more likely to be engaged than disengaged; this finding is important in indicating that both settings supported peer interaction. However, as predicted, there was a greater degree of engagement in the kitchen setting and a greater degree of disengagement in the toy setting.

These analyses indicate that although both types of toys encouraged engagement, the amount and type of engagement varied across settings. The kitchen setting encouraged a greater amount of engagement overall. Furthermore, the engagement encouraged by the kitchen setting tended to involve shared goals, whereas engagement in the toy setting did not. These findings can be accounted for in terms of the relation between the toys in each setting and the children's representations of how to use them. Although both settings contained objects or "tools" that mediated activity, the objects in the kitchen prescribed certain activities that collectively imply social goals. The kitchen setting has sociocultural meanings attached to it that imply social events and social goals (e.g., preparing and sharing meals). Social interaction, then, is one of the meanings associated with the kitchen setting (as is the conversation that generally accompanies social interaction). Taken individually, the toys in the athematic collection may also have sociocultural meanings. However, taken as a group they do not prescribe a specific type of social interaction. Children may attach a wide range of meanings to their play with these toys, some of which do not require social interaction or support the achievement of social goals.

Amount of talk and MLU

The utterances produced by each child in each setting were tallied.[3]
The average number of utterances was 82.6 in the kitchen setting
and 47.6 in the toy setting. These results are in accord with the
original expectation that the children would talk more in the kitchen
than in the toy setting. The average MLU was virtually identical
across settings: 3.31 in the kitchen setting and 3.35 in the toy setting. Essentially, these results suggest that syntactic level (as measured by MLU at least) is not affected by the variations in setting
that we introduced. This is not surprising, because there would be
no reason to expect that setting would affect the length of a sentence a child could generate or the range of inflections and other
grammatical morphemes at her disposal. Furthermore, there do not
appear to be any differences between these two free-play situations
that would affect discourse expectations having to do with the appropriate length of utterances.

Cohesion

Cohesion refers to the ways that language is used to establish and
maintain reference. Reference to preceding language, that is, to the
discourse itself, is considered to be *endophoric;* such reference may
involve such devices as repetition, pronomial reference, substitution, ellipsis, collocation, continuatives, and conjunctions (Halliday
& Hasan, 1976). Reference to something apparent in the situational
context but not mentioned in the preceding discourse (e.g., "It's hot
in here," or "Can you give me that?") is considered *exophoric.*

   The relative frequency of endophoric and exophoric reference varies across situations, with, for example, a formal lecture containing
more endophoric reference and a conversation during the viewing
of a ballgame containing more exophoric reference. Although endophoric and exophoric references are equally essential for communication, endophoric reference is in some ways more sophisticated from the perspectives of cohesion and development. If one
looks at text *qua* text, a text with a higher proportion of endophoric
reference would be considered more cohesive than one with a higher
proportion of exophoric reference. From a developmental perspective, endophoric reference is a later achievement than exophoric reference. That is, children refer to objects or events in the physical

Table 13.3. *Mean number of utterances by setting and reference type*

| Setting | Reference type[a] | |
	Endophoric	Exophoric
Kitchen	63	15
Toy	33	14

[a]Utterances directed toward adults and those that were uninterpretable are excluded. The frequency of such utterances did not differ across settings.

environment earlier than they refer to the content of their own or another speaker's utterances. Hickmann (1985) refers to the child becoming able to use language in relation to linguistically constituted reality as well as nonlinguistic reality.

There has been very little work on children's mastery of the forms and functions of cohesive devices in oral language. However, we predicted that the support provided by the kitchen setting in terms of suggesting and providing the means of enacting shared thematic knowledge would lead to more endophoric reference, and hence to more cohesive discourse in this setting relative to the toy setting.

As an initial approach to considering cohesion, each utterance was coded as endophoric or exophoric. Utterances containing both types of reference were coded as endophoric in order to credit the speakers with the higher level of reference attained. The mean number of endophoric and exophoric utterances in each setting is shown in Table 13.3. There was more endophoric than exophoric talk in both settings, indicating that the children genuinely conversed with one another. That is, in each setting the children tended to maintain a discourse topic by linking their utterances to their own and their partner's prior utterances. The means shown in Table 13.3 indicate that there was substantially more endophoric reference in the kitchen than in the toy setting.

Summary

The preliminary results from the six dyads indicate that this experimental study will bear out our observations in naturalistic settings, that the quality of conversations between young children varies with the physical setting in which they take place. These findings are in accord with our claim that the transition from talking with conversationally skilled adult partners to talking with conversationally inept child partners is accomplished in part through selection and reliance on physical contexts that elicit and support the enactment of shared knowledge. This shared knowledge serves as conversational presuppositions and thereby supports emergent conversational skills.

Interdependence of language and thought

An essential argument throughout this chapter, and the hypothesis behind our current program of research, is that a central, if not determining, factor in young preschoolers' (ages 2 to 3) ability to communicate with their peers is the underlying knowledge base (referred to as a "cognitive context" by Nelson and Gruendel, 1981) they can activate and draw upon. In its most straightforward form, the claim is that when children take *shared* event knowledge as the topic of their play interactions, they use (and therefore practice and gain fluency in) more complex conversational skills. This is particularly true when children are in physical settings that cue, and then provide a means of enacting, the event knowledge. As illustrated in the scenario in which Eddie and Danielle "drove the jungle gym" in search of missing parents, it is possible for children to evoke shared knowledge through verbal means. However, without physical reminders of the topic, and without props to extend the topic, Eddie and Danielle's conversation was very simple and repetitive.

Whether elicited through physical or verbal means, shared knowledge between interlocutors can reduce the disruptions to communication caused by young children's difficulties in establishing presuppositions and taking one another's perspective. Shared knowledge, about typical kitchen activities, for example, enables children to make appropriate and comprehensible verbal contributions, to interpret potentially ambiguous contributions made by their partners, and to maintain topic even when verbal contingency is not maintained due to inattentiveness, failure to respond to questions, and so forth. The scenario in which Eddie and Jared "played kitchen" although they never talked directly to one another and were rarely spoken to by the girls offers an extreme illustration of how the physical and cognitive contexts can compensate for inadequate conversational partners in supporting appropriate talk. In many ways, a setting that elicits shared event knowledge serves some of the same conversational functions as does a skilled conversational partner such as a parent.

In short, the hypothesis underlying our research is that physical settings that elicit shared knowledge and hence shared presuppositions facilitate young children's communications with one another. Successful communication always involves shared meaning; drawing some of this shared meaning from environmental sources reduces the demands on the linguistic channel and makes communication easier and more likely.

We make the further assumption that children learn to communicate by communicating. That is, children develop the skills that underlie successful perspective taking and presupposition establishing as they have more, and more extended, verbal interactions with one another. In a case study drawn from the sample of 16 children in the partner-setting study described earlier, the subject used more sophisticated conversation maintenance devices (e.g., questions and turnabouts) with her peer partner than with her mother (French, Sobel, & Boynton, 1985). Although this intriguing finding awaits replication, it suggests that in talking to relatively inept conversational partners children have an opportunity to practice conversational skills that are infrequently needed when they interact with their conversationally skilled and supportive parent partners.

Thus far, we have discussed how thought – instantiated here as shared event representations – influences language – instantiated here as the talk that accompanies play interactions. How is thought influenced by language? Obviously there are myriad answers to this question! Here we focus on only two, again restricting ourselves to a communicative perspective. First, when people converse, they often learn new things or new ways of thinking about familiar things. Second, when people attempt to formulate thoughts so that they can be communicated to others via language, they translate the thoughts from a private form to one that can be socially shared; this process undoubtedly has important implications for the status of those thoughts. Each of these points will be elaborated briefly.

With reference to the types of peer discourse situations described in this chapter, children who enact a theme such as making breakfast will probably learn new things about breakfast from what their partners say. For example, a child who proposes waffles as a suitable breakfast food may find herself describing waffles and how they are prepared (communicating new knowledge to the interlocutor) or defending their function as breakfast rather than supper food (extending old knowledge for the interlocutor). During the preschool and early school years, verbal communication (i.e., language) gradually replaces enactment and observation as the dominant means of learning new material. Even children's earliest communications with one another are likely to lead to the acquisition of new knowledge for all participants in an exchange.

Language is a symbolization process that in addition to making thought communicable to others, imposes a particular structure on thought. Translating thought into language may involve gains (possibly in terms of communicability and access to consciousness) as well as losses (possibly in terms of diminished richness and flexibility). Our general question of how children learn to communicate with peers can be redefined in terms of how children in a particular setting manage to translate the meanings they are independently generating and operating with into meanings that are shared among participants in a play interaction. The assumption underlying our program of research is that whereas adults can accomplish such translation entirely through linguistic means, young preschoolers (i.e., novice communicators) necessarily rely on the physical setting for some portion of the translation and use language to supplement meaning, rather than to create meaning de novo. With experience in peer communication, children presumably decrease their reliance on setting to convey meaning and increase their ability to encapsulate and communicate meaning via language. This accomplishment is twofold in that it involves symbolizing thought or knowledge as language as well as taking account of the knowledge of others involved in the communicative exchange.

Conclusion

This chapter has raised the question of how children acquire the ability to communicate with their peers. Original data have been presented from observations of play interactions in preschool classrooms and in children's homes. These data are in accord with our claim that the transition from talking with skilled conversational partners (such as mothers) to talking with conversationally inept partners (such as peers) is accomplished in part through reliance on physical contexts that elicit, and provide the means of enacting, shared knowledge about familiar events. In this way, children are able to practice talking with one another while bypassing their difficulties in taking the perspective of the other and establishing shared presuppositions to support the interpretation of utterances. In the course of interacting (talking and playing), they will occasionally encounter situations that require these emergent skills, and they will be able to practice them within a context in which they are generally aware of their interlocutor's perspective and in which communication often can be reestablished easily in cases of breakdown.

Notes

1. In this chapter, the term *language* generally refers to talk, rather than to the underlying linguistic knowledge that supports, and is evident in, talking.
2. Others have recently pointed out that children differ along many dimensions and that the word *peer* may imply equality where none exists (e.g., Cooper & Cooper, 1984; Kanner, 1989). In this chapter, *peer* refers simply to children of approximately the same age.
3. In this and the subsequent analyses reported here, only those utterances that were both acoustically interpretable and directed toward the peer were included.

References

Bates, E. (1975). Peer relations and the acquisition of language. In M. Lewis & L. A. Rosenblum (Eds.), *Friendship and peer relations* (pp. 259–292). New York: Wiley.

Bates, E. (1976). *Language and context: The acquisition of pragmatics.* New York: Academic Press.

Bates, E., Camioni, L., & Volterra, V. (1979). The acquisition of performatives before speech. In E. Ochs & B. Schieffelin (Eds.), *Developmental pragmatics* (pp. 111–130). New York: Academic Press.

Boynton, M. (1990). *The representation of shared meaning.* Unpublished doctoral dissertation, University of Rochester, Rochester, NY.

Boynton, M., & French, L. (1983, October). *Holding it together: Preverbal children's play in a scripted setting.* Paper presented at the Eighth Annual Boston University Conference on Language Development.

Brenner, J., & Mueller, E. (1982). Shared meaning in boy toddlers' peer relations. *Child Development, 53,* 380–391.

Bruner, J. (1975). The ontogenesis of speech acts. *Journal of Child Language, 2,* 1–20.

Bruner, J. (1981). The social context of language acquisition. *Language and Cognition, 1,* 155–178.

Bruner, J. (1983). *Child's talk: Learning to use language.* New York: Norton.

Bruner, J., & Sherwood, V. (1976). Early rule structure: The case of peek-aboo. In J. S. Bruner, A. Jolly, & K. Sylva (Eds.), *Play: Its role in evolution and development* (pp. 277–285). New York: Basic Books.

Clark, H. H., & Clark, E. V. (1977). *Psychology and language: An introduction to psycholinguistics.* New York: Harcourt Brace Jovanovich.

Cooper, C. R., & Cooper, R. G. (1984). Skill in peer learning discourse: What develops? In S. A. Kuczaj (Ed.), *Discourse development: Progress in cognitive development research* (pp. 77–97). New York: Springer.

DeLoache, J., & DeMendoza, O. A. T. (1987). Joint picturebook reading of mothers and one-year-old children. *British Journal of Developmental Psychology, 5,* 111–123.

Ervin-Tripp, S. (1979). Children's verbal turn-taking. In E. Ochs & B. B. Schieffelin (Eds.), *Developmental pragmatics* (pp. 392–414). New York: Academic Press.

French, L. (1985). Real-world knowledge as the basis for social and cogjnitive development. In J. B. Pryor & J. D. Day (Eds.), *Social and developmental perspectives on social cognition* (pp. 179–209). New York: Springer.

French, L., & Boynton, M. (1984, March). *The effects of classroom setting on child–child speech.* Paper presented at the Fifth Annual University of Pennsylvania Ethnography in Education Research Forum, Philadelphia.

French, L., Lucariello, J., Seidman, S., & Nelson, K. (1985). The influence of discourse content and context on preschoolers' use of language. In L. Galda & A. D. Pellegrini (Eds.), *Play, language, and stories: The development of children's literate behavior* (pp. 1–27). Norwood, NJ: Ablex.

French, L., & Nelson, K. (1982). Taking away the supportive context: Preschoolers talk about the "then and there." *Quarterly Newsletter of the Laboratory of Comparative Human Cognition, 4,* 1–6.

French, L., & Nelson, K. (1983). More talk about then and there. *Quarterly Newsletter of the Laboratory of Comparative Human Cognition, 5,* 25–27.

French, L., Sobel, K., & Boynton, M. (1985). *Partner and setting: Important discourse variables.* Paper presented at the annual meeting of the American Educational Research Association, Chicago.

Garvey, C. (1974). *Play.* Cambridge, MA: Harvard University Press.

Garvey, C. (1984). *Children's talk.* Cambridge, MA: Harvard University Press.

Garvey, C., & Hogan, R. (1973). Social speech and social interaction: Egocentrism revisited. *Child Development, 44,* 562–568.

Gleason, J. B. (1973). Code-switching in children's language. In T. E. Moore (Ed.), *Cognitive development and the acquisition of language* (pp. 159–167). New York: Academic Press.

Halliday, M. A. K., & Hasan, R. (1976). *Cohesion in English.* London: Longman Group.

Hickmann, M. (1985). The implications of discourse skills in Vygotsky's developmental theory. In J. W. Wertsch (Ed.), *Culture, communication, and cognition* (pp. 236–257). Cambridge University Press.

Hodapp, R. M., Goldfield, E. C., & Boyatzis, C. J. (1984). The use and effectiveness of maternal scaffolding in mother–infant games. *Child Development, 55,* 772–781.

Kanner, B. G. (1989, June). *When are peers not peers: Implications for investigating the effects of peer interactions on conceptual development.* Paper presented at the 19th Annual Symposium of the Jean Piaget Society, Philadelphia.

Keenan, E. O. (1977). Making it last: Repetition in children's discourse. In S. Ervin-Tripp & C. Mitchell-Kernan (Eds.), *Child discourse* (pp. 125–138). New York: Academic Press.

Lucariello, J. (1987). Spinning fantasy: Themes, structure, and the knowledge base. *Child Development, 58,* 434–442.

Maratsos, M. (1974). Preschool children's use of definite and indefinite articles. *Child Development, 45,* 446–455.

Mueller, E. (1972). The maintenance of verbal exchanges between young children. *Child Development, 43,* 930–938.

Mueller, E., Bleier, M., Krakow, J., Hededus, K., & Cournoyer, P. (1977). The development of peer interaction among two-year-old boys. *Child Development, 48,* 284–287.

Mueller, E. C., & Brenner, J. (1977). The origins of social skills and interaction among playgroup toddlers. *Child Development, 48,* 854–861.

Mueller, E., & Cooper, C. R. (1986). On conceptualizing peer research. In E. Mueller & C. Cooper (Eds.), *Process and outcome in peer relationships* (pp. 3–24). New York: Academic Press.

Mueller, E., & Lucas, T. (1975). A developmental analysis of peer interaction among toddlers. In M. Lewis & L. A. Rosenblum (Eds.), *Friendship and peer relations* (pp. 223–257). New York: Wiley.

Mueller, E., & Rich, A. (1976). Clustering and socially directed behaviors in a playgroup of 1-year-old boys. *Journal of Child Psychology and Psychiatry, 17,* 315–322.

Nelson, K., et al. (1986). *Event knowledge: Structure and function in development.* Hillsdale, NJ: Erlbaum.

Nelson, K., & Gruendel, J. (1979). At morning it's lunchtime: A scriptal view of children's dialogue. *Discourse Processes, 2,* 73–94.

Nelson, K., & Gruendel, J. (1981). General event representations: Basic building blocks of cognitive development. In M. Lamb & A. L. Brown (Eds.), *Advances in developmental psychology* (Vol. 1, pp. 131–158). Hillsdale, NJ: Erlbaum.

Nelson, K., & Seidman, S. (1984). Playing with scripts. In I. Bretherton (Ed.), *Symbolic play* (pp. 45–71). New York: Academic Press.

Ninio, A., & Bruner, J. S. (1978). The achievements and antecedents of labeling. *Journal of Child Language, 5,* 1–16.

Ochs, E., & Schieffelin, B. (1976). Topic as a discourse notion: A study of topic in the conversations of children and adults. In C. Li (Ed.), *Subject and topic* (pp. 335–384). New York: Academic Press.

Parten, M. (1932). Social participation among preschool children. *Journal of Abnormal and Social Psychology, 27,* 243–269.

Pellegrini, A. D. (1983). Sociolinguistic contexts of the preschool. *Journal of Applied Developmental Psychology, 4,* 389–397.

Phyfe-Perkins, E. (1980). Children's behavior in preschool settings: A review of research concerning the influence of the physical environment. In L. G. Katz (Ed.), *Current topics in early childhood education* (Vol. 3, pp. 91–125). Norwood, NJ: Ablex.

Piaget, J. (1955). *The language and thought of the child.* New York: Meridian. (Original work published 1926.)

Ratner, N., & Bruner, J. S. (1978). Games, social exchange, and the acquisition of language. *Journal of Child Language, 5,* 391–402.

Sachs, J. (1983). Talking about the there and then in parent–child discourse. In K. E. Nelson (Ed.), *Children's language* (Vol. 4, pp. 1–28). New York: Gardner Press.

Shatz, M. (1983). Communication. In J. H. Flavell & E. M. Markman (Eds.), *Cognitive Development* (Vol. 3, pp. 841–889 of P. H. Mussen [Ed.], *Handbook of child psychology*). New York: Wiley.

Shatz, M., & Gelman, R. (1973). The development of communication skills: Modifications in the speech of young children as a function of listener. *Monographs of the Society for Research on Child Development, 38*(5, Serial No. 152).

Shugar, G. (1981). Early child discourse analyzed in the dyadic unit. *International Journal of Psycholinguistics, 8,* 55–78.

Snow, C. E. (1977). The development of conversation between mothers and babies. *Journal of Child Language, 4,* 1–22.

Snow, C. E. (1979). Conversations with children. In P. Fletcher & M. Garman (Eds.), *Language acquisition: Studies in first language development* (pp. 363–376). Cambridge University Press.

Snow, C. E. (1985). Literacy and language: Relationships during the preschool years. *Harvard Educational Review, 55,* 165–189.

Snow, C. E., & Goldfield, B. (1983). Turn the page please: Situation-specific language acquisition. *Journal of Child Language, 10,* 551–569.

Vygotsky, L. S. (1978). *Mind in society.* Cambridge, MA: MIT Press.

Wells, G., Montgomery, M., & MacLure, M. (1979). Adult–child discourse: Outline of a model of analysis. *Journal of Pragmatics, 3,* 3–4.

Wertsch, J. (1979). From social interaction to higher psychological processes: A clarification and application of Vygotsky's theory. *Human Development, 22,* 1–22.

Wertsch, J., McNamee, G. D., McLane, J. B., & Budwig, N. A. (1980). The adult–child dyad as a problem-solving system. *Child Development, 51,* 1215–1221.

Author index

Abbot, V., 38
Abramovitch, R., 381, 383, 384, 428
Adams, A. K., 133, 285, 459, 467, 468, 469, 473, 477
Allan, K., 135
Anderson, A. R., 371
Anderson, E. N., 114
Anderson, J. R., 251, 359
Anderson, R. C., 284
Andersson, L. G., 361
Anglin, J. M., 46, 60, 116, 118, 119, 136, 205, 212, 225, 256, 459
Antinucci, F., 292
Aristotle, 198
Armstrong, S., 116
Arns, F. J., 454
Arter, J. A., 228, 230
Asch, S. E., 197
Atran, S., 152, 158
Au, T. K., 18, 44, 77, 89, 91, 92, 139, 282
Augustine, Saint, 281
Austin, G. A., 111, 118, 149
Azmitia, M., 455

Backhouse, A. E., 36
Backscheider, A., 76, 78, 79, 98
Baduini, C., 85, 86
Bailey, F. L., 114
Bailey, L. M., 44, 45
Baillargeon, R., 120, 174, 190, 236, 237, 238, 239, 240, 249, 356
Baker, C. L., 323, 341
Baker, E., 120, 188, 408, 478
Balcom, P. A., 39

Baldwin, D. A., 44, 76, 77, 82, 98, 183, 443
Banigan, R. L., 94, 460, 461, 477
Baratz, D., 77
Barrett, M. D., 37, 46
Barsalou, L. W., 113, 150, 446, 455, 479
Bartlett, E. J., 64, 88, 304
Bartsch, R., 61
Bates, E., 19, 81, 82, 279, 355, 371, 375, 385, 416, 421, 486, 487, 488
Batterman, N., 162, 208, 388
Bauer, P. J., 78, 79, 236, 299
Beeghly, M., 408
Beeghly-Smith, M., 81
Behrend, D., 175, 341
Bellugi, U., 117, 327, 328, 329, 332
Belnap, N. D., 371
Benedict, H., 323
Benveniste, L., 124
Bereiter, C., 387
Berk, L. E., 20
Berko Gleason, J., 381, 382, 383, 384
Berlin, B., 38, 112, 114, 115, 116, 117, 135
Berman, R. A., 39, 47, 49, 51, 52, 53, 56, 59, 65, 254, 292
Bickerton, D., 269
Biderman, C. A., 179
Biederman, I., 181
Bierwisch, N., 282
Billeter, J., 228
Billman, D. O., 231, 327, 328, 329
Billow, R. M., 230, 231
Bjorklund, D. F., 415

511

518   *Author index*

Subject index